Tubulointerstitial Nephritis

Mohamed G. Atta • Mark A. Perazella
Editors

Tubulointerstitial Nephritis

Springer

Editors
Mohamed G. Atta
Division of Nephrology
Johns Hopkins University
Baltimore, MD, USA

Mark A. Perazella
Section of Nephrology
Department of Internal Medicine
Yale University
New Haven, CT, USA

ISBN 978-3-030-93437-8 ISBN 978-3-030-93438-5 (eBook)
https://doi.org/10.1007/978-3-030-93438-5

This Springer imprint is published by the registered company Springer Nature Switzerland AG
The registered company address is: Gewerbestrasse 11, 6330 Cham, Switzerland

Contents

Contributors

Medha Airy The Selzman Institute of Kidney Health, Section of Nephrology, Department of Medicine, Baylor College of Medicine, Houston, TX, USA

Abinet M. Aklilu Yale University School of Medicine, Section of Nephrology, Department of Internal Medicine, New Haven, CT, USA

Shuchi Anand Center for Tubulointerstitial Kidney Disease, Stanford University School of Medicine, Palo Alto, CA, USA

Abraham W. Aron Section of Nephrology, Yale University School of Medicine, New Haven, CT, USA

Mohamed G. Atta Division of Nephrology, Johns Hopkins University, Baltimore, MD, USA

Serena Bagnasco Department of Pathology, Johns Hopkins University School of Medicine, Baltimore, MD, USA

Megan L. Baker Section of Nephrology, Department of Internal Medicine, Yale University, New Haven, CT, USA

Laurence Beck Department of Medicine, Nephrology Section, Boston Medical Center and Boston University School of Medicine, Boston, MA, USA

Lena Berchtold Service of Nephrology, Department of Medicine, University Hospital of Geneva, Geneva, Switzerland

Whitney Besse Section of Nephrology, Yale School of Medicine, New Haven, CT, USA

Anthony J. Bleyer Section in Nephrology, Wake Forest School of Medicine, Winston-Salem, NC, USA

Daniel C. Brennan Division of Nephrology, Department of Medicine, Johns Hopkins University School of Medicine, Baltimore, MD, USA

Comprehensive Transplant Center, Johns Hopkins University School of Medicine, Baltimore, MD, USA

Alessia Buglioni Division of Anatomic Pathology, Department of Laboratory Medicine and Pathology, Mayo Clinic, Rochester, MN, USA

Fernando Caravaca-Fontán Department of Nephrology, Hospital Universitario 12 de Octubre, Madrid, Spain

Clara Cases-Corona Hospital Universitario Fundación Alcorcón, Madrid, Spain

Tiffany Caza Arkana Laboratories, Little Rock, AR, USA

Carmen Elena Cervantes Division of Nephrology, Johns Hopkins University, Baltimore, MD, USA

Cody Cobb Division of Renal Diseases and Hypertension, McGovern Medical School at University of Texas – Houston, Houston, TX, USA

Lynn D. Cornell Division of Anatomic Pathology, Department of Laboratory Medicine and Pathology, Mayo Clinic, Rochester, MN, USA

Neera K. Dahl Section of Nephrology, Yale School of Medicine, New Haven, CT, USA

Bianca Davidson Department of Nephrology and Hypertension, Kidney Research Unit, Groote Schuur Hospital, University of Cape Town, Cape Town, Western Cape, South Africa

Dries Deleersnijder Department of Microbiology, Immunology and Transplantation, Laboratory of Molecular Immunology, Rega Institute, KU Leuven, Leuven, Belgium

Division of Nephrology, University Hospitals Leuven, Leuven, Belgium

Garabed Eknoyan The Selzman Institute of Kidney Health, Section of Nephrology, Department of Medicine, Baylor College of Medicine, Houston, TX, USA

Francesco Emma Department of Pediatric Subspecialties, Division of Nephrology, Bambino Gesù Children's Hospital – IRCCS, Rome, Italy

Gema Fernández-Juárez Hospital Universitario Fundación Alcorcón, Madrid, Spain

Pablo Garcia Stanford University School of Medicine, Division of Nephrology, Stanford, CA, USA

Marvin Gonzalez-Quiroz Research Centre on Health, Work and Environment (CISTA), National Autonomous University of Nicaragua, León, Nicaragua

Centre for Nephrology, University College London, London, UK

Facultad de Ciencias Médicas, Edificio C (CISTA), León, Nicaragua

Jean Hou Department of Pathology, Cedars-Sinai Medical Center, Los Angeles, CA, USA

Bernard G. Jaar Division of Nephrology, Department of Medicine, Johns Hopkins University School of Medicine, Baltimore, MD, USA

Department of Epidemiology, Johns Hopkins Bloomberg School of Public Health, Baltimore, MD, USA

Welch Center for Prevention, Epidemiology and Clinical Research, Johns Hopkins University, Baltimore, MD, USA

Nephrology Center of Maryland, Baltimore, MD, USA

Bojan Jelakovic Department of Nephrology, Hypertension, Dialysis and Transplantation, University Hospital Centre Zagreb, Zagreb, Croatia

School of Medicine, University of Zagreb, Zagreb, Croatia

Sam Kant Division of Nephrology, Department of Medicine, Johns Hopkins University School of Medicine, Baltimore, MD, USA

Comprehensive Transplant Center, Johns Hopkins University School of Medicine, Baltimore, MD, USA

Joshua King Department of Medicine, University of Maryland, Baltimore, MD, USA

Department of Pharmacy, University of Maryland, Baltimore, MD, USA

Maryland Poison Center, Baltimore, MD, USA

Ravi Kodali Section of Nephrology, Department of Internal Medicine, Yale School of Medicine, New Haven, CT, USA

Namrata Krishnan Section of Nephrology, Yale University School of Medicine, New Haven, CT, USA

Elena Levtchenko Department of Pediatric Nephrology and Development and Regeneration, University Hospitals Leuven, Leuven, Belgium

Randy L. Luciano Yale University School of Medicine, Section of Nephrology, Department of Internal Medicine, New Haven, CT, USA

Blaithin A. McMahon Department of Medicine, Division of Nephrology, Medical University of South Carolina, Charleston, SC, USA

Dennis G. Moledina Section of Nephrology, Department of Internal Medicine, Yale School of Medicine, New Haven, CT, USA

Clincal and Translational Research Accelerator, Department of Internal Medicine, Yale School of Medicine, New Haven, CT, USA

Cynthia C. Nast Department of Pathology, Cedars-Sinai Medical Center, Los Angeles, CA, USA

Oana Nicoara Department of Pediatrics, Division of Nephrology, MUSC Children's Hospital, Charleston, SC, USA

Joëlle L. Nortier Department of Nephrology-Dialysis, Brugmann University Hospital, Université libre de Bruxelles (ULB), Brussels, Belgium

Laboratory of Experimental Nephrology, Faculty of Medicine, Université libre de Bruxelles (ULB), Brussels, Belgium

Mark A. Perazella Section of Nephrology, Department of Internal Medicine, Yale University, New Haven, CT, USA

Emmanuelle Plaisier Department of Nephrology -AURA Paris Plaisance, Paris, France

Rare and Common Kidney Diseases: From Molecular Mechanisms to Personalized Medicine Unit, INSERM UMRS 1155, Sorbonne Université, Paris, France

Manuel Praga Department of Nephrology, Hospital Universitario 12 de Octubre, Madrid, Spain

Maria Prendecki Centre for Inflammatory Disease, Department of Immunology and Inflammation, Imperial College London, Hammersmith Campus, London, UK

Charles D. Pusey Centre for Inflammatory Disease, Department of Immunology and Inflammation, Imperial College London, Hammersmith Campus, London, UK

J. Nelson Reed Department of Medicine, Medical University of South Carolina, Charleston, SC, USA

Pierre Ronco Rare and Common Kidney Diseases: From Molecular Mechanisms to Personalized Medicine Unit, INSERM UMRS 1155, Sorbonne Université, Paris, France

Department of Nephrology, Centre Hospitalier du Mans, Le Mans, France

Beatriz Sanchez-Alamo Hospital Universitario Fundación Alcorcón, Madrid, Spain

Sophie de Seigneux Service of Nephrology, Department of Medicine, University Hospital of Geneva, Geneva, Switzerland

Sanjeev Sethi Division of Anatomic Pathology, Department of Laboratory Medicine and Pathology, Mayo Clinic, Rochester, MN, USA

Anushree C. Shirali Section of Nephrology, Yale University School of Medicine, New Haven, CT, USA

Ben Sprangers Department of Microbiology, Immunology and Transplantation, Laboratory of Molecular Immunology, Rega Institute, KU Leuven, Leuven, Belgium

Division of Nephrology, University Hospitals Leuven, Leuven, Belgium

Hernando Trujillo Department of Nephrology, Hospital Universitario 12 de Octubre, Madrid, Spain

Jean-Louis Vanherweghem Department of Nephrology, Erasme University Hospital, Université libre de Bruxelles (ULB), Brussels, Belgium

Nicola Wearne Department of Nephrology and Hypertension, Kidney Research Unit, Groote Schuur Hospital, University of Cape Town, Cape Town, Western Cape, South Africa

Matthias T. F. Wolf Pediatric Nephrology, University of Texas Southwestern Medical Center, Dallas, TX, USA

Part I
History and Epidemiology

Tubulointerstital Nephritis: A History of Its Conceptual Evolution

Garabed Eknoyan and Medha Airy

For most of their history the kidneys were considered parenchymatous secretory glandular organs subservient to the nutritional needs of the body in eliminating excess fluidities, a function they shared with other constitutional emunctory organs. As for their importance, "The kidneys are not present for necessity in animals ..." asserted Aristotle (384–322 BC) in the 4th century BC, an unfortunate notion that prevailed for the next 20 centuries. It was only in the nineteenth century that the importance of the kidney began to be appreciated when it was identified as a site of disease by Richard Bright (1789–1858) in 1827 and its functions in maintaining the '*milieu intérieur*' substantiated by Claude Bernard (1813–1878) in the 1850s. The studies that followed unraveled the misconceptions that had shrouded the kidney in ambiguity over the past and gradually elucidated its central role in maintaining not just water balance but that of total body homeostasis; finally justifying the concluding statement of Aristotle about the kidneys, "... but have the function of perfecting the animal itself." It is within this evolving framework of accruing renal knowledge that tubulointerstitial nephritis emerged as a pathogenetic destructive process that accounts for the acute onset of some and the progression of most chronic diseases of the kidney.

G. Eknoyan (✉) · M. Airy
The Selzman Institute of Kidney Health, Section of Nephrology, Department of Medicine, Baylor College of Medicine, Houston, TX, USA
e-mail: geknoyan@bcm.edu; airy@bcm.edu

M. G. Atta, M. A. Perazella (eds.), *Tubulointerstitial Nephritis*,
https://doi.org/10.1007/978-3-030-93438-5_1

1 Foundations

Unfolding the structural features of the kidney in health and disease were as much a product of advances in the basic sciences and progress in experimental medicine as they were a result of technological improvements in tissue processing, the magnifying power of available observational tools and ultimately the advent of kidney biopsy in the 1950s (Fig. 1). The foundation of studies of kidney disease derives from the initial 1827 report of Richard Bright who considered his eponymous disease to be due to inflammation, hence the term "nephritis", and his classification of the diseased kidney based on its gross appearance into: (1) a large white kidney, (2) a red granular kidney and (3) a contracted scirrhous small kidney. Their respective microscopic features were then classified in 1858 by Rudolf Virchow (1821–1902) as: (1) a degenerative process of the tubules or "parenchymatous nephritis", (2) an inflammatory process of the non-tubular renal tissue or "interstitial nephritis", both of which could coexist in the same kidney and either could eventuate in (3) a small cirrhotic kidney. Glomerular lesions received increasing attention after 1869 when Edwin Klebs (1834–1913) described "glomerulo-nephritis", while vascular lesions received increasing attention after William Gull (1816–1890) and Henry Sutton (1837–1891) reported in 1872 the "arterio-capillary fibrosis" of hypertension as a cause of the small contracted kidneys of Bright's disease. Subsequent studies confirmed that the lesions of the small renal vessels were due to hypertension that occurred independent of kidney disease resulting in the term "nephrosclerosis", introduced by John S. Billings (1838–1913) in 1890 (Fig. 1). To classify kidney disease whose pathology was not distinctly evident or was a combination of degeneration and inflammation the term "nephropathy" was introduced by Émile Achard (1860–1944) in 1895, and to differentiate the degenerative renal tubular changes from those of inflammatory nephritis, the term "nephrosis" was introduced by Friedrich Müller (1858–1941) in 1905.

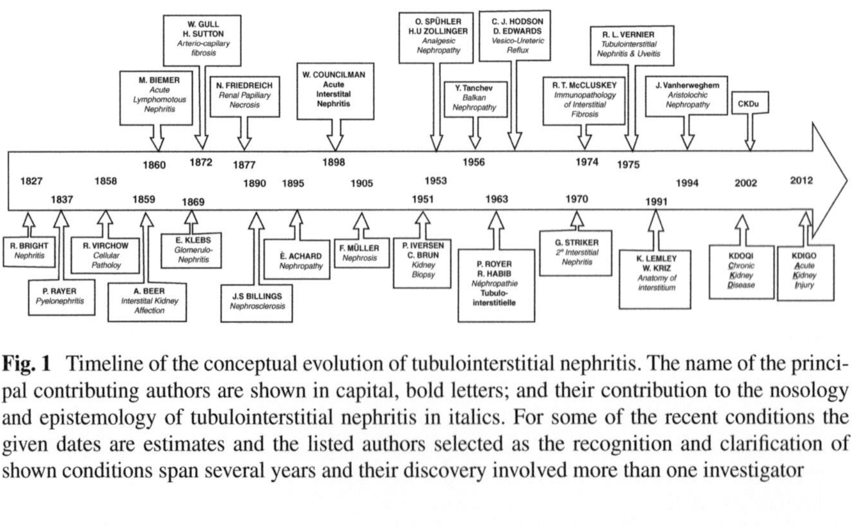

Fig. 1 Timeline of the conceptual evolution of tubulointerstitial nephritis. The name of the principal contributing authors are shown in capital, bold letters; and their contribution to the nosology and epistemology of tubulointerstitial nephritis in italics. For some of the recent conditions the given dates are estimates and the listed authors selected as the recognition and clarification of shown conditions span several years and their discovery involved more than one investigator

Renal interstitial tissue, distinct from its vasculature, tubules and glomeruli was recognized but considered to be limited principally to the renal medulla. In his classic 1842 report on the glomerular capsule William Bowman (1816–1892) does refer to "a sort of matrix ... in which the convoluted tubules and vessels are embedded in" but its pathology went unexplored. Attention to the renal interstitial supporting tissue as a distinct site of disease was highlighted in 1859 by a student of Virchow, Arnold Beer (1835–1880) who used the term "*interstitielle Nierenaffection*" or "interstitial kidney affection" to characterize the hyperplastic interstitial renal tissue changes he had observed in cases of infection, notably in scarlet fever.

1.1 Acute Interstitial Nephritis

Report of the first case of acute interstitial nephritis is credited to another trainee of Virchow, Michael Biermer (1827–1892) who in 1860 reported the case of a 5.5-year-old boy with scarlet fever who became anuric and died, whose kidneys at autopsy were grossly enlarged due to interstitial infiltration with lymphoid cells. Subsequent reports of similar cases led to a diagnosis of "acute lymphomatous nephritis" in the 1880s. William Councilman (1854–1933), a pathologist at Harvard with an interest in infectious diseases, introduced the term "acute interstitial nephritis" (AIN) as a distinct entity in 1898 based on his review of 42 cases of "non-suppurative inflammatory interstitial lesions" predominantly in cases of diphtheria, scarlet fever, and measles. His classic description of the pathology summarizes the lesions of AIN as lucidly and succinctly as they have ever been as: "an acute inflammation of the kidney characterized by cellular and fluid exudation in the interstitial tissue, accompanied but not dependent on, degeneration of the epithelium; the exudation is not purulent in character, and the lesions may be both diffuse and focal." He identified the infiltrating cells as mononuclear plasma cells that had migrated from the circulation and multiplied locally. He localized the inflammatory foci to the boundary zones of the pyramids, the subcapsular region of the cortex, and around the glomeruli.

As might be expected, some of the cases reported as AIN then were likely those of acute tubular necrosis (ATN) due to septic shock. Difficulty in differentiating the clinical and morphological features of these two entities (AIN *vs.* ATN), now considered as pathological variants of tubulointerstitial nephritis, persists; hence the need of a kidney biopsy to establish the diagnosis of AIN. Clinically, this diagnostic conundrum is now circumvented by use of the inclusive term of 'acute kidney injury' (AKI). With eradication of infections and increased interest in ATN during and after World War II, coupled with the rather limited interest in AIN its further diagnostic consideration literally faded away by the 1940s. Ironically, the entity was resurrected in the late 1950s because of the dramatic increased occurrence of AIN due the very chemotherapeutic agents that had eradicated infections. Since then, drug-induced in general and antibiotic-induced, in particular, continue to be the leading cause of AIN.

The broader descriptive term "tubulointerstitial" entered the parlance of nephrology in the early 1960s in French as "*néphropathie tubulo-interstitielle*" in describing an inherited form of chronic kidney disease (CKD) of children. It soon became evident that in AIN as well variable degrees of tubular injury were usually present, that the tubules had a major role in the pathogenesis of the interstitial lesions, and that tubular dysfunction preceded the fall in glomerular filtration rate and was usually clinically detectable well before the onset of azotemia and oliguria in AIN leading to the introduction and preferential use of the term of 'acute tubulointerstitial nephritis' (ATIN).

1.2 Chronic Tubulointerstitial Nephritis

Much of the early interest of CKD centered around the glomeruli, tubules and vasculature of the kidneys. Lesions of chronic tubulointerstitial nephritis (CTIN) were traditionally attributed to pyelonephritis. That this is not the actual case became evident after the availability of kidney biopsy. The two diseases to attract attention to CTIN as a primary cause of CKD, in which the glomeruli and vasculature are initially spared, were analgesic nephropathy in the 1950s and vesico-ureteral reflux (VUR) in the 1960s. Since then, a growing number of a motley group of diseases have been implicated as a cause of primary CTIN. Most recent on this expanding list are those of "aristolochic acid nephropathy", now recognized as what had been reported as Balkan nephropathy and Chinese Herbal nephropathy; and what was initially considered Mesoamerican nephropathy but is now more appropriately referred to as CKD of Unknown etiology (CKDu).

What actually increased interest and contributed much more to the understanding of tubulointerstitial lesions was the appreciation of their role in the progression of CKD of any etiology. Tubulointerstitial changes were noted early in cases of Bright's disease, but interest in the glomeruli, vasculature and tubules detracted from their further consideration. It was the advent of kidney biopsy that revived interest in CTIN when interstitial injury and fibrosis were noted to be the best correlates of the severity and progression to kidney failure in cases of glomerulonephritis in 1968 and documented by morphometric studies correlating them to measured glomerular filtration rate in 1970.

Since then, the interstitium has been precisely delineated as "the intertubular, extraglomerular, extracellular space of the kidney bounded by tubular and vascular basement membrane" and its residual cellular and fibrillar components identified. Also, the interstitium has become the center of exponentially increasing studies that have determined its function in generating renin-angiotensin and erythropoietin in addition to elucidating its role in the pathogenesis of interstitial fibrosis as a principal determinant of progressive kidney failure. Advances in the understanding of the mechanisms of interstitial fibrosis in CKD notwithstanding, the functions of the normal renal interstitium in health remain to be elucidated.

Suggested Reading

Anumudu S, Eknoyan G. Pyelonephritis. A historical reappraisal. J Am Soc Nephrol. 2019;30:914–7.

Beer A. Die Binddesubstang der menschlichen Niere in gesunden und krankhaften Zustande. Berlin: Verlag von August Hirschwald; 1859.

Councilman WT. Acute interstitial nephritis. J Exp Med. 1898;3:393–420.

DeBroe ME, Elseviers MM. Analgesic nephropathy. N Engl J Med. 1998;338:446–52.

Eknoyan G, Airy M, Anumudu S. On the evolution of the language of nephrology. Nephrol Dial Transplant. 2021;37:1–5.

Eknoyan G, McDonald MA, Appel D, Truong LD. Chronic tubulo-interstitial nephritis: correlation between structural and functional findings. Kidney Int. 1996;38:736–43.

Eknoyan G. On the etymology of nephritis: a historical appraisal of its origins. J Am Soc Nephrol. 2020;31:1170–3.

Eknoyan G. On the origins of experimental renal physiology. Nephrol Dial Transplant. 2021;36:392–5.

Greenwood M, Russell WT. Bright's disease, nephritis and arteriosclerosis: a contribution to the history of medical statistics. Biometrika. 1938;29:249–76.

Grollman AP. Aristolochic acid nephropathy: harbinger of a global iatrogenic disease. Environ Mol Mutagen. 2013;54:1–7.

Hewiston TD, Holt SG, Smith ER. Progression of tubulointerstitial fibrosis and chronic kidney disease phenotype – role of risk factors and epigenetics. Front Pharmacol. 2017;8(520):1–8.

Hewiston TD. Renal interstitial fibrosis: common but never simple. Am J Physiol Renal Physiol. 2009;296:F1239–44.

Hodson CJ, Edwards D. Chronic pyelonephritis and vesico-ureteric reflux. Clin Radiol. 1960;11:219–31.

Humphreys BD. Mechanism of renal fibrosis. Annu Rev Physiol. 2018;80:309–26.

Johnson RJ, Wesseling C, Newman LS. Chronic kidney disease of unknown cause in agricultural communities. N Engl J Med. 2019;380:1843–52.

Lemley KV, Kirz W. Anatomy of the renal interstitium. Kidney Int. 1991;39:370–81.

Oertel H. The anatomic histological processes of Bright's disease and their relation to the functional changes. Philadelphia: W. B. Saunders Co.; 1917.

Raghavan R, Eknoyan G. Acute interstitial nephritis – a reappraisal and update. Clin Nephrol. 2014;84:149–62.

Rastegar A, Kashgarian M. The clinical spectrum of tubulointerstitial nephritis. Kidney Int. 1998;54:313–27.

Royer P, Habib R, Mathieu H, Courtecuisse V. Les néphropathies tubulointerstitielles chroniques idiopathiques de l'enfant. Ann Pediatr. 1963;10:620–38.

Saundby R. Lectures on Bright's disease. Bristol: John Wright & Co.; 1889.

Schainuck LI, Striker GE, Cutler RE, Bendit EF. Structural-functional correlates in renal disease. Part II correlations. Hum Pathol. 1970;1:631–41.

Zeisberg M, Kallun R. Physiology of the renal interstitium. Clin J Am Soc Nephrol. 2015;10:1831–40.

Epidemiology of Tubulointerstitial Nephritis

Sophie de Seigneux and Lena Berchtold

1 Introduction

Interstitial nephritis (IN) is characterized by an inflammatory infiltrate in the kidney interstitium, usually leading to a decline in kidney function. Its diagnosis therefore requires performing a kidney biopsy. Acute interstitial nephritis (AIN) refers to the acute form of the disease with a rapid decline in kidney function, whereas chronic interstitial nephritis (CIN) has a more protracted course with more fibrosis detected by histology. The definite diagnosis of AIN or CIN is thus histological since no reliable non-invasive marker allows its confirmation or exclusion. Thus, the exact incidence of AIN and CIN are difficult to establish given differences in prevalence and etiologies worldwide, and mostly given the differences in kidney biopsies policies. The frequency of this type of lesion is likely underestimated since it may either go unrecognized if moderate, or diagnosed without a biopsy, particularly in the case of drug-induced AIN. Most epidemiological data available refers to AIN epidemiology.

2 Incidence of Interstitial Nephritis

Several series of biopsies have described the prevalence of IN worldwide. In Europe, the prevalence varies between 1% and 4.7% in different biopsy registries (Fig. 1). In The US, an incidence of 2.4–4% was reported. In Africa, the frequency of IN was reported from 1.4% up to 7.3% in Morocco. In different Asian series the prevalence

S. de Seigneux (✉) · L. Berchtold
Service of Nephrology, Department of Medicine, University Hospital of Geneva, Geneva, Switzerland
e-mail: Sophie.deseigneux@hcuge.ch

M. G. Atta, M. A. Perazella (eds.), *Tubulointerstitial Nephritis*,
https://doi.org/10.1007/978-3-030-93438-5_2

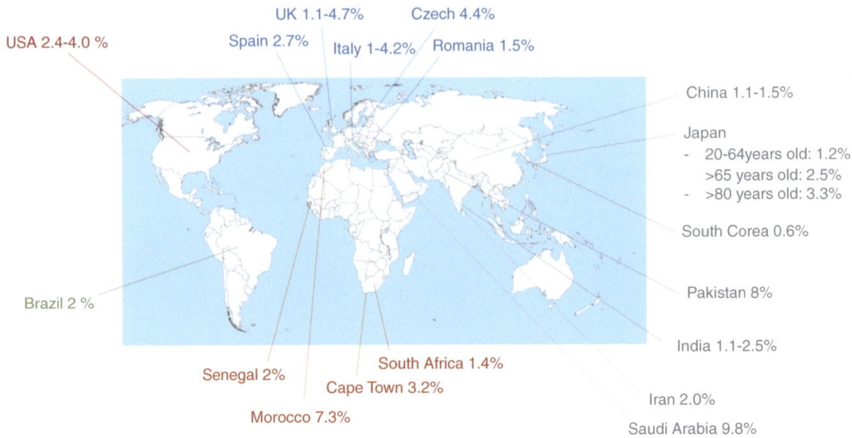

Fig. 1 Prevalence of Interstitial Nephritis worldwide (as % of biopsies in registries)

of IN among biopsies were from 0.6% in South Korea to 9.8% in Saudi Arabia, with 8% in Pakistan (5% AIN, 3% CIN). In Brazil, a large registry of kidney biopsies reported 2% of IN.

IN prevalence appears to increase with time, and in a Spanish registry, this prevalence increased form 3.6% in the first 4 years of the registry (1994–1998) to 10.5% in the last 4 years (2005–2009), with an increased incidence that was mostly noticeable in elderly patients (from 1.6% to 12.3%). This may reflect raise in disease prevalence depending on expositions to specific agents or predispositions, but also percentage augmentation of kidney biopsies, with for example more biopsies performed in older patients over the recent years.

Specific populations display higher incidence of IN. Among 290 biopsies performed in HIV positive patients in Baltimore, 11% revealed IN, which was also confirmed in a French series with approximately 13% of IN among kidney biopsies of HIV patients. Thus, IN prevalence worldwide in kidney biopsies oscillates between 1% and 5% in the general population and in up to 11% in specific populations.

When focusing on biopsies performed for the investigation of AKI, the incidence of IN, here AIN, is notably higher. In a Spanish registry, prevalence of AIN among biopsies performed in the investigation for AKI was 12.9%. This was also confirmed in two registries of biopsies performed for AKI in older adults, where AIN was diagnosed in 15.5% and 18.6% of the cases and in a European registry of biopsies. In patients with impaired kidney function and kidneys of normal size, IN was reported in 27% of the cases. Thus, AIN remains an important etiology of AKI.

Granulomatous interstitial nephritis is a rarer subtype of IN that is observed in 0.5–0.9% of native kidney biopsies.

Chronic interstitial nephritis (CIN) incidence is less documented than AIN and is probably less frequent and often unrecognized. Most etiologies are similar between AIN and CIN, with toxic and genetic causes being more specific for

Table 1 Genetic causes of autosomal dominant tubulointerstitial kidney disease (ADTKD)

Name	Causal gene	Chromosome	Clinical manifestation
ADTKD-UMOD	UMOD Uromodulin	16p12.3	Early gout, occasional renal cysts
ADTKD-MUC1	MUC1 Mucin-1	1q22	Occasional renal cysts
ADTKD-REN	REN Renin	1q32.1	Mild hypertension, increased risk for AKI, anemia
ADTKD-HNF1β	HNF1β Hepatocyte nuclear factor 1- β	17q12	MODY, few bilateral renal cysts,
ADTKD-NOS	Not otherwise specified		

CIN. Among genetic causes, Autosomal Dominant tubulointerstitial Kidney Disease (ADTKD) is a disease characterized by progressive tubulointerstitial fibrosis and progression to end stage kidney disease (ESKD). ADTKD involves mutations of genes encoding uromodulin (*UMOD*), hepatocyte nuclear factor-1β (*HNF1B*), renin (*REN*), and mucin-1 (*MUC1*) (Table 1). The exact prevalence of these mutations is unknown and is likely underestimated. UMOD mutations were recently described as a relatively frequent kidney genetic disease with an estimated prevalence of 9/million. Cystinuria may also lead to interstitial kidney disease with an estimated prevalence of 1 per 10,000 in the US. CKD of unknown origin (CKDu) is another type of CIN with prevalence that are highly variable, as discussed later. Altogether CIN epidemiology is not well established and would deserve more studies.

3 Etiology of AIN

The causes of AIN vary according to patient's age, time period, and geography. In 133 North American biopsy proven AIN cases collected between 1993 and 2011, 71% were drug-induced, whereas immunological and infectious causes explained 20% and 4% of the cases respectively (Table 2). In three collected European series with 128 AIN patients from 1968 to 2001, 71.1% were drug-related, 15.6% were infectious, 7.8% were idiopathic, and only 5% were immunologically mediated. Thus, the frequency of infection mediated AIN likely decreases over time in Europe and the US, whereas the frequency of drug-induced AIN increases reaching almost 90% in more recent reports.

HIV positive patients are at higher risk of IN. In this population, drug-induced cases were also most common in the US (around 70%), whereas this proportion was lower (26.7%) in a French series of HIV positive patients, where infectious (16.7%) and idiopathic cases (15.7%) were more prevalent. In HIV positive patients co-infected with tuberculosis, drugs were incriminated in 70% of the cases, whereas infections in 14.8%.

Table 2 Acute interstitial nephritis etiology

Medication 71–90%
Antibiotics: Beta Lactams, quinolones, rifampicin, sulfonamides, vancomycin, tetracycline, isoniazid
NSAIDS
Proton pump inhibitors
Others: Allopurinol, acyclovir, furosemide, thiazides, phenytoin, carbamazepine
Immunological 5–20%
Sarcoidosis
Sjögren
TINU
IgG4
ANCA vasculitis
Systemic lupus erythematosus
Infectious 4–17%
Virus: Cytomegalovirus, Epstein-Barr, hantavirus, human immunodeficiency virus, polyomavirus
Bacteria: Brucella, campylobacter, Escherichia coli, Legionella, Salmonella, Streptococcus, Staphylococcus, Yersinia, Leptospira, Syphilis, Yersinia, Diphtheria
Other: Tuberculosis, Toxoplasmosis, Mycoplasma

Age may be an independent determinant of the etiology of AIN. Drug-induced AIN was responsible for 64% of cases in patients younger than 64 years versus 88% in older patients in the US, whereas auto-immune diseases were responsible for 27% in younger and 7% in older patients, and infectious nephritis were rare with 4.5% versus 2% in younger versus older patients, respectively. Thus, drugs are much more frequent causes of AIN in older patients, likely related to the higher frequency of polypharmacy in this age group.

Among auto-immune cases, sarcoidosis is usually more frequent than Sjögren syndrome, followed by TINU and IgG4 related disease, and more rarely ANCA vasculitis. Among infectious cases, bacteria are rarely causative nowadays given the wide antibiotic availability, whereas virus and infections such as toxoplasma, mycoplasma and tuberculosis are more frequent causes of AIN particularly in immunocompromised patients.

Granulomatous IN is a specific and rare type of IN. Drug-induced granulomatous IN are still most often reported, followed by sarcoidosis in western countries. In a series of granulomatous nephritis in HIV patients in Cape Town, tuberculosis explained 60% of the cases, followed by drugs (20%), which was confirmed in India.

Altogether drug-induced AIN is the most common type of AIN worldwide, followed by immunologic causes and infections. Depending on the population studied, the proportion of infectious cases may display more variability.

4 Drug Induced AIN

Drug induced AIN is by far the most frequent etiology of the disease in most series. The first cases of drug induced AIN were described in 1968 followed by several reports and case series. Among incriminated drugs, antibiotics (mainly penicillin) and NSAIDs are associated to the highest risk. More recently proton pump inhibitors (PPIs) were incriminated, with the first case reported in 1992. Since then, the role of PPI in AIN has been increasingly recognized. In the US case series of 133 biopsy proven AIN, antibiotics were responsible for 49% of drug-induced cases, whereas proton pumps inhibitors (PPIs) and NSAIDS were involved in 14% and 11% respectively. Among antibiotics, penicillin was most often incriminated, followed by quinolones and cephalosporins. The causative drugs also vary according to specific populations. In older patients, antibiotics and proton pump inhibitors were more frequently identified than NSAIDs. This may reflect an increased exposure of older patients to PPIs and antibiotics, or a higher susceptibility of this population to these molecules. In HIV positive patients, NSAIDS and trimethoprim/sulfamethoxazole were the most frequent offending agents in a US series, whereas Indinavir was more often reported in France and Rifampicin in patients from Cape-Town with tuberculosis co-infection.

In more recent series, the emergence of IN related to checkpoints inhibitors is increasing in oncological patients, and PPI seem to play an important predisposing factor. These drugs are peculiar since they probably enhance the risk of AIN related to other causes and drugs. The prevalence of the complication is likely underestimated because of variable biopsy policies.

Thus, AIN causative drugs are usually found among antibiotics, PPIs and NSAIDs, with varying prevalence depending mostly on exposure.

5 Endemic Nephritis

When considering IN epidemiology, endemic nephritis deserves a specific mention. Also named Chronic kidney disease of unknown origin (CKDu) or chronic interstitial nephritis in agricultural communities (CINAC), these epidemic nephritides can occur worldwide and are usually related to a toxic or environmental factors, identified or not (Table 3). CKDu is a diagnosis of exclusion in patients with CKD according to KDIGO criteria, without evidence of a recognized cause such as diabetes, hypertension or glomerulonephritis and is usually related to interstitial disease. These diseases appear responsible for an important increase in CKD incidence over the past 20 years in low to middle income countries and are restricted to specific geographical areas. For example, "Itai-Itai disease" was attributed to cadmium

Table 3 Endemic nephritis

Name	Endemic areas	Etiology confirmed	Risk factors
Itai-Itai disease	Japan	Cadmium	Water – Crops- Mining pollution
Balkan endemic nephropathy (BEN) Or Chinese herb nephropathy	Serbia Bulgaria Croatia Romania Bosnia	Aristocholic acid	Wheat
Meso-american nephropathy (MEN)	Nicaragua El Salvador Costa Rica	Unexplained	Sugarcane, heat stress, agrochemical exposure, heavy metals exposure, genetic predisposition, alcohol "LIJA" consumption
Sri Lanka CKDu	Sri Lanka	Unexplained	Agricultural works, heat stress, agrochemical exposure, heavy metals exposure, genetic predisposition, alcohol/betel/tobacco
India CKDu (Uddanam Nephropathy)	India	Unexplained	Agricultural workers Heat stress Agrochemical exposure Heavy metals Genetic predisposition

intoxication and "Chinese herb nephropathy", and "Balkan nephropathy" were attributed to aristocholic acid. More recently, the Meso-American nephritis and CKDu were described extensively in some parts of El Salvador, Nicaragua, Sri-Lanka, and India. CKDu prevalence is largely unknown. In El Savador between 1990 and 2009, CKD prevalence increased to 18% of the population, with a 7-fold increase in CKD related mortality. Similarly, a 3-fold increase in mortality was described in Nicaragua. In North Central Sri Lanka, in the same period of time, a prevalence of 13% in females and 17% in males of CKDu was reported. A similar high prevalence of CKDu was described in India in 2010, explaining up to 40% of reported CKD cases depending on regions. In Egyptian dialysis centers, up to 27% percent of ESRD are attributed to CKDu. The pathophysiology of these endemic nephritis is not completely resolved but heavy metals, pesticides, heat-induced dehydration, and some infections have been linked to these cases, characterized by a high prevalence restricted to some geographic areas.

6 Conclusion

Overall, AIN is a frequent cause of AKI, with an incidence increasing with time. Although immunological diseases and infections are important causes of the disease, most cases are nowadays driven by drugs or toxic exposure. This explains variations with time and with the studied population. The epidemiology of CIN is less well described and would certainly deserve more studies.

Suggested Reading

Abdou N, Boucar D, El Hadj Fary KA, Mouhamadou M, Abdoulaye L, Mamadou Mourtala KA, et al. Histopathological profiles of nephropathies in Senegal. Saudi J Kidney Dis Transpl. 2003;14(2):212–4. PubMed PMID: 18209451.

Agrawal V, Kaul A, Prasad N, Sharma K, Agarwal V. Etiological diagnosis of granulomatous tubulointerstitial nephritis in the tropics. Clin Kidney J. 2015;8(5):524–30. PubMed PMID: 26413276. Pubmed Central PMCID: 4581389.

Baker RJ, Pusey CD. The changing profile of acute tubulointerstitial nephritis. Nephrol Dial Transplant. 2004;19(1):8–11. PubMed PMID: 14671029.

Baldwin DS, Levine BB, McCluskey RT, Gallo GR. Renal failure and interstitial nephritis due to penicillin and methicillin. N Engl J Med. 1968;279(23):1245–52. PubMed PMID: 4176988.

Blank ML, Parkin L, Paul C, Herbison P. A nationwide nested case-control study indicates an increased risk of acute interstitial nephritis with proton pump inhibitor use. Kidney Int. 2014;86(4):837–44. PubMed PMID: 24646856. Pubmed Central PMCID: 4184187.

Brewster UC, Perazella MA. Proton pump inhibitors and the kidney: critical review. Clin Nephrol. 2007;68(2):65–72. PubMed PMID: 17722704.

Buysen JG, Houthoff HJ, Krediet RT, Arisz L. Acute interstitial nephritis: a clinical and morphological study in 27 patients. Nephrol Dial Transplant. 1990;5(2):94–9. PubMed PMID: 2113219.

Cortazar FB, Kibbelaar ZA, Glezerman IG, Abudayyeh A, Mamlouk O, Motwani SS, et al. Clinical features and outcomes of immune checkpoint inhibitor-associated AKI: a multicenter study. J Am Soc Nephrol. 2020;31(2):435–46. PubMed PMID: 31896554. Pubmed Central PMCID: 7003302.

Davidson B, Nel D, Jones ESW, Manning K, Spies R, Bohmer R, et al. Granulomatous interstitial nephritis on renal biopsy in human immunodeficiency virus positive patients: prevalence and causes in Cape Town, South Africa. Nephrology. 2019;24(7):681–8. PubMed PMID: 30663206.

Davison AM, Jones CH. Acute interstitial nephritis in the elderly: a report from the UK MRC Glomerulonephritis Register and a review of the literature. Nephrol Dial Transplant. 1998;13(Suppl 7):12–6. PubMed PMID: 9870431.

Devuyst O, Olinger E, Weber S, Eckardt KU, Kmoch S, Rampoldi L, et al. Autosomal dominant tubulointerstitial kidney disease. Nat Rev Dis Primers. 2019;5(1):60. PubMed PMID: 31488840.

Eckardt KU, Alper SL, Antignac C, Bleyer AJ, Chauveau D, Dahan K, et al. Autosomal dominant tubulointerstitial kidney disease: diagnosis, classification, and managementDOUBLEHYPHENA KDIGO consensus report. Kidney Int. 2015;88(4):676–83. PubMed PMID: 25738250.

Farrington K, Levison DA, Greenwood RN, Cattell WR, Baker LR. Renal biopsy in patients with unexplained renal impairment and normal kidney size. Q J Med. 1989;70(263):221–33. PubMed PMID: 2602535.

Gifford FJ, Gifford RM, Eddleston M, Dhaun N. Endemic nephropathy around the world. Kidney Int Rep. 2017;2(2):282–92. PubMed PMID: 28367535. Pubmed Central PMCID: 5362147.

Goicoechea M, Rivera F, Lopez-Gomez JM, Spanish Registry of G. Increased prevalence of acute tubulointerstitial nephritis. Nephrol Dial Transplant. 2013;28(1):112–5. PubMed PMID: 22759386.

Gubelmann C, Waszak SM, Isakova A, Holcombe W, Hens K, Iagovitina A, et al. A yeast one-hybrid and microfluidics-based pipeline to map mammalian gene regulatory networks. Mol Syst Biol. 2013;9:682. PubMed PMID: 23917988. Pubmed Central PMCID: 3779800.
Haas M, Spargo BH, Wit EJ, Meehan SM. Etiologies and outcome of acute renal insufficiency in older adults: a renal biopsy study of 259 cases. Am J Kidney Dis. 2000;35(3):433–47. PubMed PMID: 10692269.
Jayatilake N, Mendis S, Maheepala P, Mehta FR, Team CKNRP. Chronic kidney disease of uncertain aetiology: prevalence and causative factors in a developing country. BMC Nephrol. 2013;14:180. PubMed PMID: 23981540.
Joss N, Morris S, Young B, Geddes C. Granulomatous interstitial nephritis. Clin J Am Soc Nephrol. 2007;2(2):222–30. PubMed PMID: 17699417.
Li LS, Liu ZH. Epidemiologic data of renal diseases from a single unit in China: analysis based on 13,519 renal biopsies. Kidney Int. 2004;66(3):920–3. PubMed PMID: 15327382.
Muriithi AK, Leung N, Valeri AM, Cornell LD, Sethi S, Fidler ME, et al. Biopsy-proven acute interstitial nephritis, 1993-2011: a case series. Am J Kidney Dis. 2014;64(4):558–66. PubMed PMID: 24927897.
Muriithi AK, Leung N, Valeri AM, Cornell LD, Sethi S, Fidler ME, et al. Clinical characteristics, causes and outcomes of acute interstitial nephritis in the elderly. Kidney Int. 2015;87(2):458–64. PubMed PMID: 25185078.
Parkhie SM, Fine DM, Lucas GM, Atta MG. Characteristics of patients with HIV and biopsy-proven acute interstitial nephritis. Clin J Am Soc Nephrol. 2010;5(5):798–804. PubMed PMID: 20338962. Pubmed Central PMCID: 2863972.
Perazella MA, Markowitz GS. Drug-induced acute interstitial nephritis. Nat Rev Nephrol. 2010;6(8):461–70. PubMed PMID: 20517290.
Pettersson E, von Bonsdorff M, Tornroth T, Lindholm H. Nephritis among young Finnish men. Clin Nephrol. 1984;22(5):217–22. PubMed PMID: 6518672.
Polito MG, de Moura LA, Kirsztajn GM. An overview on frequency of renal biopsy diagnosis in Brazil: clinical and pathological patterns based on 9,617 native kidney biopsies. Nephrol Dial Transplant. 2010;25(2):490–6. PubMed PMID: 19633091.
Praga M, Gonzalez E. Acute interstitial nephritis. Kidney Int. 2010;77(11):956–61. PubMed PMID: 20336051.
Preston RA, Stemmer CL, Materson BJ, Perez-Stable E, Pardo V. Renal biopsy in patients 65 years of age or older. An analysis of the results of 334 biopsies. J Am Geriatr Soc. 1990;38(6):669–74. PubMed PMID: 2358629.
Qureshi R, Imtiaz S, Dhrolia M, Ahmad A. Frequency and etiology of tubulo-interstitial nephritis in an adult renal biopsies in a tertiary renal care hospital: a single-center study. Saudi J Kidney Dis Transpl. 2020;31(2):335–41. PubMed PMID: 32394905.
Ruffenach SJ, Siskind MS, Lien YH. Acute interstitial nephritis due to omeprazole. Am J Med. 1992;93(4):472–3. PubMed PMID: 1341422.
Sarwal D, D'Cruz S, Singh Punia RP, Minz RW. The spectrum of renal diseases observed in native renal biopsies in a single North Indian tertiary care center. Saudi J Kidney Dis Transpl. 2019;30(2):492–500. PubMed PMID: 31031385.
Schena FP. Survey of the Italian Registry of Renal Biopsies. Frequency of the renal diseases for 7 consecutive years. The Italian Group of Renal Immunopathology. Nephrol Dial Transplant. 1997;12(3):418–26. PubMed PMID: 9075118.
Vervaet BA, Nast CC, Jayasumana C, Schreurs G, Roels F, Herath C, et al. Chronic interstitial nephritis in agricultural communities is a toxin-induced proximal tubular nephropathy. Kidney Int. 2020;97(2):350–69. PubMed PMID: 31892415.

Yokoyama H, Sugiyama H, Sato H, Taguchi T, Nagata M, Matsuo S, et al. Renal disease in the elderly and the very elderly Japanese: analysis of the Japan Renal Biopsy Registry (J-RBR). Clin Exp Nephrol. 2012;16(6):903–20. PubMed PMID: 23053590.

Zaidan M, Lescure FX, Brocheriou I, Dettwiler S, Guiard-Schmid JB, Pacanowski J, et al. Tubulointerstitial nephropathies in HIV-infected patients over the past 15 years: a clinico-pathological study. Clin J Am Soc Nephrol. 2013;8(6):930–8. PubMed PMID: 23430209. Pubmed Central PMCID: 3675854.

Zajjari Y, Montasser D, Sobhi A, Aatif T, Azizi M, Alayoud A, et al. Acute interstitial nephritis in the military hospital of Morocco: clinical features and renal outcomes. Saudi J Kidney Dis Transpl. 2019;30(6):1407–14. PubMed PMID: 31929288.

Part II
Pathogenesis

Pathogenesis of Acute Tubulointerstitial Nephritis

Abraham W. Aron, Namrata Krishnan, and Anushree C. Shirali

1 Introduction

General immunology concepts will be reviewed in order to provide an understanding of the inflammatory mechanisms underlying the specific etiologies of acute tubulointerstitial nephritis (ATIN). Subsequently, the mechanisms underlying specific etiologies will be discussed in greater depth.

The immune system has classically been defined as having two subsystems of innate and adaptive immunity. The innate immune system governs an antigen-independent response generated by dendritic cells (DCs) and other antigen-presenting cells (APC) recognizing non-self- ligands. After processing antigen, APC are capable of activating T cells and B cells in an antigen-specific, major histocompatibility (MHC) restricted manner. In particular, DCs reside in all tissue types and are involved in immune surveillance and tolerance. DCs probe their environment via stellate projections and take up antigen-containing extracellular fluid via phagocytosis, pinocytosis, and receptor mediated endocytosis. Processed antigens are expressed on the DC surface via MHC II after which DCs migrate to lymph nodes and interact with naive CD4+ T cells.

Kidney DCs are restricted to the tubulointerstitial compartment where they form a contiguous surveillance network and closely associate with renal tubular epithelial cells (RTEC). DCs express the pattern recognition receptor (PRR), toll-like receptor (TLR), which recognize pathogen associated molecular patterns (PAMPs) and damage associated molecular patterns (DAMPs) allowing for rapid initiation of an immune response. As the name suggests, PAMPs are associated with specific molecules expressed on various pathogens whereas DAMPs are intracellular molecules released by damaged cells.

A. W. Aron (✉) · N. Krishnan · A. C. Shirali
Section of Nephrology, Yale University School of Medicine, New Haven, CT, USA
e-mail: Abraham.aron@yale.edu; namrata.krishnan@yale.edu; anushree.shiral@yale.edu

M. G. Atta, M. A. Perazella (eds.), *Tubulointerstitial Nephritis*,
https://doi.org/10.1007/978-3-030-93438-5_3

TLR activation initiates an intracellular signaling cascade via MyD88, which activates the transcription factor NF-κB leading to the expression of pro-inflammatory cytokines including TNF-α and IL-6. In addition, PAMPs and DAMPs acting as TLR ligands can lead to the activation of inflammasomes. Inflammasomes are an assembly of scaffolding proteins that allow the activation to caspase-1 and signaling via IL-β and IL-18, leading to pyroptosis (inflammatory cell death). Importantly, IL-1β increases nuclear translocation of NF-κB and increases the chemoattractant, MCP-1.

In an inflammatory milieu, renal tubular epithelial cells (RTECs) can also present antigens via MHC II, allowing identification by infiltrating CD4+ T cells. Interferon-γ (INF-γ), which is released by activated T cells, can increase expression of MHC II on RTECs. Additionally, RTECs can produce inflammatory cytokines such as IL-1, TNF-α and IL-6 in addition to cell adhesion molecules and chemoattractants including MCP-1, further promoting immune cell infiltration and inflammation.

With prolonged inflammation, the tubulointerstitial compartment can undergo fibrosis via epithelial to mesenchymal transformation (EMT), characterized by the transformation of epithelial cells into fibroblasts (Fig. 1). EMT is involved in organogenesis, tumor development, and fibrosis. EMT is regulated by TGF-β which, through signaling via Smad, MAPK and PI3k/Akt, leads to the translation of profibrotic and apoptotic genes. A hallmark of EMT is the reduced expression of cell adhesion molecules (E-cadherin) by epithelial cells and an increased expression of mesenchymal markers (α-SMA, vimentin and fibronectin). This is followed by actin

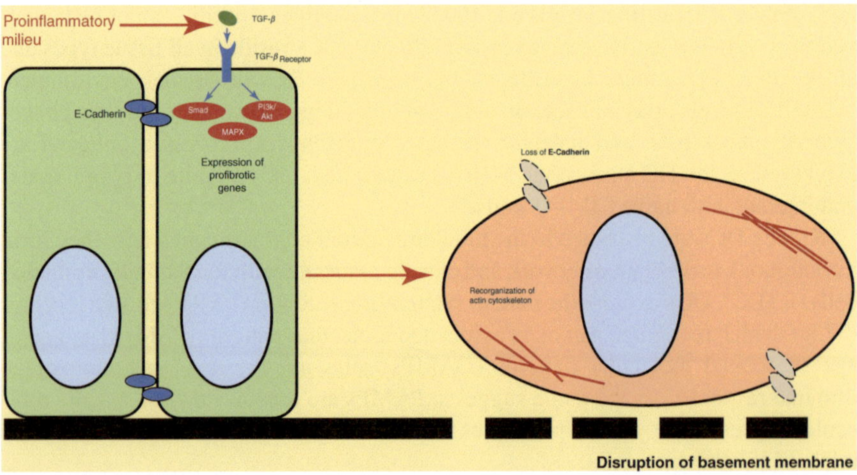

Fig. 1 Simplified schematic of epithelial to mesenchymal transformation (EMT). Pro-inflammatory milieu leads to expression of multiple pro-inflammatory cytokines including TGF-Upon binding to the TGF- Receptor various signaling pathways including Smad, MAPK and PI3K/Akt are activated which leads to the loss of epithelial markers such as E-Cadherin and loss of cell-cell adhesion. In addition, there is expression of profibrotic genes and mesenchymal markers leading to a morphological transformation and eventual fibrosis

reorganization, disruption of the tubular basement membrane, increased cell migration, and invasion to the surrounding tissue. TLR signaling, TNF-α, INF-γ, IL-6 and IL-1β can all stimulate TGF-β transcription and TGF-β receptor expression on RTEC and stabilize the profibrotic transcription factor Snail via NF-κB.

Cell lineage studies demonstrate that 36% of renal fibroblasts are derived from proximal tubule cells. This reduction in epithelial phenotype and increased fibroblast phenotype has also been observed in human kidney biopsy specimens. Antigen-sensitized T lymphocytes can induce fibroblast proliferation and collagen formation. Interstitial matrix can be laid down with fibrosis evident in as little as 3 weeks after the onset of inflammation.

2 Immune ATIN

With its large blood supply and concentrating ability, the kidney is exposed to circulating self and non-self antigens. Filtered proteins are taken up by the megalin/cubulin complex in the proximal tubule, broken down into peptides and released into the circulation.

Antigens are processed by DC and expressed on their cell surface via MHC II allowing them to interact with CD4+ T cells in local lymph nodes (Fig. 2). In a process known as peripheral tolerance, no immune response is elicited without the proper inflammatory costimulatory mileu, which prevents the activation of T cells when APC presents native or innocuous proteins and their fragments. The immune system has regulatory "checkpoints" including inhibitory receptors on T cells including programmed death protein-1 (PD-1) and CTLA-4 to prevent activation by autoantigens.

Effector T cells become tolerized via several pathways including binding of PD-1 to its cognate ligand PD-L1 on DC. Regulatory T cells (Treg) are essential in this process as they inhibit the maturation of renal DC and expression of proinflammatory cytokines in a CTLA-4 dependent fashion. Experiments in mouse models of AKI demonstrate that Treg depletion leads to a significant increase in inflammatory response after ischemia reperfusion injury. Drugs can interfere with this process of antigen presentation, recognition, and tolerance, which can lead to immune cell infiltration of the renal parenchyma.

When immature DC sense danger signals via PRR or process non-self antigens, they are activated and undergo maturation, resulting in the secretion of pro-inflammatory cytokines including TNF- α, interferons and IL-6. DC co-stimulatory molecule expression is enhanced which allows for CD4+ T cell activation once they are in close proximity to local lymph nodes. CCR7 expression is also increased in T cell rich areas of local lymph nodes which allows for DC migration. Activated CD4+ T cells then leave their lymph node, enter the circulation, and search out their antigen.

The hallmark lesions of ATIN on kidney biopsy are tubulitis and interstitial inflammation with edema. The infiltrate is composed of mostly mononuclear cells

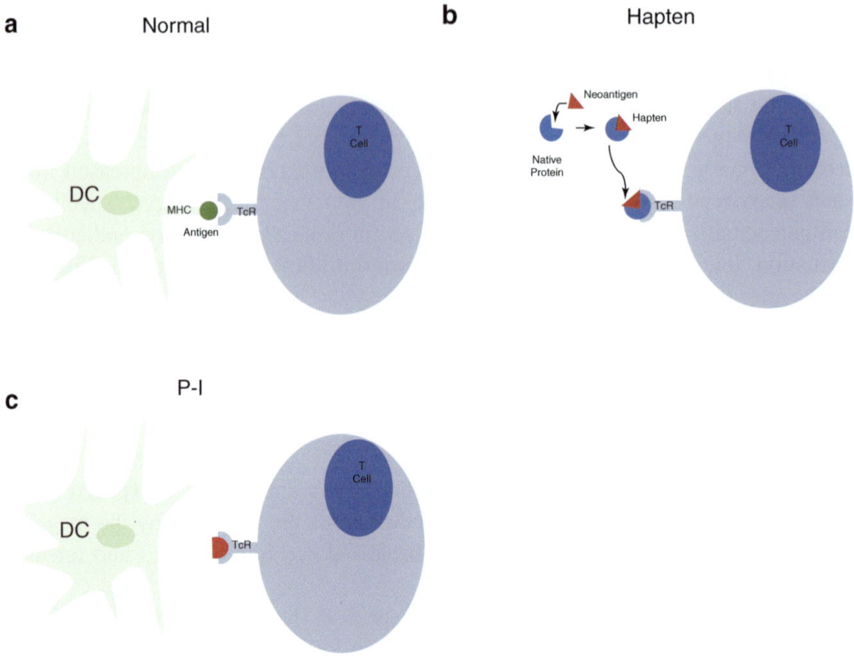

Fig. 2 Simple schematic of T Cell activation in drug induced ATIN. (**a**) Normal response. DC processes foreign antigen and expresses it to T cells via MHC II, binding to the TcR and eliciting a response. (**b**) Hapten response. Drug or foreign substance acts as a neoantigen, binding to a native protein creating a hapten which can bind to and activate the TcR. (**c**) P-I concept. Drug or foreign substance can bind directly to and activate the TcR without any need for modification. Please note, this is a simplified diagram, co-stimulatory molecules have been purposely omitted for simplicity. Abbreviations: DC= dendritic cell. TcR= T cell receptor MHC = Major histocompatibility complex

with CD4+ T cells comprising the majority cell type. Monocytes, B cells, eosinophils, and plasma cells can also be found in smaller numbers. The number of these infiltrating immune cells in kidney biopsy specimens correlates inversely to kidney function.

3 Allergic ATIN

Allergic ATIN is commonly referred to as allergic interstitial nephritis (AIN) and is caused by a hypersensitivity reaction to an exogenous substance, such as a medication or infection. This substance can be recognized as an antigen via molecular mimicry to a kidney antigen or be modified after its metabolism to elicit an immune response.

Drug-induced allergic ATIN is a Type B idiosyncratic immune reaction, described as a delayed type IV hypersensitivity reaction with typical onset around 7–10 days after exposure. For a drug to be recognized by the immune system as an allergen, it usually must first undergo modification.

Covalent binding of a neoantigen to protein causes a conformational change leading to its immune recognition (Fig. 2). This neoantigen-protein complex is known as a hapten. Haptens can elicit an antibody-mediated reaction through direct recognition or molecular mimicry via structural similarity to a native antigen. β-lactam antibiotics form haptens by binding lysine residues on albumin where molecular mimicry against a renal tubular basement membrane antigen is induced by methicillin.

Allergens can act as pro-haptens that are processed in the liver to haptens via the insertion or demasking of functional groups (Phase I reaction) or conjugation with small molecules such as glucuronic acid, glutathione, acetate or sulfate (Phase II reaction). The drug sulfamethoxazole is metabolized to nitroso-sulfamethoxazole, which acts as a hapten after binding to cysteine residues on host proteins. Genetic polymorphisms of phase II reaction enzymes may determine adverse drug reactions in certain populations. In a cohort of patients with sulfonamide induced Stevens-Johnson syndrome, 90% were found to have a slow acetylation phenotype.

An allergen may also directly stimulate T cells by binding to and activating the T cell receptor (TcR) or MHC directly, bypassing traditional processing in what is known as the p-i concept (Fig. 2). This is seen in carbamazepime hypersensitivity.

T cells that react against a specific drug can be identified in-vitro via a lymphocyte transformation test (LTT) where patient T cells are exposed to disks impregnated with candidate drugs and inflammatory cytokines are measured. Drug specific T cells are found circulating in patients with ATIN. Based on T cell receptor phenotype, subpopulations of circulating drug reactive T cells were found in kidney biopsy T cell infiltrates suggesting that the culprit drug or its associated hapten is present within the kidney.

NSAIDs, in addition to acting as haptens may cause ATIN via other immune mechanisms. NSAIDs inhibit cyclooxygenase and subsequently shift the conversion of arachidonic acid from prostaglandins to the chemoattractant leukotrienes possibly explaining the T cell predominant infiltrate often seen on biopsy.

ATIN has been well described in patients receiving immune check point inhibitors (ICI). which inhibit CTLA-4, PD-1, or PD-L1 and allow activation of antitumor T cell immunity. As mentioned previously, both CTLA-4 and PDL-1 are integral in maintaining tolerance to innocuous antigens within the kidney. Interestingly, ATIN from ICI can have a significant delay from initial exposure (21–245 days) and can occur up to 63 days from drug discontinuation. This is significantly different from the typical course of traditional drug induced ATIN and suggests that ICIs uniquely exert their adverse effect through loss of tolerance to antigens processed by the kidney.

Table 1 Pathogenesis, histology and systemic involvement of toxic interstitial nephropathies

Disorder	Pathogenesis	Renal histological characteristics	Other organ involvement
Chinese Herbal Nephropathy/ Balkan Endemic Nephropathy	Acute or chronic poisoning by aristolochic acid leading to oxidative stress, inflammation and fibrosis.	Chronic interstitial nephritis. Interstitial fibrosis. Variable cellular infiltration.	Urothelial carcinoma
Cadmium and Lead Nephropathy	Depletion of intracellular antioxidants (i.e. metallothionein) leading to oxidative stress. Disruption of cell adhesion molecules and calcium homeostasis.	Proximal tubular injury. Intranuclear inclusion bodies. Nonspecific interstitial nephritis	Abdominal pain. Arthralgia/myalgia. Anemia. Gout (Lead). Osteomalacia/ osteoporosis (Cadmium)
Lithium Nephropathy	Inhibition of the enzyme GSK3 involved in epithelial cell function and cell cycle progression. Also disrupts microtubules involved in AQ2 trafficking leading to cyst formation	Distal tubule/collecting duct microcysts. Interstitial fibrosis/ tubular atrophy. Glomerulosclerosis	Nephrogenic diabetes insipidus. Tremor/ataxia/ confusion.

Abbreviations: *AQ2* aquaporin, *GSK3* glycogen synthase kinase 3

4 Toxic ATIN

Most of the world uses botanicals as medicinals and some have been linked to nephrotoxicity. Environmental pollutants such as heavy metals can contaminate the surrounding soil or directly expose workers who are in contact with these substances (Table 1).

4.1 Aristolochic Acid

4.1.1 Cellular Toxicity and Inflammation and Fibrosis

Aristolochic acid (AA) is the cause of both Chinese herbal nephropathy and Balkan endemic nephropathy; characterized by severe tubulointerstitial disease. The former may develop acutely with large ingestions of AA leading to rapid development of CKD while the latter has a more indolent course due to longer duration of low level exposure. AA nephropathy pathogenesis can be divided into 3 main phases: cellular toxicity, inflammation, and fibrosis.

4.2 Cellular Toxicity

AA are compounds found in plants from the genus *Aristolochia* which contain more than 500 species and have long been used for medicinal purposes. Several hepatic enzymes are involved in AAs metabolism including NADPH, NQO1, and CYP

P450. AA undergo aerobic and anaerobic metabolism and are reduced to aristolactam I (AAI) and aristolactam II (AAII) respectively. AAI and AAII are then transported out of the liver and reabsorbed by the kidney via organic anion transporters (OATs) in the proximal tubule.

AA metabolites cause oxidative stress by depletion of the intracellular antioxidant glutathione,. In cell culture studies, AA induces endoplasmic reticulum stress, mitochondrial dysfunction, and apoptosis. Pretreatment with antioxidants N-acetylcysteine and glutathione inhibit AA induced apoptosis suggesting an important role of reactive oxygen species (ROS) in the pathogenesis of AA nephropathy.

4.3 *Inflammation and Fibrosis*

With 3 days of AA administration, rats demonstrate proximal tubulopathy and tubulitis with monocytic and macrophage infiltration as well as increased expression of inflammatory cytokines and activation of the inflammasome. This is in contrast to the acellular infiltration typically seen in human biopsy specimens, though this may be reflective of delayed presentation in the disease course.

Both mouse and cell culture models have demonstrated increased expression of the profibrotic cytokine, TGF-β after exposure to AA resulting in profibrotic gene expression (α-SMA and vimentin) which also suggests the presence of EMT (5, 129, 150, 154).

4.4 *Heavy Metals*

People are exposed to heavy metals as environmental pollutants and occupational hazards. While many heavy metals can cause kidney injury; the divalent metals, cadmium (Cd) and lead (Pb) are the most well-described causes of tubulointerstitial disease.

4.5 *Transport and Uptake*

Cd is absorbed in the small intestine via the divalent metal transporter (DMT-1), which displays high affinity for other divalent. Once absorbed, Cd binds primarily to albumin and is transported to the liver where it increases the transcription of metallothionein (MT), a cysteine-rich protein that protects against heavy metal toxicity by intracellular sequestration. In normal hepatocyte turn over or injury, Cd-MT complexes are released into the circulation, freely filtered at the glomerulus and subsequently reabsorbed by the megalin/cubulin complex in the proximal tubule (PT). MT knockout mice still demonstrate Cd uptake into the PT suggesting that Cd also circulates in a MT-independent manner. These forms of circulating Cd are also filtered and reabsorbed along the nephron likely via ZnT1 (Zinc transporter 1), DMT-1 and ATP-binding cassette (ABC) type transporter family suggesting that zinc may be able to outcompete Cd uptake.

Pb is also absorbed by DMT-1 in the intestine where it is quickly transported by erythrocytes bound to δ-aminolevulinic acid dehydratase (ALAD); higher concentrations of Pb can induce the expression of Pb binding protein. The exact mechanism of PT uptake of Pb has yet to be elucidated but may involve receptor-mediated endocytosis or utilization of calcium channels. Pb inclusion bodies in PT are often seen on biopsy, potentially representing Pb-protein complexes with proteins such as α-microglobulin, diazepine-binding inhibitor and thymosin β-4.

4.6 Toxicity

Heavy metals can cause cellular injury through oxidative stress, mitochondrial damage, and alterations in intracellular calcium homeostasis leading to inflammation and fibrosis.

Cd can cause proximal tubulopathy via disruption of cadherin cell adhesion molecules by binding to the extracellular calcium binding domain and interfering with intracellular signaling of β-catenin, influencing control of the cell cycle and apoptosis. This leads to the loss of epithelial cell polarity and basolateral specificity of the Na/K ATPase. Cd and Pb binding to intracellular thiol containing substances deplete antioxidants MT and glutathione and generate ROS leading to oxidative stress and apoptosis which can be attenuated by the administration of N-acetyl-cysteine in-vitro.

Intracellular Cd and Pb accumulation leads to mitochondrial damage via alterations in intracellular calcium homeostasis, likely through interactions with the CaSR and calmodulin. Intracellular Cd and Pb can also modulate the activity of MAP Kinases involved in regulation of apoptosis.

Furthermore, exposure to Pb and Cd can increase expression of pro-inflammatory and fibrotic cytokines including NF-κB and TGF-β; mice exposed to Cd demonstrate an increase transcription in genes involved in EMT.

4.7 Lithium

Lithium (Li) is effective treatment for bipolar disorder though chronic use is associated with nephrogenic diabetes insipidus and chronic tubulointerstitial disease. Additionally, microcysts originating from distal tubules and collecting ducts are common.

Li is freely filtered at the glomerulus, >80% is reabsorbed at the PT by the sodium hydrogen antiporter, NHE3 and the remainder is taken up by epithelial sodium channel (ENaC) in the distal nephron. ENaC has a higher affinity for Li than sodium, allowing Li to accumulate to toxic levels in the RTEC. The basolateral Na/K ATPase has low affinity for Li which further hinders its exit from the cell.

Li inhibits the enzyme GSK3, which is involved in regulation of epithelial function, cell survival, and cell cycle progression. GSK3 interacts with the microtubules involved in ciliary function and interferes with aquaporin 2 water channel trafficking which is suggested to be the mechanism of Li-induced microcyst formation. In addition, Li can affect cell signaling pathways involved in fibrosis and EMT.

5 Metabolic ATIN

Many metabolic end products are filtered and excreted by the kidney though these substances are not always innocuous. Under normal conditions, they are primarily located intracellularly and their release into the extracellular space can be recognized as a danger signal in the proper inflammatory milieu, leading to activation of the immune system (Table 2).

Table 2 Pathogenesis, histology and systemic involvement in metabolic interstitial nephropathies

Disorder	Pathogenesis	Renal histological characteristics	Other organ involvement
Urate Nephropathy	Oxidative stress causing endothelial dysfunction leading to vasoconstriction, glomerular hypertension and increased renin/ AII. Activation of TLRs. Possible direct DC stimulation and TcR activation.	Interstitial fibrosis. Focal interstitial inflammation with giant cells	Gout. Nephrolithiasis.
Oxalate Nephropathy	Deposition as calcium oxalate. Activation of inflammasome.	Oxalate crystal deposition (+birefringence with polarized light) with giant cell reaction. Non-specific tubular atrophy and interstitial fibrosis.	Systemic deposition of calcium oxalate if primary oxalosis is underlying etiology. Nephrolithiasis.
Kaliopenic Nephropathy	Increased renin/AII leading to increased fibrosis. Increased ammoniagenesis may lead to direct activation of alternative complement pathway via direct activation of C3 by ammonia.	Vacuolization of proximal and distal tubules. Lymphocytic infiltrate. Interstitial fibrosis. Kidney cysts.	Dependent upon cause of hypokalemia (malnutrition, spurious diuretic use).

Abbreviations: *AII* angiotensin II, *DC* dendritic cell, *TcR* T cell receptor, *TLR* toll-like receptor

5.1 Uric Acid

Uric acid (UA), a product of purine metabolism, has long been implicated as a cause of crystal nephropathy and CKD. An autopsy study in the 1960s demonstrated 50% of patients with gout had evidence of glomerular, vascular or tubulointerstitial lesions in their kidneys. However, asymptomatic, severe hyperuricemia in healthy subjects is associated with development of hypertension and CKD, suggesting a mechanism of injury outside of UA crystal deposition. The majority of UA is filtered by the glomerulus where it is reabsorbed in the proximal tubule via the urate anion transporter 1 (URAT1).

UA causes kidney injury via two main mechanisms: **a.** hemodynamic/endothelial injury and **b.** activation of the innate and adaptive immunity. In animal models, hyperuricemia has been shown to increase renal cortical vasoconstriction, glomerular hypertension, afferent arteriolar thickening and increase renin and angiotensin II levels. This occurs via activation of NADPH oxidase leading to the generation of ROS and reduction in nitric oxide production causing endothelial dysfunction through mitochondrial damage. Interestingly, this is in direct opposition to UA's role in the serum where it functions as an antioxidant.

Most UA is intracellular, though it can be released into the extracellular space by damaged cells where it acts as a DAMP and TLR ligand and subsequently activates the inflammasome. Activation leads to further expression of inflammatory cytokines. In addition, the generation of ROS leads to increased apoptosis via MAPK signaling in PT cells. Blockade of TLR2, TLR4 and their adaptor protein MyD88 can blunt the expression of these proinflammatory cytokines and reduce macrophage infiltration whereas blockade of NADPH oxidase, administration of the antioxidant NAC and inhibition of UA uptake via probenecid and losartan, can reduce ROS, proinflammatory cytokine production and apoptosis.

This proinflammatory environment induced by UA leads to the expression the chemoattractant MCP-1 and subsequent T cells and macrophages infiltration of the kidney. Furthermore, UA can directly stimulate DC maturation and TcR activation suggesting independent activation of the adaptive immune system.

Through increased expression of NF-κB and transcription factors Snail/Slug, UA has been able to induce EMT and fibrosis. Interestingly, manipulation of histone methylation has been shown to augment inflammation and fibrosis in response to UA suggesting a potential role for epigenic modifications in chronic hyperuricemia.

5.2 Oxalate

Hyperoxaluria can be primary (due to genetic mutations affecting enzymes involved in oxalate and glyoxylate metabolism) or secondary (due to increased oxalate consumption or intestinal absorption). Oxalate can complex with calcium leading to systemic deposition, inflammation, and fibrosis in organs including the kidney (oxalate nephropathy).

Circulating oxalate is excreted by the PT via the OAT, SCL26a6, where it forms calcium oxalate and crystalizes around proteins such as osteopontin that then bind to CD44 leading to endocytosis and expression of the TNF-receptor. Once endocytosed, calcium oxalate can lead to ROS generation, necrosis, and release of ATP, which acts as DAMPs and activate the inflammasome. Additionally, interstitial calcium oxalate phagocytosed by resident DC can also lead to inflammasome activation.

5.3 Hypokalemia

Early pathologic studies of patients with chronic hypokalemia and CKD described vacuolization of the proximal and distal tubules, significant interstitial fibrosis with lymphocytic infiltrate, juxtaglomerular apparatus hypertrophy (JGA) and development of kidney cysts.

Animals fed low potassium diets demonstrate increased renin, prostaglandin, intrarenal ACE, and angiotensin II expression as well as increased capillary loss, inflammatory cytokine expression and macrophage infiltration on biopsy. Angiotensin II and aldosterone are known to mediate activation of TGF-ß, which may explain the increased fibrosis associated with chronic hypokalemia. Lastly, hypokalemia-induced ammoniagenesis may lead to activation of the alternative complement pathway by ammonia's ability to interact with C3's reactive thiolester bond, which may explain the increased tubular C3 deposition on biopsy. Although the exact mechanism of kaliopenic nephropathy remains elusive, existing data suggest that chronic hypokalemia activates the RAAS system and ammoniagenesis; responses that become maladaptive over time.

6 Genetic ATIN

6.1 Karyomegalic Interstitial Nephritis

Karyomegalic interstitial nephritis (KIN) is a rare cause of hereditary chronic interstitial nephritis, characterized by the presence of enlarged, hyperchromatic and dysplastic nuclei in proximal and distal RTE cells (Table 3). Liver and lung involvement is seen in half of the cases, with skin, brain and digestive tissues less frequently involved. The kidney manifestations tend to be the most severe leading to tubular degeneration, interstitial fibrosis, and CKD. Tubular karyomegaly is also seen with viral infections (cytomegalovirus, adenovirus, polyoma virus), medications (ifosfamide, cisplatin) and mycotoxins such as Ochratoxin.

Pathogenesis of KIN has been linked to bi-allelic autosomal recessive mutations in the Fanconi anemia-associated nuclease 1 (*FAN1*) gene, which is an important DNA inter-strand crosslink repair gene in the Fanconi anemia DNA damage response pathway. Despite its name, *FAN1* gene mutation is not associated with a

Table 3 Genetic defects, pathogenesis and histology in genetic interstitial nephropathies

Disorder	Genetic defect	Pathogenesis	Renal histological characteristics	Other organ involvement
Karyomegalic Interstitial Nephritis	Bi-allelic autosomal recessive mutations in the Fanconi anemia-associated nuclease 1 (*FAN1*) gene	Mutations in *FAN1*, an endonuclease that facilitates DNA crosslink repair, increase susceptibility of RTECs to DNA damage (ploidy)	Enlarged, hyperchromatic and dysplastic nuclei in RTECs (tubular karyomegaly), tubular degeneration, interstitial fibrosis, and CKD	Liver, lung, skin involvement. Linked to hereditary colorectal cancer, microcephaly, and bone marrow failure.
Familial Nephronophthisis	AR (*NPHP1-20 genes*) that encode nephrocystin protein. *NPHP1* homozygous deletion most frequent (~20%).	Defects in Nephrocystin which is involved in primary cilia, centrosome, and basal body functions, result in a ciliopathy and defective cellular signaling.	Corticomedullary kidney cysts, chronic tubulointerstitial nephritis (TIN), tubular basement membrane disruption, and tubular atrophy	Retinitis pigmentosa, hepatic fibrosis, situs inversus, skeletal and cardiac defects, cerebellar hypoplasia, and mental retardation
TINU syndrome	Linkage to several HLA genes (detailed in text suggests genetic susceptibility.	Immune-mediated injury (cell and humoral) in response to an environmental trigger	Predominantly lymphocytic and monocytic interstitial infiltrate (indicative of a cell mediated process). Modified CRP may be a target antigen for antibody mediated injury	Bilateral anterior uveitis
ADTKD-UMOD	Autosomal dominant gene mutations in *UMOD.*	ADTKD-UMOD mutations result in misfolded proteins that activate an ER stress response resulting in mitochondrial and cellular dysfunction and inflammation and interstitial fibrosis	Progressive tubulointerstitial damage and fibrosis without glomerular involvement and ultimate progression to ESKD	Gout

Abbreviations: *ADTKD* autosomal dominant tubulointerstitial kidney disease, *AR* autosomal recessive, *CKD* chronic kidney disease, *ER* endoplasmic reticulum, *ESKD* end stage kidney disease, *NPNH* Nephronophthisis, *RTECs* renal tubular epithelial cells, *TINU* tubulointerstitial nephritis and uveitis, *UMOD* uromodulin

Fanconi anemia phenotype as its role in DNA crosslink repair is distinct from the other genes implicated in Fanconi anemia pathogenesis. *FAN1* is an endonuclease that prevents genotoxin induced polyploidy by facilitating DNA crosslink repair. Given the kidney's role as a systemic filter, *FAN1* mutations could increase the susceptibility of RTE cells to environmental genotoxin-induced renal DNA damage (ploidy) resulting in KIN. High doses of cisplatin at 20 mg/kg resulted in development of AKI in wild type mice as well as $FAN1^{-/-}$ knockout mice. However, chronic injection of cisplatin at 2 mg/kg induced KIN in $FAN1^{-/-}$ mice within 5 weeks but not in wild type mice, suggesting the role of *FAN1* in genotoxin induced DNA repair process in the kidney and development of KIN. In addition to KIN, *FAN1* gene mutations have been linked to hereditary colorectal cancer, developmental defects such as microcephaly and bone marrow failure.

6.2 *Familial Nephronophthisis*

Nephronophthisis (NPHP) is the most common monogenic cause of end-stage kidney disease (ESKD) in patients <30 years of age and is histologically marked by corticomedullary kidney cysts, chronic tubulointerstitial nephritis (TIN), tubular basement membrane disruption, and tubular atrophy (Table 3). NPHP is an autosomal recessive, genetically heterogenous disorder, linked to over 20 genes (*NPHP1-20*) that encode nephrocystin protein involved in primary cilia, centrosome, and basal body functions. *NPHP1* homozygous deletion is the most frequently implicated in this disorder (~20%) while the other mutations account for <3% each. In the remainder (~30%), genetic defect may be unknown. Primary cilium is a sensory organelle that regulates intracellular signaling, cell polarity, cell cycle and function. Genes linked to NPHP result in a ciliopathy and defects in cellular signaling pathways such as noncanonical Wnt and sonic hedgehog pathways. In the kidney, the inability of ciliary mechanosensors to accurately assess tubular luminal flow rates results in dysregulated tissue growth and kidney cyst formation.

NPHP displays phenotypic variability ranging from urinary concentrating defects and bland urinalysis to kidney cysts progressing to kidney atrophy and ESKD. Extra-renal manifestations are prevalent (~23% in *NPHP1* and ~66% in those without *NPHP1*), and include retinitis pigmentosa, hepatic fibrosis, situs inversus, skeletal and cardiac defects, cerebellar hypoplasia, and mental retardation. Due to the non-specific clinical and biopsy findings as well as significant overlap with other ciliopathies, precise diagnosis may require genetic analysis. Although NPHP is categorized alongside medullary cystic kidney disease, the latter is an autosomal dominant disorder with onset of ESKD in adulthood.

6.3 *Tubulointerstitial-Uveitis Syndrome (TINU)*

TINU syndrome is a multisystem autoimmune disease that primarily manifests as bilateral anterior uveitis and TIN (Table 3). Initially described in 1975, around 200 cases of TINU have been reported worldwide since. Both genetic and environmental factors have been linked to its pathogenesis. TINU has been reported with certain infections (Campylobacter jejuni, Epstein-Barr virus, Human T-lymphotropic virus type 1, etc.) and chemical exposures (non- steroidal anti-inflammatory drugs, herbal formulation Goreisan). Reports of familial clustering of the disease and linkage to several HLA genes such as HLA DRB1*14, DQA1*01:04, DQA1*04:01, DRB1*14, DRB1*0102 suggests genetic susceptibility. Immune-mediated injury (cell and humoral) in response to an environmental trigger is central to the pathogenesis of TINU. The predominantly lymphocytic and monocytic interstitial infiltrate found in the kidney interstitium of patients with TINU is indicative of a cell mediated process. High levels of antibodies against modified C-reactive protein (CRP) have been detected in patients with TINU. Interestingly, these antibodies co-localize in kidney and ocular tissue leading to the theory that modified CRP may be a target antigen in the disease. Other antibodies such as anti-nuclear, anti-neutrophil cytoplasmic, and anti-glomerular basement membrane antibody have been detected in patients with TINU, however their significance is unclear. TINU has several overlapping features with sarcoidosis and Sjogren's syndrome which may make the diagnosis challenging.

6.4 Autosomal Dominant Tubulointerstitial Kidney Disease (ADTKD)

In recent years, ~5% of monogenic causes of CKD have been attributed to ADTKD, a group of disorders characterized by progressive tubulointerstitial damage and fibrosis without glomerular involvement and ultimate progression to ESKD (Table 3). Mutations in at least five different genes including *UMOD*, *MUC1*, *REN*, *HNF1B* and, more rarely, *SEC61A1* have been implicated. These proteins have several renal and extra-renal functions. Pathogenesis of ADTKD-UMOD is the most extensively studied and will be briefly described here. UMOD encodes uromodulin, a kidney-specific protein secreted by the RTEC of the thick ascending loop and early distal convoluted tubule. UMOD mutations result in misfolded proteins that accumulate within the endoplasmic reticulum (ER) in large amounts, activating an ER stress response that leads to impaired autophagy, mitochondrial and cellular dysfunction and ultimately, inflammation and interstitial fibrosis. For a detailed discussion of ADTKD, the reader is referred to an excellent review on the topic.

7 Infiltrative ATIN

While all cases of ATIN involve infiltration of the tubulointerstitium by inflammatory cells, certain systemic diseases associated with multi-organ pathology appear to induce inflammatory infiltration in kidney, via putative autoimmune mechanisms. Among these, Sjogrens syndrome, sarcoidosis, systemic lupus erythematosus (SLE), and IgG4-related disease (IgG4-RD). Hematological malignancies such as leukemia can also cause infiltrative ATIN but we will limit this discussion to autoimmune systemic diseases (Table 4).

Table 4 Pathogenesis, histology, and systemic involvement in infiltrative interstitial nephropathies

Disorder	Pathogenesis	Renal histological characteristics	Other organ involvement
Sjogren's syndrome	Environmental triggers expose neoantigens in salivary gland that activate lymphocytes in genetically susceptible patients. These activated lymphocytes cause kidney injury.	Interstitial infiltrate rich in T and B-cells and plasma cells, interstitial fibrosis and CKD	Salivary glands
Sarcoidosis	? Environmental trigger (i.e. bacterial infection); Vimentin has been implicated as an autoantigen. A variety of immune cells including antigen presenting cells and CD4+ cells are involved.	Non-caseating granulomas with lymphoplasmacytic interstitial infiltrate	Eye, skin, lung
Systemic Lupus Erythematosus	Multiple mechanisms including antibody mediated injury against an in-situ antigen (e.g. anti-vimentin antibodies); innate immunity via toll-like receptors; cytokine mediated injury (IFN-α,IL-6). Binding of anti-ds-DNA to RTECs has been implicated in some of these processes.	Plasma and B-cell rich interstitial infiltrate	Multi-organ involvement including brain, lungs, liver, skin
IgG4 disease	Clonal expansion of self-reactive B cells results in activation of CD4+ T cells and recruitment of other immune cells (macrophages, follicular helper T cells, fibroblasts) and IgG4+ isotype switching resulting in direct cytotoxicity, and cytokine mediated injury	IgG4+ plasma cells scattered throughout the interstitium and often, IgG4+ immune complex deposition in tubular basement membranes. Storiform fibrosis is a characterizing feature.	Multi-organ involvement including liver, gastrointestinal tract, lymph nodes

Abbreviations: *CKD* chronic kidney disease, *RTECs* renal tubular epithelial cells

7.1 Sjogren's Syndrome

TIN in Sjogren's syndrome involves an infiltrate rich in T and B-cells and plasma cells, that eventually leads to fibrosis and CKD. These infiltrates resemble those seen in the salivary glands and other organs more typically affected by Sjogren's. The inciting factor for kidney involvement likely occurs outside the kidney, with factors as diverse as viral and bacterial infections exposing epithelial neoantigens in salivary glands of genetically susceptible individuals. Glandular epithelia in Sjogren's have also been shown to express HLA-DR, potentially highlighting a role of antigen presentation by epithelial cells to T-cells and B-cells. These activated lymphocytes access the general circulation and deposit in various organs including the kidney. Additional kidney injury may result from autoantibodies binding to transporters common to salivary gland and kidney epithelia, such as H^+/ATPase. This can cause local destruction of kidney tissue and release novel kidney antigens targeted by T and B-cells.

7.2 Sarcoidosis

Kidney sarcoidosis is characterized by granulomatous ATIN. Non-caseating granulomas are also present in other organs including lung, skin, and eyes. The trigger is unclear though bacterial infections have been implicated in pulmonary sarcoid. A variety of immune cells are critical to granuloma formation including antigen presenting cells and CD4+ T-cells. The inciting antigens are not definitively identified but in pulmonary sarcoid, increasing attention has been focused on vimentin, a filament protein. Vimentin is also expressed in kidney tubules and interstitium and is upregulated in states of regeneration, repair and even EMT, making it conceivable that as with pulmonary sarcoid, it acts as an autoantigen in kidney sarcoidosis. Tumor necrosis factor (TNF) may also play a role in the pathogenesis of kidney sarcoidosis, as demonstrated by anti-TNF therapy inducing granulomatous changes similar to sarcoidosis.

7.3 Systemic Lupus Erythematosus (SLE) Nephritis

While primarily thought of as a glomerular disease, SLE nephritis (LN) may also involve the tubulointerstitium and lupus TIN is associated with progressive kidney disease. In contrast to glomerulonephritis, lupus TIN is characterized by a plasma and B-cell rich infiltrate. Germinal center-like as well as B and T cell aggregates have been noted within these infiltrates, leading to the idea of in situ antigen driving the inflammatory response. Indeed, cytoplasmic antibodies have been detected in patients with lupus TIN that show local rather than circulating clonal expansion. These antibodies display antigen specificity for vimentin, suggesting that as with kidney sarcoidosis, a protein expressed in the tubulointerstitium stimulates inflammation.

Innate immunity via toll-like receptors (TLRs) may also play a role in lupus TIN. TLR9 expression on RTECs is upregulated in experimental murine models of lupus TIN and in kidney biopsies from patients with lupus TIN. Antibodies against double stranded (ds) DNA reflect disease activity in patients with lupus and bind directly to RTECs. Notably, dsDNA binding activates TLR9, suggesting another pathway for a pathogenic role in lupus TIN.

Cytokine activation may also be involved in lupus TIN. Type 1 interferons (IFN), particularly IFN-α, are recognized as central inflammatory mediators in SLE and are secreted by RTECs, but a specific role in lupus TIN is not defined. However, anti-dsDNA antibody binding to RTECs results in IL-6 secretion and higher levels of IL-6 tubulointerstitial staining correlates with worsening TIN scores. Similarly, TNF expression in proliferative LN is associated with worsening TIN as well as glomerulonephritis.

7.4 IgG4 Disease

IgG4 related disease (IgG4RD) has a heterogeneous presentation ranging from solid mass formation to lymphoplasmacytic cell infiltration in various organ systems, including the kidney. In IgG4 TIN, the disease is defined by IgG4+ plasma cells scattered throughout the interstitium and often, IgG4+ immune complex deposition in tubular basement membranes. The interstitial infiltrate can occur on a background of swirl-like fibrosis known as storiform fibrosis.

The proposed mechanism behind IgG4RD centers around the clonal expansion of self-reactive B cells. Antigen-specific B cell expansion is critical for antigen presentation to and activation of CD4+ T cells with activity in various tissues, including the kidney. In addition to cytotoxic effector functions that lead to direct tissue damage, these activated T cells also stimulate a cytokine rich environment that can recruit other immune cells, including macrophages. Furthermore, other cytokines can act on resident fibroblasts to create local fibrosis.

Other immune cells that are involved in the pathogenesis of IgG4RD include follicular helper T (T_{fh}) cells, which are found in extra-lymphoid or ectopic germinal centers (EGCs). EGCs have been described in IgG4RD affecting salivary glands but have also been less commonly noted in kidney IgG4RD. T_{fh} cells interact with antigen-specific B cells in EGCs to encourage affinity maturation and IgG4+ isotype switching, both of which are also critical to clonal expansion of B-cells and plasma cells.

Suggested Reading

Airik R, Schueler M, Airik M, Cho J, Porath JD, Mukherjee E, et al. A FANCD2/FANCI-associated nuclease 1-knockout model develops karyomegalic interstitial nephritis. J Am Soc Nephrol. 2016;27(12):3552–9.

Alsady M, Baumgarten R, Deen PM, de Groot T. Lithium in the kidney: friend and foe? J Am Soc Nephrol. 2016;27(6):1587–95.

Anger EE, Yu F, Li J. Aristolochic acid-induced nephrotoxicity: molecular mechanisms and potential protective approaches. Int J Mol Sci. 2020;21(3):1157.

Austyn JM, Hankins DF, Larsen CP, Morris PJ, Rao AS, Roake JA. Isolation and characterization of dendritic cells from mouse heart and kidney. J Immunol. 1994;152(5):2401–10.
Bajema IM, Wilhelmus S, Alpers CE, Bruijn JA, Colvin RB, Cook HT, et al. Revision of the International Society of Nephrology/Renal Pathology Society classification for lupus nephritis: clarification of definitions, and modified National Institutes of Health activity and chronicity indices. Kidney Int. 2018;93(4):789–96.
Baldwin DS, Levine BB, McCluskey RT, Gallo GR. Renal failure and interstitial nephritis due to penicillin and methicillin. N Engl J Med. 1968;279(23):1245–52.
Barbier O, Jacquillet G, Tauc M, Cougnon M, Poujeol P. Effect of heavy metals on, and handling by, the kidney. Nephron Physiol. 2005;99(4):105–10.
Benigni A, Caroli C, Longaretti L, Gagliardini E, Zoja C, Galbusera M, et al. Involvement of renal tubular Toll-like receptor 9 in the development of tubulointerstitial injury in systemic lupus. Arthritis Rheum. 2007;56(5):1569–78.
Bishop GA, Waugh JA, Hall BM. Expression of HLA antigens on renal tubular cells in culture. II. Effect of increased HLA antigen expression on tubular cell stimulation of lymphocyte activation and on their vulnerability to cell-mediated lysis. Transplantation. 1988;46(2):303–10.
Border WA, Lehman DH, Egan JD, Sass HJ, Glode JE, Wilson CB. Antitubular basement-membrane antibodies in methicillin-associated interstitial nephritis. N Engl J Med. 1974;291(8):381–4.
Border WA, Noble NA. Interactions of transforming growth factor-beta and angiotensin II in renal fibrosis. Hypertension. 1998;31(1 Pt 2):181–8.
Bossini N, Savoldi S, Franceschini F, Mombelloni S, Baronio M, Cavazzana I, et al. Clinical and morphological features of kidney involvement in primary Sjögren's syndrome. Nephrol Dial Transplant. 2001;16(12):2328–36.
Braga TT, Forni MF, Correa-Costa M, Ramos RN, Barbuto JA, Branco P, et al. Soluble uric acid activates the NLRP3 inflammasome. Sci Rep. 2017;7:39884.
Bridges CC, Zalups RK. Molecular and ionic mimicry and the transport of toxic metals. Toxicol Appl Pharmacol. 2005;204(3):274–308.
Chang SY, Weber EJ, Sidorenko VS, Chapron A, Yeung CK, Gao C, et al. Human liver-kidney model elucidates the mechanisms of aristolochic acid nephrotoxicity. JCI Insight. 2017;2(22):e95978.
Charen E, Harbord N. Toxicity of herbs, vitamins, and supplements. Adv Chronic Kidney Dis. 2020;27(1):67–71.
Chen JQ, Szodoray P, Zeher M. Toll-like receptor pathways in autoimmune diseases. Clin Rev Allergy Immunol. 2016;50(1):1–17.
Christensen EI, Birn H. Megalin and cubilin: synergistic endocytic receptors in renal proximal tubule. Am J Physiol Renal Physiol. 2001;280(4):F562–73.
Chuang SM, Wang IC, Yang JL. Roles of JNK, p38 and ERK mitogen-activated protein kinases in the growth inhibition and apoptosis induced by cadmium. Carcinogenesis. 2000;21(7):1423–32.
Clark MR, Trotter K, Chang A. The pathogenesis and therapeutic implications of tubulointerstitial inflammation in human lupus nephritis. Semin Nephrol. 2015;35(5):455–64.
Clive DM, Vanguri VK. The syndrome of tubulointerstitial nephritis with uveitis (TINU). Am J Kidney Dis. 2018;72(1):118–28.
Cochat P, Rumsby G. Primary hyperoxaluria. N Engl J Med. 2013;369(7):649–58.
Conn JW, Johnson RD. Kaliopenic nephropathy. Am J Clin Nutr. 1956;4(5):523–8.
Cortazar FB, Kibbelaar ZA, Glezerman IG, Abudayyeh A, Mamlouk O, Motwani SS, et al. Clinical features and outcomes of immune checkpoint inhibitor-associated AKI: a multicenter study. J Am Soc Nephrol. 2020;31(2):435–46.
Cortazar FB, Marrone KA, Troxell ML, Ralto KM, Hoenig MP, Brahmer JR, et al. Clinicopathological features of acute kidney injury associated with immune checkpoint inhibitors. Kidney Int. 2016;90(3):638–47.
Cortazar FB, Stone JH. IgG4-related disease and the kidney. Nat Rev Nephrol. 2015;11(10):599–609.
Crişan TO, Cleophas MC, Oosting M, Lemmers H, Toenhake-Dijkstra H, Netea MG, et al. Soluble uric acid primes TLR-induced proinflammatory cytokine production by human primary cells via inhibition of IL-1Ra. Ann Rheum Dis. 2016;75(4):755–62.

Crow MK. Type I interferon in the pathogenesis of lupus. J Immunol. 2014;192(12):5459–68.
Davis J, Desmond M, Berk M. Lithium and nephrotoxicity: a literature review of approaches to clinical management and risk stratification. BMC Nephrol. 2018a;19(1):305.
Davis J, Desmond M, Berk M. Lithium and nephrotoxicity: unravelling the complex pathophysiological threads of the lightest metal. Nephrology (Carlton). 2018b;23(10):897–903.
Devuyst O, Olinger E, Weber S, Eckardt KU, Kmoch S, Rampoldi L, et al. Autosomal dominant tubulointerstitial kidney disease. Nat Rev Dis Primers. 2019;5(1):60.
Dobrin RS, Vernier RL, Fish AL. Acute eosinophilic interstitial nephritis and renal failure with bone marrow-lymph node granulomas and anterior uveitis. A new syndrome. Am J Med. 1975;59(3):325–33.
Dong X, Swaminathan S, Bachman LA, Croatt AJ, Nath KA, Griffin MD. Antigen presentation by dendritic cells in renal lymph nodes is linked to systemic and local injury to the kidney. Kidney Int. 2005;68(3):1096–108.
Ebbo M, Daniel L, Pavic M, Sève P, Hamidou M, Andres E, et al. IgG4-related systemic disease: features and treatment response in a French cohort: results of a multicenter registry. Medicine (Baltimore). 2012;91(1):49–56.
Enomoto A, Kimura H, Chairoungdua A, Shigeta Y, Jutabha P, Cha SH, et al. Molecular identification of a renal urate anion exchanger that regulates blood urate levels. Nature. 2002;417(6887):447–52.
Faurskov B, Bjerregaard HF. Evidence for cadmium mobilization of intracellular calcium through a divalent cation receptor in renal distal epithelial A6 cells. Pflugers Arch. 2002;445(1):40–50.
Ferguson CJ, Wareing M, Ward DT, Green R, Smith CP, Riccardi D. Cellular localization of divalent metal transporter DMT-1 in rat kidney. Am J Physiol Renal Physiol. 2001;280(5):F803–11.
Fervenza FC, Rabkin R. The role of growth factors and ammonia in the genesis of hypokalemic nephropathy. J Ren Nutr. 2002;12(3):151–9.
Finkelstein A, Fraley DS, Stachura I, Feldman HA, Gandy DR, Bourke E. Fenoprofen nephropathy: lipoid nephrosis and interstitial nephritis. A possible T-lymphocyte disorder. Am J Med. 1982;72(1):81–7.
François H, Mariette X. Renal involvement in primary Sjögren syndrome. Nat Rev Nephrol. 2016;12(2):82–93.
Frangogiannis N. Transforming growth factor-β in tissue fibrosis. J Exp Med. 2020;217(3):e20190103.
Fujishiro H, Yano Y, Takada Y, Tanihara M, Himeno S. Roles of ZIP8, ZIP14, and DMT1 in transport of cadmium and manganese in mouse kidney proximal tubule cells. Metallomics. 2012;4(7):700–8.
Garrick MD, Dolan KG, Horbinski C, Ghio AJ, Higgins D, Porubcin M, et al. DMT1: a mammalian transporter for multiple metals. Biometals. 2003;16(1):41–54.
Gobe G, Crane D. Mitochondria, reactive oxygen species and cadmium toxicity in the kidney. Toxicol Lett. 2010;198(1):49–55.
Gonick HC. Nephrotoxicity of cadmium & lead. Indian J Med Res. 2008;128(4):335–52.
Gould TD, Manji HK. Glycogen synthase kinase-3: a putative molecular target for lithium mimetic drugs. Neuropsychopharmacology. 2005;30(7):1223–37.
Griem P, Wulferink M, Sachs B, González JB, Gleichmann E. Allergic and autoimmune reactions to xenobiotics: how do they arise? Immunol Today. 1998;19(3):133–41.
Grünfeld JP, Rossier BC. Lithium nephrotoxicity revisited. Nat Rev Nephrol. 2009;5(5):270–6.
Guo H, Callaway JB, Ting JP. Inflammasomes: mechanism of action, role in disease, and therapeutics. Nat Med. 2015;21(7):677–87.
Haller H, Bertram A, Nadrowitz F, Menne J. Monocyte chemoattractant protein-1 and the kidney. Curr Opin Nephrol Hypertens. 2016;25(1):42–9.
Hart BA, Lee CH, Shukla GS, Shukla A, Osier M, Eneman JD, et al. Characterization of cadmium-induced apoptosis in rat lung epithelial cells: evidence for the participation of oxidant stress. Toxicology. 1999;133(1):43–58.

He L, Wang B, Hay EB, Nebert DW. Discovery of ZIP transporters that participate in cadmium damage to testis and kidney. Toxicol Appl Pharmacol. 2009;238(3):250–7.
Hildebrandt F, Attanasio M, Otto E. Nephronophthisis: disease mechanisms of a ciliopathy. J Am Soc Nephrol. 2009;20(1):23–35.
Hong S, Healy H, Kassianos AJ. The emerging role of renal tubular epithelial cells in the immunological pathophysiology of lupus nephritis. Front Immunol. 2020;11:578952.
Isnard Bagnis C, Deray G, Baumelou A, Le Quintrec M, Vanherweghem JL. Herbs and the kidney. Am J Kidney Dis. 2004;44(1):1–11.
Isnard P, Rabant M, Labaye J, Antignac C, Knebelmann B, Zaidan M. Karyomegalic interstitial nephritis: a case report and review of the literature. Medicine. 2016;95(20):e3349.
Iwano M, Plieth D, Danoff TM, Xue C, Okada H, Neilson EG. Evidence that fibroblasts derive from epithelium during tissue fibrosis. J Clin Invest. 2002;110(3):341–50.
Iyer SS, Pulskens WP, Sadler JJ, Butter LM, Teske GJ, Ulland TK, et al. Necrotic cells trigger a sterile inflammatory response through the Nlrp3 inflammasome. Proc Natl Acad Sci U S A. 2009;106(48):20388–93.
Jevnikar AM, Wuthrich RP, Takei F, Xu HW, Brennan DC, Glimcher LH, et al. Differing regulation and function of ICAM-1 and class II antigens on renal tubular cells. Kidney Int. 1990;38(3):417–25.
Jin T, Lu J, Nordberg M. Toxicokinetics and biochemistry of cadmium with special emphasis on the role of metallothionein. Neurotoxicology. 1998;19(4-5):529–35.
John R, Nelson PJ. Dendritic cells in the kidney. J Am Soc Nephrol. 2007;18(10):2628–35.
Kalita-De Croft P, Bedford JJ, Leader JP, Walker RJ. Amiloride modifies the progression of lithium-induced renal interstitial fibrosis. Nephrology (Carlton). 2018;23(1):20–30.
Kamekura R, Takano K, Yamamoto M, Kawata K, Shigehara K, Jitsukawa S, et al. Cutting edge: a critical role of lesional T follicular helper cells in the pathogenesis of IgG4-related disease. J Immunol. 2017;199(8):2624–9.
Kaneko K, Nishii S, Izumi Y, Yasuda M, Yamanobe T, Fukuuchi T, et al. Proteomic analysis after sequential extraction of matrix proteins in urinary stones composed of calcium oxalate monohydrate and calcium oxalate dihydrate. Anal Sci. 2015;31(9):935–42.
Kanellis J, Watanabe S, Li JH, Kang DH, Li P, Nakagawa T, et al. Uric acid stimulates monocyte chemoattractant protein-1 production in vascular smooth muscle cells via mitogen-activated protein kinase and cyclooxygenase-2. Hypertension. 2003;41(6):1287–93.
Kang DH, Park SK, Lee IK, Johnson RJ. Uric acid-induced C-reactive protein expression: implication on cell proliferation and nitric oxide production of human vascular cells. J Am Soc Nephrol. 2005;16(12):3553–62.
Kemter E, Fröhlich T, Arnold GJ, Wolf E, Wanke R. Mitochondrial dysregulation secondary to endoplasmic reticulum stress in autosomal dominant tubulointerstitial kidney disease – UMOD (ADTKD-UMOD). Sci Rep. 2017;7:42970.
Khosla UM, Zharikov S, Finch JL, Nakagawa T, Roncal C, Mu W, et al. Hyperuricemia induces endothelial dysfunction. Kidney Int. 2005;67(5):1739–42.
Kimura O, Endo T, Hotta Y, Sakata M. Effects of P-glycoprotein inhibitors on transepithelial transport of cadmium in cultured renal epithelial cells, LLC-PK1 and LLC-GA5-COL 150. Toxicology. 2005;208(1):123–32.
Kinloch AJ, Chang A, Ko K, Henry Dunand CJ, Henderson S, Maienschein-Cline M, et al. Vimentin is a dominant target of in situ humoral immunity in human lupus tubulointerstitial nephritis. Arthritis Rheumatol. 2014;66(12):3359–70.
Kinsey GR, Sharma R, Huang L, Li L, Vergis AL, Ye H, et al. Regulatory T cells suppress innate immunity in kidney ischemia-reperfusion injury. J Am Soc Nephrol. 2009;20(8):1744–53.
Kinsey GR, Sharma R, Okusa MD. Regulatory T cells in AKI. J Am Soc Nephrol. 2013;24(11):1720–6.
Klaassen CD, Liu J, Choudhuri S. Metallothionein: an intracellular protein to protect against cadmium toxicity. Annu Rev Pharmacol Toxicol. 1999;39:267–94.

Klassen RB, Crenshaw K, Kozyraki R, Verroust PJ, Tio L, Atrian S, et al. Megalin mediates renal uptake of heavy metal metallothionein complexes. Am J Physiol Renal Physiol. 2004;287(3):F393–403.
Knauf F, Asplin JR, Granja I, Schmidt IM, Moeckel GW, David RJ, et al. NALP3-mediated inflammation is a principal cause of progressive renal failure in oxalate nephropathy. Kidney Int. 2013;84(5):895–901.
Kobayashi Y, Honda M, Yoshikawa N, Ito H. Immunohistological study in sixteen children with acute tubulointerstitial nephritis. Clin Nephrol. 1998;50(1):14–20.
König J, Kranz B, König S, Schlingmann KP, Titieni A, Tönshoff B, et al. Phenotypic spectrum of children with nephronophthisis and related ciliopathies. Clin J Am Soc Nephrol. 2017;12(12):1974–83.
Kosiba AA, Wang Y, Chen D, Wong CKC, Gu J, Shi H. The roles of calcium-sensing receptor (CaSR) in heavy metals-induced nephrotoxicity. Life Sci. 2020;242:117183.
Krishnan N, Perazella MA. Drug-induced acute interstitial nephritis: pathology, pathogenesis, and treatment. Iran J Kidney Dis. 2015;9(1):3–13.
Kurts C. Dendritic cells: not just another cell type in the kidney, but a complex immune sentinel network. Kidney Int. 2006;70(3):412–4.
Kuwabara M, Niwa K, Hisatome I, Nakagawa T, Roncal-Jimenez CA, Andres-Hernando A, et al. Asymptomatic hyperuricemia without comorbidities predicts cardiometabolic diseases: five-year Japanese cohort study. Hypertension. 2017;69(6):1036–44.
Lachaud C, Slean M, Marchesi F, Lock C, Odell E, Castor D, et al. Karyomegalic interstitial nephritis and DNA damage-induced polyploidy in Fan1 nuclease-defective knock-in mice. Genes Dev. 2016;30(6):639–44.
Lebeau C, Debelle FD, Arlt VM, Pozdzik A, De Prez EG, Phillips DH, et al. Early proximal tubule injury in experimental aristolochic acid nephropathy: functional and histological studies. Nephrol Dial Transplant. 2005;20(11):2321–32.
Lee JW, Kim HJ, Sung SH, Lee SJ. A case of tubulointerstitial nephritis and uveitis syndrome with severe immunologic dysregulation. Pediatr Nephrol (Berlin, Germany). 2005;20(12):1805–8.
Levinson RD, Park MS, Rikkers SM, Reed EF, Smith JR, Martin TM, et al. Strong associations between specific HLA-DQ and HLA-DR alleles and the tubulointerstitial nephritis and uveitis syndrome. Invest Ophthalmol Vis Sci. 2003;44(2):653–7.
Li C, Su T, Chu R, Li X, Yang L. Tubulointerstitial nephritis with uveitis in Chinese adults. Clin J Am Soc Nephrol. 2014;9(1):21–8.
Linas SL, Dickmann D. Mechanism of the decreased renal blood flow in the potassium-depleted conscious rat. Kidney Int. 1982;21(5):757–64.
Liu F, Li ZF, Wang ZY, Wang L. Role of subcellular calcium redistribution in regulating apoptosis and autophagy in cadmium-exposed primary rat proximal tubular cells. J Inorg Biochem. 2016;164:99–109.
Liu H, Xiong J, He T, Xiao T, Li Y, Yu Y, et al. High uric acid-induced epithelial-mesenchymal transition of renal tubular epithelial cells via the TLR4/NF-kB signaling pathway. Am J Nephrol. 2017;46(4):333–42.
Liu J, Kadiiska MB, Corton JC, Qu W, Waalkes MP, Mason RP, et al. Acute cadmium exposure induces stress-related gene expression in wild-type and metallothionein-I/II-null mice. Free Radic Biol Med. 2002;32(6):525–35.
Liu Y. New insights into epithelial-mesenchymal transition in kidney fibrosis. J Am Soc Nephrol. 2010;21(2):212–22.
Liu-Bryan R, Scott P, Sydlaske A, Rose DM, Terkeltaub R. Innate immunity conferred by Toll-like receptors 2 and 4 and myeloid differentiation factor 88 expression is pivotal to monosodium urate monohydrate crystal-induced inflammation. Arthritis Rheum. 2005;52(9):2936–46.
Lucas GNC, Leitão ACC, Alencar RL, Xavier RMF, Daher EF, Silva Junior GBD. Pathophysiological aspects of nephropathy caused by non-steroidal anti-inflammatory drugs. J Bras Nefrol. 2019;41(1):124–30.

Luciano RL, Perazella MA. Aristolochic acid nephropathy: epidemiology, clinical presentation, and treatment. Drug Saf. 2015;38(1):55–64.
Lukacs-Kornek V, Burgdorf S, Diehl L, Specht S, Kornek M, Kurts C. The kidney-renal lymph node-system contributes to cross-tolerance against innocuous circulating antigen. J Immunol. 2008;180(2):706–15.
Lumlertgul N, Siribamrungwong M, Jaber BL, Susantitaphong P. Secondary oxalate nephropathy: a systematic review. Kidney Int Rep. 2018;3(6):1363–72.
Macconi D, Chiabrando C, Schiarea S, Aiello S, Cassis L, Gagliardini E, et al. Proteasomal processing of albumin by renal dendritic cells generates antigenic peptides. J Am Soc Nephrol. 2009;20(1):123–30.
Mamlouk O, Selamet U, Machado S, Abdelrahim M, Glass WF, Tchakarov A, et al. Nephrotoxicity of immune checkpoint inhibitors beyond tubulointerstitial nephritis: single-center experience. J Immunother Cancer. 2019;7(1):2.
Manchanda T, Hess D, Dale L, Ferguson SG, Rieder MJ. Haptenation of sulfonamide reactive metabolites to cellular proteins. Mol Pharmacol. 2002;62(5):1011–26.
Markowitz GS, Radhakrishnan J, Kambham N, Valeri AM, Hines WH, D'Agati VD. Lithium nephrotoxicity: a progressive combined glomerular and tubulointerstitial nephropathy. J Am Soc Nephrol. 2000;11(8):1439–48.
Martin P, Boulukos KE, Poggi MC, Pognonec P. Long-term extracellular signal-related kinase activation following cadmium intoxication is negatively regulated by a protein kinase C-dependent pathway affecting cadmium transport. FEBS J. 2009;276(6):1667–79.
Martin-Higueras C, Ludwig-Portugall I, Hoppe B, Kurts C. Targeting kidney inflammation as a new therapy for primary hyperoxaluria? Nephrol Dial Transplant. 2019;34(6):908–14.
Martinez Valenzuela L, Draibe J, Fulladosa X, Torras J. New biomarkers in acute tubulointerstitial nephritis: a novel approach to a classic condition. Int J Mol Sci. 2020;21(13):4690.
Martinon F, Pétrilli V, Mayor A, Tardivel A, Tschopp J. Gout-associated uric acid crystals activate the NALP3 inflammasome. Nature. 2006;440(7081):237–41.
Mazzali M, Hughes J, Kim YG, Jefferson JA, Kang DH, Gordon KL, et al. Elevated uric acid increases blood pressure in the rat by a novel crystal-independent mechanism. Hypertension. 2001;38(5):1101–6.
Menke J, Lucas JA, Zeller GC, Keir ME, Huang XR, Tsuboi N, et al. Programmed death 1 ligand (PD-L) 1 and PD-L2 limit autoimmune kidney disease: distinct roles. J Immunol. 2007;179(11):7466–77.
Miyanaga T, Mizuguchi K, Hara S, Zoshima T, Inoue D, Nishioka R, et al. Tertiary lymphoid tissue in early-stage IgG4-related tubulointerstitial nephritis incidentally detected with a tumor lesion of the ureteropelvic junction: a case report. BMC Nephrol. 2021;22(1):34.
Mulay SR, Eberhard JN, Desai J, Marschner JA, Kumar SV, Weidenbusch M, et al. Hyperoxaluria requires TNF receptors to initiate crystal adhesion and kidney stone disease. J Am Soc Nephrol. 2017;28(3):761–8.
Mulay SR, Kulkarni OP, Rupanagudi KV, Migliorini A, Darisipudi MN, Vilaysane A, et al. Calcium oxalate crystals induce renal inflammation by NLRP3-mediated IL-1β secretion. J Clin Invest. 2013;123(1):236–46.
Naisbitt DJ, Britschgi M, Wong G, Farrell J, Depta JP, Chadwick DW, et al. Hypersensitivity reactions to carbamazepine: characterization of the specificity, phenotype, and cytokine profile of drug-specific T cell clones. Mol Pharmacol. 2003;63(3):732–41.
Najafian B, Fogo AB, Lusco MA, Alpers CE. AJKD atlas of renal pathology: IgG4-related tubulointerstitial nephritis. Am J Kidney Dis. 2017;69(4):e19–20.
Nast CC. Medication-induced interstitial nephritis in the 21st century. Adv Chronic Kidney Dis. 2017;24(2):72–9.
Nath KA, Hostetter MK, Hostetter TH. Pathophysiology of chronic tubulo-interstitial disease in rats. Interactions of dietary acid load, ammonia, and complement component C3. J Clin Invest. 1985;76(2):667–75.
Neilson EG. Pathogenesis and therapy of interstitial nephritis. Kidney Int. 1989;35(5):1257–70.

Neilson EG, Jimenez SA, Phillips SM. Cell-mediated immunity in interstitial nephritis. III. T lymphocyte-mediated fibroblast proliferation and collagen synthesis: an immune mechanism for renal fibrogenesis. J Immunol. 1980;125(4):1708–14.

Nielsen R, Christensen EI, Birn H. Megalin and cubilin in proximal tubule protein reabsorption: from experimental models to human disease. Kidney Int. 2016;89(1):58–67.

Noonan SC, Savage GP. Oxalate content of foods and its effect on humans. Asia Pac J Clin Nutr. 1999;8(1):64–74.

Olbrich H, Fliegauf M, Hoefele J, Kispert A, Otto E, Volz A, et al. Mutations in a novel gene, NPHP3, cause adolescent nephronophthisis, tapeto-retinal degeneration and hepatic fibrosis. Nat Genet. 2003;34(4):455–9.

Orr SE, Bridges CC. Chronic kidney disease and exposure to nephrotoxic metals. Int J Mol Sci. 2017;18(5):1039.

Oskarsson A, Squibb KS, Fowler BA. Intracellular binding of lead in the kidney: the partial isolation and characterization of postmitochondrial lead binding components. Biochem Biophys Res Commun. 1982;104(1):290–8.

Peräsaari J, Saarela V, Nikkilä J, Ala-Houhala M, Arikoski P, Kataja J, et al. HLA associations with tubulointerstitial nephritis with or without uveitis in Finnish pediatric population: a nationwide study. Tissue Antigens. 2013;81(6):435–41.

Perazella MA, Markowitz GS. Drug-induced acute interstitial nephritis. Nat Rev Nephrol. 2010;6(8):461–70.

Perazella MA, Shirali AC. Immune checkpoint inhibitor nephrotoxicity: what do we know and what should we do? Kidney Int. 2020;97(1):62–74.

Perugino CA, Stone JH. IgG4-related disease: an update on pathophysiology and implications for clinical care. Nat Rev Rheumatol. 2020;16(12):702–14.

Pichler WJ, Tilch J. The lymphocyte transformation test in the diagnosis of drug hypersensitivity. Allergy. 2004;59(8):809–20.

Ponticelli C, Podestà MA, Moroni G. Hyperuricemia as a trigger of immune response in hypertension and chronic kidney disease. Kidney Int. 2020;98(5):1149–59.

Porile JL, Bakris GL, Garella S. Acute interstitial nephritis with glomerulopathy due to nonsteroidal anti-inflammatory agents: a review of its clinical spectrum and effects of steroid therapy. J Clin Pharmacol. 1990;30(5):468–75.

Posser T, de Aguiar CB, Garcez RC, Rossi FM, Oliveira CS, Trentin AG, et al. Exposure of C6 glioma cells to Pb(II) increases the phosphorylation of p38(MAPK) and JNK1/2 but not of ERK1/2. Arch Toxicol. 2007;81(6):407–14.

Pozdzik AA, Salmon IJ, Debelle FD, Decaestecker C, Van den Branden C, Verbeelen D, et al. Aristolochic acid induces proximal tubule apoptosis and epithelial to mesenchymal transformation. Kidney Int. 2008a;73(5):595–607.

Pozdzik AA, Salmon IJ, Husson CP, Decaestecker C, Rogier E, Bourgeade MF, et al. Patterns of interstitial inflammation during the evolution of renal injury in experimental aristolochic acid nephropathy. Nephrol Dial Transplant. 2008b;23(8):2480–91.

Prozialeck WC. Evidence that E-cadherin may be a target for cadmium toxicity in epithelial cells. Toxicol Appl Pharmacol. 2000;164(3):231–49.

Prozialeck WC, Edwards JR. Cell adhesion molecules in chemically-induced renal injury. Pharmacol Ther. 2007;114(1):74–93.

Prozialeck WC, Lamar PC, Appelt DM. Differential expression of E-cadherin, N-cadherin and beta-catenin in proximal and distal segments of the rat nephron. BMC Physiol. 2004;4:10.

Qi X, Cai Y, Gong L, Liu L, Chen F, Xiao Y, et al. Role of mitochondrial permeability transition in human renal tubular epithelial cell death induced by aristolochic acid. Toxicol Appl Pharmacol. 2007;222(1):105–10.

Qu W, Diwan BA, Reece JM, Bortner CD, Pi J, Liu J, et al. Cadmium-induced malignant transformation in rat liver cells: role of aberrant oncogene expression and minimal role of oxidative stress. Int J Cancer. 2005;114(3):346–55.

Quiroz JA, Gould TD, Manji HK. Molecular effects of lithium. Mol Interv. 2004;4(5):259–72.

Raghavan R, Shawar S. Mechanisms of drug-induced interstitial nephritis. Adv Chronic Kidney Dis. 2017;24(2):64–71.
Raghavan SR, Culver BD, Gonick HC. Erythrocyte lead-binding protein after occupational exposure. I. Relationship to lead toxicity. Environ Res. 1980;22(1):264–70.
Rani A, Kumar A, Lal A, Pant M. Cellular mechanisms of cadmium-induced toxicity: a review. Int J Environ Health Res. 2014;24(4):378–99.
Rastaldi MP, Ferrario F, Giardino L, Dell'Antonio G, Grillo C, Grillo P, et al. Epithelial-mesenchymal transition of tubular epithelial cells in human renal biopsies. Kidney Int. 2002;62(1):137–46.
Reddy AK, Hwang YS, Mandelcorn ED, Davis JL. HLA-DR, DQ class II DNA typing in pediatric panuveitis and tubulointerstitial nephritis and uveitis. Am J Ophthalmol. 2014;157(3):678–86.e1–2.
Rees A. Cross dendritic cells anger T cells after kidney injury. J Am Soc Nephrol. 2009;20(1):3–5.
Reungjui S, Roncal CA, Sato W, Glushakova OY, Croker BP, Suga S, et al. Hypokalemic nephropathy is associated with impaired angiogenesis. J Am Soc Nephrol. 2008;19(1):125–34.
Riemenschneider T, Bohle A. Morphologic aspects of low-potassium and low-sodium nephropathy. Clin Nephrol. 1983;19(6):271–9.
Romanov V, Whyard TC, Waltzer WC, Grollman AP, Rosenquist T. Aristolochic acid-induced apoptosis and G2 cell cycle arrest depends on ROS generation and MAP kinases activation. Arch Toxicol. 2015;89(1):47–56.
Romero CA, Remor A, Latini A, De Paul AL, Torres AI, Mukdsi JH. Uric acid activates NRLP3 inflammasome in an in-vivo model of epithelial to mesenchymal transition in the kidney. J Mol Histol. 2017;48(3):209–18.
Rovin BH, Dickerson JA, Tan LC, Hebert CA. Activation of nuclear factor-kappa B correlates with MCP-1 expression by human mesangial cells. Kidney Int. 1995;48(4):1263–71.
Rubin-Kelley VE, Jevnikar AM. Antigen presentation by renal tubular epithelial cells. J Am Soc Nephrol. 1991;2(1):13–26.
Rubinstein M, Dvash E. Leukotrienes and kidney diseases. Curr Opin Nephrol Hypertens. 2018;27(1):42–8.
Rui HL, Wang YY, Cheng H, Chen YP. JNK-dependent AP-1 activation is required for aristolochic acid-induced TGF-β1 synthesis in human renal proximal epithelial cells. Am J Physiol Renal Physiol. 2012;302(12):F1569–75.
Ryu ES, Kim MJ, Shin HS, Jang YH, Choi HS, Jo I, et al. Uric acid-induced phenotypic transition of renal tubular cells as a novel mechanism of chronic kidney disease. Am J Physiol Renal Physiol. 2013;304(5):F471–80.
Sakthivel P, Bruder D. Mechanism of granuloma formation in sarcoidosis. Curr Opin Hematol. 2017;24(1):59–65.
Salido E, Pey AL, Rodriguez R, Lorenzo V. Primary hyperoxalurias: disorders of glyoxylate detoxification. Biochim Biophys Acta. 2012;1822(9):1453–64.
Samarakoon R, Helo S, Dobberfuhl AD, Khakoo NS, Falke L, Overstreet JM, et al. Loss of tumour suppressor PTEN expression in renal injury initiates SMAD3- and p53-dependent fibrotic responses. J Pathol. 2015;236(4):421–32.
Sánchez-Lozada LG, Lanaspa MA, Cristóbal-García M, García-Arroyo F, Soto V, Cruz-Robles D, et al. Uric acid-induced endothelial dysfunction is associated with mitochondrial alterations and decreased intracellular ATP concentrations. Nephron Exp Nephrol. 2012;121(3-4):e71–8.
Sánchez-Lozada LG, Soto V, Tapia E, Avila-Casado C, Sautin YY, Nakagawa T, et al. Role of oxidative stress in the renal abnormalities induced by experimental hyperuricemia. Am J Physiol Renal Physiol. 2008;295(4):F1134–41.
Sánchez-Lozada LG, Tapia E, Santamaría J, Avila-Casado C, Soto V, Nepomuceno T, et al. Mild hyperuricemia induces vasoconstriction and maintains glomerular hypertension in normal and remnant kidney rats. Kidney Int. 2005;67(1):237–47.
Sánchez-Sánchez N, Riol-Blanco L, Rodríguez-Fernández JL. The multiple personalities of the chemokine receptor CCR7 in dendritic cells. J Immunol. 2006;176(9):5153–9.

Sautin YY, Nakagawa T, Zharikov S, Johnson RJ. Adverse effects of the classic antioxidant uric acid in adipocytes: NADPH oxidase-mediated oxidative/nitrosative stress. Am J Physiol Cell Physiol. 2007;293(2):C584–96.

Scholz SS, Vukadinović D, Lauder L, Ewen S, Ukena C, Townsend RR, et al. Effects of arteriovenous fistula on blood pressure in patients with end-stage renal disease: a systematic meta-analysis. J Am Heart Assoc. 2019;8(4):e011183.

Schoop R, Wahl P, Le Hir M, Heemann U, Wang M, Wüthrich RP. Suppressed T-cell activation by IFN-gamma-induced expression of PD-L1 on renal tubular epithelial cells. Nephrol Dial Transplant. 2004;19(11):2713–20.

Segerer S, Heller F, Lindenmeyer MT, Schmid H, Cohen CD, Draganovici D, et al. Compartment specific expression of dendritic cell markers in human glomerulonephritis. Kidney Int. 2008;74(1):37–46.

Segerer S, Schlöndorff D. B cells and tertiary lymphoid organs in renal inflammation. Kidney Int. 2008;73(5):533–7.

Setyaningsih WAW, Arfian N, Suryadi E, Romi MM, Tranggono U, Sari DCR. Hyperuricemia induces Wnt5a/Ror2 gene expression, epithelial-mesenchymal transition, and kidney tubular injury in mice. Iran J Med Sci. 2018;43(2):164–73.

Sevanian A, Davies KJ, Hochstein P. Serum urate as an antioxidant for ascorbic acid. Am J Clin Nutr. 1991;54(6 Suppl):1129s–34s.

Shi H, Feng JM. Aristolochic acid induces apoptosis of human umbilical vein endothelial cells in vitro by suppressing PI3K/Akt signaling pathway. Acta Pharmacol Sin. 2011;32(8):1025–30.

Shi Y, Evans JE, Rock KL. Molecular identification of a danger signal that alerts the immune system to dying cells. Nature. 2003;425(6957):516–21.

Shi Y, Xu L, Tao M, Fang L, Lu J, Gu H, et al. Blockade of enhancer of zeste homolog 2 alleviates renal injury associated with hyperuricemia. Am J Physiol Renal Physiol. 2019;316(3):F488–f505.

Shirali AC, Perazella MA, Gettinger S. Association of acute interstitial nephritis with programmed cell death 1 inhibitor therapy in lung cancer patients. Am J Kidney Dis. 2016;68(2):287–91.

Shrestha A, Che RC, Zhang AH. Role of aldosterone in renal fibrosis. Adv Exp Med Biol. 2019;1165:325–46.

Simons M, Gloy J, Ganner A, Bullerkotte A, Bashkurov M, Krönig C, et al. Inversin, the gene product mutated in nephronophthisis type II, functions as a molecular switch between Wnt signaling pathways. Nat Genet. 2005;37(5):537–43.

Smeets B, Boor P, Dijkman H, Sharma SV, Jirak P, Mooren F, et al. Proximal tubular cells contain a phenotypically distinct, scattered cell population involved in tubular regeneration. J Pathol. 2013;229(5):645–59.

Soos TJ, Sims TN, Barisoni L, Lin K, Littman DR, Dustin ML, et al. CX3CR1+ interstitial dendritic cells form a contiguous network throughout the entire kidney. Kidney Int. 2006;70(3):591–6.

Spanou Z, Keller M, Britschgi M, Yawalkar N, Fehr T, Neuweiler J, et al. Involvement of drug-specific T cells in acute drug-induced interstitial nephritis. J Am Soc Nephrol. 2006;17(10):2919–27.

Stiborová M, Hudeček J, Frei E, Schmeiser HH. Contribution of biotransformation enzymes to the development of renal injury and urothelial cancer caused by aristolochic acid: urgent questions, difficult answers. Interdiscip Toxicol. 2008;1(1):8–12.

Strowig T, Henao-Mejia J, Elinav E, Flavell R. Inflammasomes in health and disease. Nature. 2012;481(7381):278–86.

Suga S, Mazzali M, Ray PE, Kang DH, Johnson RJ. Angiotensin II type 1 receptor blockade ameliorates tubulointerstitial injury induced by chronic potassium deficiency. Kidney Int. 2002;61(3):951–8.

Suga SI, Phillips MI, Ray PE, Raleigh JA, Vio CP, Kim YG, et al. Hypokalemia induces renal injury and alterations in vasoactive mediators that favor salt sensitivity. Am J Physiol Renal Physiol. 2001;281(4):F620–9.

Sun X, Wang Y, Jiang T, Yuan X, Ren Z, Tuffour A, et al. Nephrotoxicity profile of cadmium revealed by proteomics in mouse kidney. Biol Trace Elem Res. 2021;199(5):1929–40.

Sutariya B, Jhonsa D, Saraf MN. TGF-β: the connecting link between nephropathy and fibrosis. Immunopharmacol Immunotoxicol. 2016;38(1):39–49.

Suzuki H, Yoshioka K, Miyano M, Maeda I, Yamagami K, Morikawa T, et al. Tubulointerstitial nephritis and uveitis (TINU) syndrome caused by the Chinese herb "Goreisan". Clin Exp Nephrol. 2009;13(1):73–6.

Swenberg JA, Short B, Borghoff S, Strasser J, Charbonneau M. The comparative pathobiology of alpha 2u-globulin nephropathy. Toxicol Appl Pharmacol. 1989;97(1):35–46.

Talbott JH, Terplan KL. The kidney in gout. Medicine (Baltimore). 1960;39:405–67.

Tan Y, Yu F, Qu Z, Su T, Xing GQ, Wu LH, et al. Modified C-reactive protein might be a target autoantigen of TINU syndrome. Clin J Am Soc Nephrol. 2011;6(1):93–100.

Thoma CR, Frew IJ, Hoerner CR, Montani M, Moch H, Krek W. pVHL and GSK3beta are components of a primary cilium-maintenance signalling network. Nat Cell Biol. 2007;9(5):588–95.

Tolins JP, Hostetter MK, Hostetter TH. Hypokalemic nephropathy in the rat. Role of ammonia in chronic tubular injury. J Clin Invest. 1987;79(5):1447–58.

Torres VE, Young WF Jr, Offord KP, Hattery RR. Association of hypokalemia, aldosteronism, and renal cysts. N Engl J Med. 1990;322(6):345–51.

Trepiccione F, Pisitkun T, Hoffert JD, Poulsen SB, Capasso G, Nielsen S, et al. Early targets of lithium in rat kidney inner medullary collecting duct include p38 and ERK1/2. Kidney Int. 2014;86(4):757–67.

Tsunawaki S, Nakamura S, Ohyama Y, Sasaki M, Ikebe-Hiroki A, Hiraki A, et al. Possible function of salivary gland epithelial cells as nonprofessional antigen-presenting cells in the development of Sjögren's syndrome. J Rheumatol. 2002;29(9):1884–96.

Ulinski T, Sellier-Leclerc AL, Tudorache E, Bensman A, Aoun B. Acute tubulointerstitial nephritis. Pediatr Nephrol. 2012;27(7):1051–7.

Verhulst A, Asselman M, Persy VP, Schepers MS, Helbert MF, Verkoelen CF, et al. Crystal retention capacity of cells in the human nephron: involvement of CD44 and its ligands hyaluronic acid and osteopontin in the transition of a crystal binding- into a nonadherent epithelium. J Am Soc Nephrol. 2003;14(1):107–15.

Verzola D, Ratto E, Villaggio B, Parodi EL, Pontremoli R, Garibotto G, et al. Uric acid promotes apoptosis in human proximal tubule cells by oxidative stress and the activation of NADPH oxidase NOX 4. PLoS One. 2014;9(12):e115210.

Villemaire M, Cartier JC, Mathieu N, Maurizi J, Pinel N, Bonaz B, et al. Renal sarcoid-like granulomatosis during anti-TNF therapy. Kidney Int. 2014;86(1):215.

Waeckerle-Men Y, Starke A, Wüthrich RP. PD-L1 partially protects renal tubular epithelial cells from the attack of CD8+ cytotoxic T cells. Nephrol Dial Transplant. 2007;22(6):1527–36.

Wahlström J, Dengjel J, Persson B, Duyar H, Rammensee HG, Stevanović S, et al. Identification of HLA-DR-bound peptides presented by human bronchoalveolar lavage cells in sarcoidosis. J Clin Invest. 2007;117(11):3576–82.

Wanchoo R, Karam S, Uppal NN, Barta VS, Deray G, Devoe C, et al. Adverse renal effects of immune checkpoint inhibitors: a narrative review. Am J Nephrol. 2017;45(2):160–9.

Wang L, Cao J, Chen D, Liu X, Lu H, Liu Z. Role of oxidative stress, apoptosis, and intracellular homeostasis in primary cultures of rat proximal tubular cells exposed to cadmium. Biol Trace Elem Res. 2009a;127(1):53–68.

Wang L, Wang H, Hu M, Cao J, Chen D, Liu Z. Oxidative stress and apoptotic changes in primary cultures of rat proximal tubular cells exposed to lead. Arch Toxicol. 2009b;83(5):417–27.

Wang S, Fan J, Mei X, Luan J, Li Y, Zhang X, et al. Interleukin-22 attenuated renal tubular injury in aristolochic acid nephropathy via suppressing activation of NLRP3 inflammasome. Front Immunol. 2019;10:2277.

Webb R, Jeffries M, Sawalha AH. Uric acid directly promotes human T-cell activation. Am J Med Sci. 2009;337(1):23–7.

Wei SC, Duffy CR, Allison JP. Fundamental mechanisms of immune checkpoint blockade therapy. Cancer Discov. 2018;8(9):1069–86.

Wing K, Onishi Y, Prieto-Martin P, Yamaguchi T, Miyara M, Fehervari Z, et al. CTLA-4 control over Foxp3+ regulatory T cell function. Science. 2008;322(5899):271–5.

Wolf MT, Hildebrandt F. Nephronophthisis. Pediatr Nephrol (Berlin, Germany). 2011;26(2): 181–94.

Wolkenstein P, Carrière V, Charue D, Bastuji-Garin S, Revuz J, Roujeau JC, et al. A slow acetylator genotype is a risk factor for sulphonamide-induced toxic epidermal necrolysis and Stevens-Johnson syndrome. Pharmacogenetics. 1995;5(4):255–8.

Woltman AM, de Fijter JW, Zuidwijk K, Vlug AG, Bajema IM, van der Kooij SW, et al. Quantification of dendritic cell subsets in human renal tissue under normal and pathological conditions. Kidney Int. 2007;71(10):1001–8.

Worcester EM, Evan AP, Coe FL, Lingeman JE, Krambeck A, Sommers A, et al. A test of the hypothesis that oxalate secretion produces proximal tubule crystallization in primary hyperoxaluria type I. Am J Physiol Renal Physiol. 2013;305(11):F1574–84.

Wu Y, Deng J, Rychahou PG, Qiu S, Evers BM, Zhou BP. Stabilization of snail by NF-kappaB is required for inflammation-induced cell migration and invasion. Cancer Cell. 2009;15(5):416–28.

Xiao J, Zhang XL, Fu C, Han R, Chen W, Lu Y, et al. Soluble uric acid increases NALP3 inflammasome and interleukin-1β expression in human primary renal proximal tubule epithelial cells through the Toll-like receptor 4-mediated pathway. Int J Mol Med. 2015;35(5):1347–54.

Xiong XY, Bai L, Bai SJ, Wang YK, Ji T. Uric acid induced epithelial-mesenchymal transition of renal tubular cells through PI3K/p-Akt signaling pathway. J Cell Physiol. 2019.

Yang H, Shu Y. Cadmium transporters in the kidney and cadmium-induced nephrotoxicity. Int J Mol Sci. 2015;16(1):1484–94.

Yang PM, Chen HC, Tsai JS, Lin LY. Cadmium induces Ca^{2+}-dependent necrotic cell death through calpain-triggered mitochondrial depolarization and reactive oxygen species-mediated inhibition of nuclear factor-kappaB activity. Chem Res Toxicol. 2007;20(3):406–15.

Yu FY, Wu TS, Chen TW, Liu BH. Aristolochic acid I induced oxidative DNA damage associated with glutathione depletion and ERK1/2 activation in human cells. Toxicol In Vitro. 2011;25(4):810–6.

Yung S, Tsang RC, Sun Y, Leung JK, Chan TM. Effect of human anti-DNA antibodies on proximal renal tubular epithelial cell cytokine expression: implications on tubulointerstitial inflammation in lupus nephritis. J Am Soc Nephrol. 2005;16(11):3281–94.

Yusufi AN, Christensen S, Dousa TP. Effect of chronic lithium treatment upon the Na(+)-coupled cotransporters in renal brush border membranes. Kidney Int. 1993;43(5):1074–80.

Zavadil J, Böttinger EP. TGF-beta and epithelial-to-mesenchymal transitions. Oncogene. 2005;24(37):5764–74.

Zhao L, Li C, Zhou B, Luo C, Wang Y, Che L, et al. Crucial role of serum response factor in renal tubular epithelial cell epithelial-mesenchymal transition in hyperuricemic nephropathy. Aging (Albany NY). 2019;11(22):10597–609.

Zhao Z, Baldo BA, Rimmer J. beta-Lactam allergenic determinants: fine structural recognition of a cross-reacting determinant on benzylpenicillin and cephalothin. Clin Exp Allergy. 2002;32(11):1644–50.

Zhou W, Otto EA, Cluckey A, Airik R, Hurd TW, Chaki M, et al. FAN1 mutations cause karyomegalic interstitial nephritis, linking chronic kidney failure to defective DNA damage repair. Nat Genet. 2012a;44(8):910–5.

Zhou Y, Fang L, Jiang L, Wen P, Cao H, He W, et al. Uric acid induces renal inflammation via activating tubular NF-κB signaling pathway. PLoS One. 2012b;7(6):e39738.

Zhu S, Wang Y, Jin J, Guan C, Li M, Xi C, et al. Endoplasmic reticulum stress mediates aristolochic acid I-induced apoptosis in human renal proximal tubular epithelial cells. Toxicol In Vitro. 2012;26(5):663–71.

Zollinger HU, Mihatsch MJ, Edefonti A, Gaboardi F, Imbasciati E, Lennert T. Nephronophthisis (medullary cystic disease of the kidney). A study using electron microscopy, immunofluorescence, and a review of the morphological findings. Helv Paediatr Acta. 1980;35(6):509–30.

Part III
Causes of Immune Mediated Tubulointerstitial Nephritis

Causes of Acute Tubulointerstitial Nephritis: Drugs

Fernando Caravaca-Fontán, Hernando Trujillo, and Manuel Praga

1 Introduction

Acute tubulointerstitial nephritis (ATIN) is an emerging cause of both acute kidney injury (AKI) and acute kidney disease (AKD). An increased incidence of ATIN has been reported in several studies, especially among older patients.

Drug-induced ATIN is the most common etiology, representing almost two-thirds of the cases. Drug-induced ATIN represents a dose-independent type IV hypersensitivity reaction that typically occurs in kidney parenchyma 7–10 days after the exposure to different agents. This hypothesis is supported by the fact that the interstitial infiltrate in ATIN is predominantly composed of T-lymphocytes, without a significant deposition of complement or immunoglobulins.

In the majority of cases, symptoms associated with ATIN are non-specific (malaise, nausea-vomiting or flank pain). The classical triad of ATIN, comprising fever, rash and eosinophilia, is rare. However, it is observed more frequently in drug-related hypersensitivity reactions, particularly when beta-lactam antibiotics are involved.

Low-grade or intermittent fever can develop, but may also be absent in ATIN caused by some drugs. Skin rash is typically maculopapular or morbilliform, although diffuse erythroderma or toxic epidermal necrolysis can also develop.

Identification of the causative drug is often challenging, especially in patients exposed to polypharmacy. In fact, in a case series of drug-induced ATIN, the culprit drug could not be clearly identified in nearly 30% of cases. Oligo-symptomatic presentations of certain drug-induced ATIN often result in delayed diagnosis, and can also make it difficult to correctly identify the culprit drug.

Numerous agents have been incriminated in ATIN, although in short, almost any drug should be considered as suspected causative agent of an ATIN. Significant

F. Caravaca-Fontán · H. Trujillo · M. Praga (✉)
Department of Nephrology, Hospital Universitario 12 de Octubre, Madrid, Spain
e-mail: mpragat@senefro.org

M. G. Atta, M. A. Perazella (eds.), *Tubulointerstitial Nephritis*,
https://doi.org/10.1007/978-3-030-93438-5_4

epidemiological changes have taken place in ATIN in recent years, due to the emergence of novel causative drugs such as proton-pump inhibitors, 5-aminosalicylates, or newer anticancer therapies. This chapter aims to provide an update on the different etiologies and pathogenic mechanisms underlying drug-induced ATIN.

2 Antimicrobials

Antibiotics (including both beta and non-beta lactams) are frequently implicated in ATIN. Table 1 summarizes the main antibiotic/antiviral drugs associated with the development of ATIN. Methicillin-induced ATIN has been considered for many years as the prototypical example of this entity, however, it is no longer used in clinical practice. Despite wider usage of other antimicrobials, cases of beta-lactam related ATIN continue to be reported. Hypersensitivity syndrome with fever, rash or eosinophilia is found in a large percentage of these cases (>75%), and the presence of leukocyturia and hematuria is also a common feature. Non-beta-lactam antibiotics such as fluoroquinolones –and especially ciprofloxacin–, are among the most common causative agents, with characteristic delayed onset of clinical manifestations, making its diagnosis a challenging task. Sulfonamides may induce ATIN more frequently in patients with human immunodeficiency virus (HIV), or immunocompromised patients such as allograft recipients. The intermittent use of rifampicin in the setting of mycobacterial infections may also cause ATIN, although, in contrast to other drugs, it occurs in a dose-dependent manner. In addition, rifampicin may also cause proximal tubular injury, and a severe kidney injury with the consequent need for dialysis. On the other hand, vancomycin may cause a variety of hypersensitivity reactions including ATIN. Antibiotics may also lead to non-necrotizing granuloma formation, with a shorter latency period compared to other medications.

HIV patients are particularly prone to ATIN and several antiviral agents have been associated with the development of this condition. When the kidney damage is

Table 1 Antibiotics and anti-retroviral drugs associated with the development of acute tubulointerstitial nephritis

Antibiotics
Penicillins: amoxicillin, ampicillin, aztreonam, benzylpenicillin, cloxacillin, methicillin, nafcillin, oxacillin, piperaciliza/tazobactam
Fluoroquinolones: ciprofloxacin, levofloxacin, moxifloxacin, norfloxacin
Cephalosporins: cefazolin, cefotaxime, cefoxitin, cefoxitin, cefuroxime, ceftriaxone, cephalexin
Sulfonamides: trimethoprim-sulfamethoxazole
Macrolides: azithromycin, clarithromycin, erythromycin, telithromycin
Others: cefepime, chloramphenicol, clindamycin, colistin, colistin, doxycycline, ethambutol, gentamicin, griseofulvin, imipenem, isoniazid, linezolid, nitrofurantoin, polymyxin B, quinine, rifampicin, teicoplanin, vancomycin
Anti-retrovirals
Abacavir, acyclovir, atazanavir, foscarnet, indinavir.

Adapted from Nast et al.

not accompanied by granuloma formation, the underlying mechanism is thought to be a hypersensitivity reaction occurring 1–4 months after exposure. However, certain antiretrovirals such as atazanavir can induce chronic tubulointerstitial nephritis with progressive chronic kidney disease (CKD).

3 Non-steroidal Anti-inflammatory Drugs

Nonsteroidal anti-inflammatory drugs (NSAIDs) are commonly used in clinical settings for the treatment of pain and several inflammatory conditions, and in most countries, they are available over-the-counter. NSAIDs are commonly implicated in the development of ATIN in both children and adults. In a large case series of drug-induced ATIN, NSAIDs represented the most frequent offending drug. Table 2 summarizes different group of drugs associated with the development of ATIN.

Table 2 Miscellaneous group of drugs associated with the development of acute tubulointerstitial nephritis

Nonsteroidal anti-inflammatory drugs
COX2 inhibitors: celecoxib, rofecoxib
Others: aceclofenac, diclofenac, fenoprofen, flurbiprofen, ibuprofen, indomethacin, ketoprofen, meloxicam, naproxen, phenylbutazone
5-aminosalicylates
Balsalazine, mesalazine, olsalazine, sulfasalazine.
Gastric secretion inhibitors
Proton pump inhibitors: esomeprazole, lansoprazole, omeprazole, pantoprazole, rabeprazole.
H2 antagonists: cimetidine, famotidine, ranitidine
Anticancer drugs
Immune checkpoint inhibitors: atezolizumab, ipilimumab, nivolumab, pembrolizumab
Tyrosine kinase inhibitors: sorafenib, sunitinib
Others: adriamycin, alendronate, azathioprine, bacillus Calmette–Guerin, bevacizumab, bortezomib, carboplatin, gemcitabine, interleukin 2, ifosfamide, lenalidomide, methotrexate, pemetrexed, vemurafenib
Diuretics
Thiazides: hydrochlorothiazide, indapamide, metolazone.
Loop of Henle diuretics: furosemide, torasemide
Potassium sparing: amiloride, triamterene
Antihypertensives
Angiotensin-converting enzyme inhibitors: captopril, lisinopril
Angiotensin receptor antagonists: candesartan, losartan
Calcium channel antagonists: amlodipine, nifedipine
Anticonvulsants
Carbamazepine, diazepam, lamotrigine, levetiracetam, phenobarbital, phenytoin, valproate
Other drugs
Allopurinol, atorvastatin, carbimazole, chlorpropamide, exenatide, febuxostat, flecainide, gemfibrozil, leflunomide, metamizole, propranolol, propylthiouracil, risedronate, sildenafil

Adapted from Nast et al.

Fewer extra-renal manifestations at the time of diagnosis, and longer latency periods from the exposure are peculiar features of NSAIDs compared with other common drug-induced ATIN. In addition, NSAID-induced ATIN can also be associated with nephrotic syndrome when concomitant minimal change disease is present. The exact mechanisms underlying this form of the disease are poorly understood, however, it is possible that the systemic release of cytokines and inflammatory factors by activated cells could alter the permselectivity of the glomerular filtration barrier.

Kidney biopsies of patients with NSAID-induced ATIN may show less intense interstitial inflammation compared to other forms of drug-induced ATIN, and eosinophils may not be present.

Finally, selective cyclooxygenase 2 (COX-2) inhibitors (such as celecoxib or rofecoxib), although associated with less gastrointestinal side effects, can induce ATIN with a similar clinical pattern to that of non-selective NSAIDs. Rofecoxib is no longer available for therapy.

4 Proton-Pump Inhibitors

Proton-pump inhibitors (PPIs) are among the most widely used medications worldwide and, as with NSAIDs, they are commonly used over-the-counter. In addition, these drugs are often used for prolonged periods of time. According to different case series, PPIs were found to be responsible for ATIN in 18–64% of the cases, especially in older patients. Indeed, a case-control epidemiological study found that current PPI users >60 years old were at higher risk of ATIN compared to younger current users. The interval between PPI initiation and the onset of kidney abnormalities can oscillate between 1 week and 9 months. However, in clinical settings it is often difficult to establish a clear correlation between PPI treatment and ATIN and therefore, it is likely that the real prevalence of this complication may be underestimated.

The clinical presentation of PPI-induced ATIN is often nonspecific including asthenia or low-grade fever, with the classical triad of fever, rash, and eosinophilia found in less than 10% of the cases. The severity of the kidney damage in this setting may be lower as compared to other drug-induced ATIN, but the longer duration of the exposure due to its delayed diagnosis may hamper the recovery of kidney function. One study found a predominance of Th1–Th17 lineage infiltration in a cohort of patients with PPI-induced ATIN, suggesting this could be the main type of cell-mediated inflammatory process, as opposed to the Th2-mediated response typically seen in "classic" allergic ATIN. Furthermore, patients carrying polymorphisms of the CYP2C19 enzyme may be more prone to develop PPI-induced ATIN due to higher blood levels of these drugs. The development of end-stage CKD in cases of PPI-induced ATIN is rare, although up to 50% of the cases may not fully recover kidney function.

5 5–Aminosalicylates

The 5-aminosalicylates (5-ASA) such as mesalazine, sulfasalazine, or olsalazine, are frequently used to control symptoms of inflammatory bowel disease (IBD). Different types of kidney involvement have been reported in patients with IBD, with IgA nephropathy and interstitial nephritis the most common. 5-ASA-induced ATIN represents an idiosyncratic drug reaction, and it is most commonly found during the first year of treatment. The estimated incidence of kidney impairment among patients taking 5-aminosalicylates is 1 in 200–500 patients, although IBD itself may be associated with the development of interstitial nephritis. Hypersensitivity symptoms such as rash, fever and eosinophilia may be present after the onset of 5-ASA, whereas other patients develop a slowly progressive CKD. Thus, close monitoring of patients receiving treatment with 5-ASA is advocated for an early recognition of kidney function impairment.

6 Anticancer Drugs

Kidney disease is a relatively frequent complication among cancer patients, and has a significant impact in clinical practice. Importantly, several chemotherapeutic agents are cleared by the kidneys, which can limit its use, while a large number of anticancer drugs have also not been tested in clinical trials in patients with kidney disease. Moreover, a number of common underlying clinical characteristics of cancer patients, such as a trend towards hypoalbuminemia, reduced muscle mass, and polymedication may predispose them to develop different types of kidney injury such as ATIN. In the following lines, the different types of anticancer drugs that can potentially elicit an ATIN are reviewed (Table 2).

6.1 Immune Checkpoint Inhibitors

Over the last years, several important advances have taken place in the field of cancer immunotherapy, which have made it possible to expand the therapeutic armamentarium and, in many cases, improved prognosis of some of these diseases. Immune checkpoint inhibitors (ICPI) such as ipilimumab (cytotoxic T-lymphocyte antigen 4 [CTLA-4] antagonist), nivolumab, pembrolizumab (programmed cell death-1 [PD-1] inhibitors), atezolizumab, and durvalumab (programmed cell death ligand 1 [PD-L1] inhibitors), have revolutionized cancer therapy. However, these advances have also brought an increased incidence in drug-related side effects. The skin, gastrointestinal tract, lungs, and endocrine system are commonly involved in the setting of ICPI therapy. In addition, ICPI may induce AKI in around 1–29% of the cases, although the true incidence may be underestimated. ATIN is the most common type of kidney disease, although other forms such as pauci-immune glomerulonephritis, podocytopathies or even C3 glomerulopathy have been reported. Hence, cancer patients with kidney impairment and/or proteinuria should undergo a careful evaluation for potential underlying causes, and a kidney biopsy should be performed when possible.

In ICPI-induced ATIN the reported interval between drug initiation and the onset of kidney-related abnormalities ranges from 1 to 24 months, and extrarenal manifestations such as hypophysitis or colitis may precede AKI. Interestingly, the concomitant use of PPI in patients under treatment with ICPIs has been associated with a higher risk of ATIN. Although the exact pathogenic mechanism has not been fully deciphered, it has been suggested that ICPI could lead to loss of immune tolerance and subsequent activation of memory T-cells, previously primed by other haptens, including medications. Of note, a failure to achieve kidney recovery after an ICPI-induced ATIN has been associated with higher mortality in some studies. Moreover, up to one-quarter of the patients in which ICPI are rechallenged may develop recurrent AKI.

6.2 Tyrosine Kinase Inhibitors

Tyrosine kinase inhibitors (TKIs) such as imatinib, gefitinib, erlotinib, sorafenib or sunitinib are a group of agents whose mechanism of action consists of a competitive inhibition of adenosine triphosphate at the catalytic binding site of tyrosine kinase. Thus, TKIs block the receptors of numerous growth factors involved in cell proliferation and reparative processes. ATIN has been described in the setting of treatment with sorafenib and sunitinib.

6.3 Platinum Agents

Nephrotoxicity is a well-known side effect of platinum agents such as cisplatin or carboplatin. Conversely, the incidence of this adverse event is less frequent with third generation agents such as oxaliplatin. Platinum agents can also induce ATIN. Several cases of oxaliplatin-related ATIN have been described, often associated with systemic symptoms such as malaise, fever or skin rash.

6.4 Ifosfamide

Ifosfamide is a broad-spectrum alkylating agent, used in both solid and hematologic malignancies. Treatment with ifosfamide has been associated with both ATIN and chronic TIN through mechanisms that are poorly understood but appear to be dose related. Remarkably, ifosfamide-induced ATIN is characterized by the presence of kariomegalic changes in tubular epithelial cells. The reported kidney prognosis is variable, although an incomplete recovery of kidney function is common.

6.5 Other Anticancer Agents

Several other anticancer drugs have also been associated with the development of ATIN. Bortezomib, a proteasome inhibitor, mainly used in multiple myeloma or monoclonal gammopathy of renal significance has exceptionally been associated with ATIN with granuloma formation.

Lenalidomide is an immunomodulatory agent, used in a wide range of tumors, but mainly in hematological diseases such as multiple myeloma or myelodysplastic syndromes. Lenalidomide has also been associated with ATIN, often associated with skin rash.

Pemetrexed is a multitargeted antifolate that inhibits different enzymes involved in DNA synthesis. Pemetrexed typically induces tubular necrosis or interstitial fibrosis, although the development of ATIN and chronic TIN has also been described.

The BRAF inhibitors, such as vemurafenib or dabrafenib, have been associated with the development of AKD within the first 3 months of treatment. It has been suggested that the concomitant presence of eosinophilia in these cases may reflect the development of an ATIN.

Finally, the intravesical instillation of bacillus Calmette–Guerin (BCG) in noninvasive transitional cell carcinoma bladder have also been associated with ATIN, with or without chronic TIN and non-necrotizing granuloma.

7 Other Drugs

Virtually any drug can potentially elicit an ATIN (Table 2). Apart from the aforementioned agents, ATIN can also develop with several antihypertensive drugs –such as captopril, losartan or nifedipine–, anticonvulsants –such as carbamazepine, levetiracetam or phenytoin–, urate lowering drugs –such as allopurinol or febuxostat–, among others. Diuretics (thiazides, loop, and potassium-sparing diuretics), apart from causing afeasibly reversible increase in serum creatinine, may rarely cause ATIN. Kidney function impairment is typically identified 4–10 weeks after the onset of diuretic treatment, and the associated symptoms may be variable. Fortunately, kidney outcomes are generally favorable.

In addition, the drug reaction with eosinophilia and systemic symptoms (DRESS syndrome), a drug-induced hypersensitivity reaction characterized by fever, rash, eosinophilia, and multiple organ involvement, can also be associated with ATIN in 10–30% of cases. Allopurinol, anticonvulsant drugs, and antibiotics are the drugs most frequently involved in this syndrome.

8 Conclusions

ATIN is a common cause of AKI and AKD. Clinicians should be aware of the possibility of a drug-induced ATIN particularly in patients exposed to multiple medications. Kidney biopsy provides the definitive diagnosis of ATIN. Early discontinuation of the culprit drug is the mainstay of therapy, although the identification of this drug is often challenging in clinical practice.

Suggested Reading

Ambruzs JM, Walker PD, Larsen CP. The histopathologic spectrum of kidney biopsies in patients with inflammatory bowel disease. Clin J Am Soc Nephrol. 2014;9(2):265–70.

Appel GB, Appel AS. Acute interstitial nephritis. In: Core concepts in parenchymal kidney disease. New York: Springer New York; 2014. p. 329–39.

Azar I, Esfandiarifard S, Sinai P, Wazir A, Foulke L, Mehdi S. Sunitinib-induced acute interstitial nephritis in a thrombocytopenic renal cell cancer patient. Case Rep Oncol Med. 2017;2017:1–4.

Baldwin DS, Levine BB, McCluskey RT, Gallo GR. Renal failure and interstitial nephritis due to penicillin and methicillin. N Engl J Med. 1968;279(23):1245–52.

Berney-Meyer L, Hung N, Slatter T, Schollum JBW, Kitching AR, Walker RJ. Omeprazole-induced acute interstitial nephritis: a possible Th1-Th17-mediated injury? Nephrology. 2014;19(6):359–65.

Blank M-L, Parkin L, Paul C, Herbison P. A nationwide nested case-control study indicates an increased risk of acute interstitial nephritis with proton pump inhibitor use. Kidney Int. 2014;86(4):837–44.

Caravaca-Fontán F, Fernández-Juárez G, Praga M. Acute kidney injury in interstitial nephritis. Curr Opin Crit Care. 2019;25(6):558–64.

Chen Y, Chang C, Cho Y, Chiu H, Chu C. Long-term sequelae of drug reaction with eosinophilia and systemic symptoms: a retrospective cohort study from Taiwan. J Am Acad Dermatol. 2012;68(3):459–65.

Cheungpasitporn W, Leung N, Rajkumar SV, Cornell LD, Sethi S, Angioi A, et al. Bortezomib-induced acute interstitial nephritis. Nephrol Dial Transplant. 2015;30(7):1225–9.

Choi Y-J, Oh K-H, Kang H-R, Lee S-J. Oxaliplatin-induced acute tubulointerstitial nephritis: two case reports. Clin Nephrol. 2018;89(02):130–4.

Cortazar FB, Kibbelaar ZA, Glezerman IG, Abudayyeh A, Mamlouk O, Motwani SS, et al. Clinical features and outcomes of immune checkpoint inhibitor-associated AKI: a multicenter study. J Am Soc Nephrol. 2020;31(2):435–46.

Cortazar FB, Marrone KA, Troxell ML, Ralto KM, Hoenig MP, Brahmer JR, et al. Clinicopathological features of acute kidney injury associated with immune checkpoint inhibitors. Kidney Int. 2016;90(3):638–47.

Díaz-Mancebo R, Costero-Fernández O, Vega-Cabrera C, Olea-Tejero T, Yébenes L, Picazo ML, et al. Dress syndrome and acute tubulointerstitial nephritis after treatment with vancomycin and beta-lactams. Case report and literature review. Nefrologia. 2012;32(5):685–7.

Esteve J-B, Launay-Vacher V, Brocheriou I, Grimaldi A, Izzedine H. COX-2 inhibitors and acute interstitial nephritis: case report and review of the literature. Clin Nephrol. 2005;63(05):385–9.

Farid S, Mahmood M, Abu Saleh OM, Hamadah A, Nasr SH, Garrigos ZE, et al. Clinical manifestations and outcomes of fluoroquinolone-related acute interstitial nephritis. Mayo Clin Proc. 2018;93(1):25–31.

Fernandez-Juarez G, Perez JV, Caravaca-Fontán F, Quintana L, Shabaka A, Rodriguez E, et al. Duration of treatment with corticosteroids and recovery of kidney function in acute interstitial nephritis. Clin J Am Soc Nephrol. 2018;13(12):1851–8.

Geevasinga N, Coleman PL, Webster AC, Roger SD. Proton pump inhibitors and acute interstitial nephritis. Clin Gastroenterol Hepatol. 2006;4(5):597–604.

Gisbert JP, González-Lama Y, Maté J. 5-Aminosalicylates and renal function in inflammatory bowel disease. Inflamm Bowel Dis. 2007;13(5):629–38.

Glassock RJ. Secondary minimal change disease. Nephrol Dial Transplant. 2003;18(90006):52vi–58.

Goicoechea M, Rivera F, López-Gómez JM. Increased prevalence of acute tubulointerstitial nephritis. Nephrol Dial Transplant. 2013;28(1):112–5.

Hara M, Suganuma A, Yanagisawa N, Imamura A, Hishima T, Ando M. Atazanavir nephrotoxicity. Clin Kidney J. 2015;8(2):137–42.

Ishizaki H. Review article: cytochrome P450 and the metabolism of proton pump inhibitors – emphasis on rabeprazole. Aliment Pharmacol Ther. 1999;13:27–36.

Izzedine H, Brocheriou I, Rixe O, Deray G. Interstitial nephritis in a patient taking sorafenib. Nephrol Dial Transplant. 2007;22(8):2411.

Izzedine H, Mathian A, Champiat S, Picard C, Mateus C, Routier E, et al. Renal toxicities associated with pembrolizumab. Clin Kidney J. 2018;12(1):81–8.

Izzedine H, Perazella MA. Anticancer drug-induced acute kidney injury. Kidney Int Rep Elsevier Inc. 2017;81:504–14.

Kheder El-Fekih R, Izzedine H. Néphrotoxicité du lénalidomide. Bull Cancer. 2016;103(5):499–506.

Kitchlu A, Jhaveri KD, Wadhwani S, Deshpande P, Harel Z, Kishibe T, et al. A systematic review of immune checkpoint inhibitor–associated glomerular disease. Kidney Int Rep. 2021;6(1):66–77.

Krishnan N, Perazella MA. Drug-induced acute interstitial nephritis: pathology, pathogenesis, and treatment. Iran J Kidney Dis. 2015;9(1):3–13.

Mamlouk O, Selamet U, Machado S, Abdelrahim M, Glass WF, Tchakarov A, et al. Nephrotoxicity of immune checkpoint inhibitors beyond tubulointerstitial nephritis: single-center experience. J Immunother Cancer. 2019;7(1):2.

Martínez-Valenzuela L, Draibe J, Fulladosa X, Gomà M, Gómez F, Antón P, et al. Acute tubulointerstitial nephritis in clinical oncology: a comprehensive review. Int J Mol Sci. 2021;22(5):1–9.

Minhas JS, Wickner PG, Long AA, Banerji A, Blumenthal KG. Immune-mediated reactions to vancomycin. Ann Allergy Asthma Immunol. 2016;116(6):544–53.

Misurac JM, Knoderer CA, Leiser JD, Nailescu C, Wilson AC, Andreoli SP. Nonsteroidal anti-inflammatory drugs are an important cause of acute kidney injury in children. J Pediatr Elsevier Ltd. 2013:1153–9.e1.

Mohammed A, Arastu Z. Emerging concepts and spectrum of renal injury following Intravesical BCG for non-muscle invasive bladder cancer. BMC Urol. 2017;17(1):114.

Moledina DG, Perazella MA. Drug-induced acute interstitial nephritis. Clin J Am Soc Nephrol. 2017;12(12):2046–9.

Moledina DG, Perazella MA. PPIs and kidney disease: from AIN to CKD. J Nephrol Springer International Publishing. 2016;29:611–6.

Muriithi AK, Leung N, Valeri AM, Cornell LD, Sethi S, Fidler ME, et al. Biopsy-proven acute interstitial nephritis, 1993–2011: a case series. Am J Kidney Dis. 2014;64(4):558–66.

Muriithi AK, Leung N, Valeri AM, Cornell LD, Sethi S, Fidler ME, et al. Clinical characteristics, causes and outcomes of acute interstitial nephritis in the elderly. Kidney Int. 2015;87(2):458–64.

Nast CC. Medication-induced interstitial nephritis in the 21st century. Adv Chronic Kidney Dis Elsevier Inc. 2017;24:72–9.

Perazella MA, Markowitz GS. Drug-induced acute interstitial nephritis. Nat Rev Nephrol Nature Publishing Group. 2010;6:461–70.

Perazella MA, Shirali AC. Immune checkpoint inhibitor nephrotoxicity: what do we know and what should we do? Kidney Int. 2020;97(1):62–74.

Perazella MA, Sprangers B. Checkpoint inhibitor therapy-associated acute kidney injury: time to move on to evidence-based recommendations. Clin Kidney J. 2021;14(5):1301–6.
Perazella MA. Drug-induced renal failure: update on new medications and unique mechanisms of nephrotoxicity. Am J Med Sci. 2003;325(6):349–62.
Pirani CL, Valeri A, D'Agati V, Appel GB. Renal toxicity of nonsteroidal anti-inflammatory drugs. Contrib Nephrol. 1987;55:159–75.
Praga M, González E. Acute interstitial nephritis. Kidney Int. 2010;77(11):956–61.
Praga M, Sevillano A, Aunon P, Gonzalez E. Changes in the aetiology, clinical presentation and management of acute interstitial nephritis, an increasingly common cause of acute kidney injury. Nephrol Dial Transplant. 2015;30:1472–9.
Seethapathy H, Zhao S, Chute DF, Zubiri L, Oppong Y, Strohbehn I, et al. The incidence, causes, and risk factors of acute kidney injury in patients receiving immune checkpoint inhibitors. Clin J Am Soc Nephrol. 2019;14(12):1692–700.
Shaaban H, Layne T, Guron G. A case of DRESS (drug reaction with eosinophilia and systemic symptoms) with acute interstitial nephritis secondary to lenalidomide. J Oncol Pharm Pract. 2014;20(4):302–4.
Shah S, Carter-Monroe N, Atta MG. Granulomatous interstitial nephritis. Clin Kidney J. 2015;8(5):516–23.
Shirali AC, Perazella MA, Gettinger S. Association of acute interstitial nephritis with programmed cell death 1 inhibitor therapy in lung cancer patients. Am J Kidney Dis. 2016;68(2):287–91.
Valluri A, Hetherington L, McQuarrie E, Fleming S, Kipgen D, Geddes CC, et al. Acute tubulointerstitial nephritis in Scotland. QJM. 2015;108(7):527–32.
Wanchoo R, Karam S, Uppal NN, Barta VS, Deray G, Devoe C, et al. Adverse renal effects of immune checkpoint inhibitors: a narrative review. Am J Nephrol. 2017;45(2):160–9.
World MJ, Stevens PE, Ashton MA, Rainford DJ. Mesalazine-associated interstitial nephritis. Nephrol Dial Transplant. 1996;11(4):614–21.

Viral-Induced Tubulointerstitial Nephritis

Emmanuelle Plaisier and Pierre Ronco

Viruses account for a substantial proportion of causes of acute interstitial nephritis (AIN). Kidney injury may be the consequence of cell damage from direct viral infection, and/or secondary to viral-induced immune response targeting the kidney tissue. Viral pathogens causing AIN are distinct between immunocompetent subjects and immunocompromised patients, resulting in distinct clinical and histopathological presentation and outcome. Nonspecific interstitial inflammation may also represent a secondary pathological feature in acute ischemic or toxic tubulopathy occurring in several viral diseases, such as Ebola, Dengue disease or COVID 19, that will not be discussed in the chapter.

1 Hantavirus Nephropathy

Hantaviruses (HV) represent the leading cause of viral-induced AIN in immunocompetent subjects, causing hemorrhagic fever with renal syndrome (HFRS) in Eurasia and cardiopulmonary syndrome in America. Puumala hantavirus serotype is endemic in Central and Northern Europe with annual cases exceeding 1000 per country and is responsible for a milder form of HFRS recognized as "nephropathia

E. Plaisier (✉)
Department of Nephrology -AURA Paris Plaisance, Paris, France

Rare and Common Kidney Diseases: From Molecular Mechanisms to Personalized Medicine Unit, INSERM UMRS 1155, Sorbonne Université, Paris, France
e-mail: emmanuelle.plaisier@auraparis.org

P. Ronco
Rare and Common Kidney Diseases: From Molecular Mechanisms to Personalized Medicine Unit, INSERM UMRS 1155, Sorbonne Université, Paris, France

Department of Nephrology, Centre Hospitalier du Mans, Le Mans, France

M. G. Atta, M. A. Perazella (eds.), *Tubulointerstitial Nephritis*,
https://doi.org/10.1007/978-3-030-93438-5_5

epidemica" (NE). NE develops after a 2–4 weeks incubation phase and is typically associated with fever, flu-like symptoms, acute kidney injury (AKI), and thrombocytopenia. One third and about half of subjects show respiratory symptoms and transient visual loss, respectively. Renal manifestations typically includes hematuria, proteinuria ranging from 1 to 4 g/day combining both albuminuria and low molecular weight proteinuria, and AKI of variable severity. Oliguria first occurs, with peak of serum creatinine typically observed after 7 days, followed by polyuria and spontaneous remission within 3 weeks. Only about 5% of patients require transient kidney replacement therapy.

Kidney biopsy typically shows large foci of interstitial hemorrhages in the medulla, which are considered the most specific pathological finding of Hantavirus nephropathy and more rarely extended to the cortex along with mild to moderate polymorphic interstitial inflammation containing lymphocytes and macrophages, and mild to diffuse acute tubular necrosis. A pathological study of 17 NE cases additionally points out to the presence of microvascular inflammation that fills the cortical peritubular capillaries and medullary vasa recta with swelling and detachment of the endothelial cells, this observation being consistent with the endothelial tropism of HV. Ultrastructural analysis may reveal focal to diffuse podocyte foot process effacement, responsible for albuminuria commonly observed in NE. Diagnosis of NE is firmly established by routine enzyme-linked immunosorbent assay test detecting IgG and IgM antibodies against HV. Treatment of NE is symptomatic as no specific antiviral drug is currently available. Large European cohorts of NE have reported excellent long-term kidney outcome regardless of the severity of AKI at presentation. By contrast to NE, severe forms of Hantavirus nephropathy are observed with other HV serotypes including Dobrava and New world in America, mostly causing multiorgan dysfunction and associated with a high mortality rate.

2 Human Immunodeficiency Virus (HIV) Infection

A spectrum of kidney diseases including AIN is observed in HIV-positive individuals, occurring as the consequence of either viral replication, immunodeficiency, opportunistic diseases including infections and malignancies, or drug toxicity. Immune reconstitution inflammatory syndrome (IRIS), and diffuse infiltrative lymphocytosis syndrome (DILS) are systemic syndromes caused by HIV-induced immune dysregulation. In both diseases, kidney involvement typically shows a histological pattern of AIN.

IRIS represents a dysregulated inflammatory response occurring shortly after antiretroviral therapy (ART) initiation in patients with severe lymphopenia (CD4 count bellow 50/mm^3) and preexisting latent or shortly treated opportunistic infection (most commonly Mycobacterium Tuberculosis, Mycobacterium Avium, cryptococcus, JC virus). Organ-limited or systemic manifestations (lymphadenopathy, organomegaly, lung disease, serositis…) with constitutional symptoms are usually observed. Most of the reported cases of AIN occurred in systemic forms of mycobacterial-related IRIS. Kidney manifestations typically include AKI, proteinuria of 1–4 g/day, and bilateral kidney enlargement. Histopathological analysis reveals acute granulomatous interstitial nephritis with dense mononuclear interstitial infiltrates mainly composed of macrophages, T lymphocytes and non-caseating granuloma. Short course of prednisone, anti-microbial therapy, and maintenance of ART are usually efficient to reverse kidney injury. Atypical presentation or outcome should prompt the search for an alternative cause of acute interstitial nephritis, in particular drug-induced AIN.

DILS is a rare syndrome characterized by CD8+ T-cell lymphocytosis with CD8+ T-cell organ infiltration, mostly affecting uncontrolled and/or untreated HIV-positive individuals, with high HIV viral load. It usually presents with sicca signs, salivary gland enlargement, lymphadenopathy, and extra-glandular organ involvement including lung, nervous systems, and digestive tract. Less than 10% of patients develop a kidney disease characterized by AKI, tubular proteinuria, leukocyturia, hematuria, and distal tubular dysfunction with metabolic acidosis, hyperkaliemia, low level of renin and aldosterone, and polyuria. Nephromegaly may also be present. Kidney biopsy shows AIN with dense interstitial mononuclear infiltrates predominantly composed of CD3+CD8+ T lymphocytes, plasma cells and monocytes, without granuloma formation. Tubulitis is commonly observed, as well as some degree of interstitial fibrosis and tubular epithelial atrophy notably affecting distal tubules. Although corticosteroids can effectively control the manifestations of DILS, incomplete recovery or relapse upon discontinuation may occur despite ART use. Table 1 displays the features of AIN in the setting of IRIS or DILS in HIV-positive patients.

Table 1 Features of AIN in IRIS and DILS in HIV-positive patients

Characteristic	IRIS	DILS
HIV status	Recent ART initiation	Uncontrolled HIV infection despite long-term ART
Predisposing factors	Exposure to infectious (typically tuberculosis) antigen before ART	HLA-DR5D4+
Clinically	Patient in the restoration phase of immunity	Sicca syndrome Parotid enlargement
Labs	Hematuria, Sterile pyuria Proteinuria (>0.3 g/day)	Hematuria, Sterile pyuria, Proteinuria (>0.3 g/day) Functional tubular disorders
Pathology and predominant infiltrating cell lineage	Noncaseous granuloma Diffuse and systemic CD4	Diffuse and systemic CD8
Treatment	Antimicrobial chemotherapy, administration of steroids ± continuation or discontinuation of ART	Administration of steroids Continuation of ART

DILS diffuse infiltrative lymphocytosis syndrome, *IRIS* immune reconstitution inflammatory syndrome, *ART* antiretroviral therapy

While mostly classified as a glomerulopathy, HIV-associated nephropathy (HIVAN) is a pan nephropathy with the interstitial inflammation being out of proportion to glomerular disease. Interstitial infiltrates in HIVAN are predominantly composed of CD4+ and CD8+ T lymphocytes, plasma cells and monocytes. In biopsy specimen with unsampled glomeruli, the presence of interstitial inflammation and microcystic tubular dilations should raise the suspicion of HIVAN in untreated and/or uncontrolled patient of African ancestry.

3 BK Virus-Associated Nephropathy

BK polyomavirus (BKV) causes frequent primary subclinical infections during childhood, spreads and infects renal tubular epithelial cells and epithelial cells of the urogenital tract, where it remains latent. Reactivation of BKV in immunocompromised individuals following solid organ transplantation (SOT) and hematopoietic stem cell transplantation (HSCT) may cause serious complications, including BKV-associated nephropathy (BKVAN) mostly in kidney allograft, ureteric stenosis, or hemorrhagic cystitis.

BKVAN is an AIN that commonly occurs in the first 2 years after kidney transplantation or following treatment of rejection. BKV viremia usually precedes the development of BKVAN by a median 8 weeks and early reduction of immunosuppression in viremic patients effectively prevent BKVAN. The 2019 American Society of Transplantation Infectious Disease Community of Practice (AST-IDCOP) guidelines established quantitative BKV PCR in blood or plasma as the reference screening method and recommends monthly screening the first 9 months and every 3 months until 2 years after kidney transplantation. Urinary cytology tests detecting infected renal tubular epithelial cells also named decoy cells, have been adopted as the first detection tests in some centers to reduce cost but are less sensitive than molecular screening, with variation due to operator-dependent performance.

BKVAN may be clinically silent or revealed by nonspecific signs including acute or progressive kidney graft dysfunction, tubular proteinuria, and hematuria. Definitive diagnosis of BKVAN is established by kidney allograft biopsy. Histologic changes include interstitial inflammatory infiltrate and tubular damage with tubulitis. While these characteristics are similar to acute cellular rejection, two findings are highly suggestive of BKVAN, namely the presence of intranuclear inclusion bodies in tubular cells and positive immunochemical staining with antibody against SV40-T Ag. The Banff Working group on Polyomavirus Nephropathy has proposed a histologic Classification System for BKVAN which combines the quantification of intrarenal BKV viral load and the Banff interstitial fibrosis of cortical area score. This classification has delineated three histologic classes which are tightly correlated with clinical presentation and kidney allograft function outcome.

Immunosuppression reduction remains the only consensual therapeutical approach in BKVAN, since no antiviral drug targeting BKV is currently available. Conversion to mTOR inhibitor has been proposed, based on experimental studies and retrospective clinical data, but its impact on allograft function outcome need to be further demonstrated. Additional therapeutic options have been tested including intravenous immunoglobulin, cidofovir or leflunomide, with conflicting results.

BKVAN has been exceptionally reported in other SOT, while HSCT recipients are more likely to experience hemorrhagic cystitis. Kidney allograft dysfunction may rarely be the consequence of hydronephrosis due ureteral BKV infection inducing ureteral epithelial cells inflammation and stenosis.

4 Adenoviral Nephritis

Adenovirus (AdV) cause epidemics of self-limited infections in healthy subjects, mostly affecting the upper and lower respiratory tract, the cornea, and gut. In immunocompromised patients, notably HSCT and SOT recipients, AdV reactivation or newly primary infection are responsible for severe and/or disseminated disease. Hemorrhagic cystitis is the most common urological manifestation in this context, presenting with fever, dysuria, and gross hematuria. AIN mostly occurs in kidney transplant recipients, more rarely in HSCT, and is suspected by the presence of hemorrhagic cystitis and acute graft dysfunction.

Allograft biopsy is required to distinguish AdV nephritis from AKI or acute rejection. AdV nephritis is associated with widespread and dense interstitial infiltrates of T-lymphocytes, plasma cells and macrophages, sometimes forming granulomatous inflammation with necrotizing foci. Acute tubular necrosis and tubulitis are commonly observed, and viral cytopathic effects may be observed in tubular cells, characterized by smudgy basophilic intranuclear inclusions with enlarged nuclei. Immunostaining for AdV shows nuclear and cytoplasmic staining of infected cells. AdV PCR testing in urine and plasma, together with histopathological analysis allow to establish the diagnosis and sequential monitoring of the AdV viral load. Similar to BKVAN, reduction of immunosuppression is the cornerstone of AdV nephritis treatment. Adjunctive therapy such as IVIg, and/or antiviral agents such as cidofovir, ribavirin or ganciclovir have also been additionally proposed. AdV nephritis is usually reversible, while disseminated infection may be life-threatening.

5 Cytomegalovirus (CMV) Interstitial Nephritis

While CMV may cause severe tissue disease in immunocompromised hosts, notably in SOT recipients, invasive CMV disease of the kidney is rare, responsible for either glomerulopathy or tubulointerstitial nephritis, mostly in the kidney allograft. Histologic findings in CMV tubulointerstitial nephritis include interstitial inflammatory infiltrate composed of plasma cells and mononuclear cells with various degree of tubular injury. Presence of typical "owl's eyes" intracellular inclusions in tubular cells or/and interstitial cells is highly suggestive of CMV nephritis, confirmed by cellular positivity for CMV by immunochemistry. Coexistence of CMV nephritis and BKVAN has been reported, and pathological differentiation with acute cellular or humoral rejection may be challenging without IHC study specially when cytopathic effect is lacking. Intravenous ganciclovir is the gold standard therapy for in CMV nephritis, commonly allowing the recovery of the graft function.

Suggested Reading

Cohen-Bucay A, Ramirez-Andrare SE, Gordon CE, Francis JM, Chitalia VC. Advences in BK virus complication in organ transplantation and beyond. Kidney Med. 2020;2:771–86.

Daugas E, Plaisier E, Boffa JJ, Guiard-Schmid JB, Pacanowski J, Mougenot B, Ronco P. Acute renal failure associated with immune restoration inflammatory syndrome. Nat Clin Pract Nephrol. 2006;2:594–8.

Gnemmi V, Verine J, Vrignaud L, Glowacki F, Ratsimbazafy A, Copin MC, et al. Microvascular inflammation and acute tubular necrosis are major histologic features of hantavirus nephropathy. Hum Pathol. 2015;46:827–35.

Hirsch HH, Randhawa PS. American Society of Transplantation Infectious Diseases Community of Practice (ASTIDCoP) BK polyomavirus in solid organ transplantation-guidelines from the American Society of Transplantation Infectious Diseases Community of Practice. Clin Transpl. 2019;33:e13528.

Nickeleit V, Singh HK, Dadhania D, Cornea V, El-Husseini A, Castellanos A, et al. The 2018 Banff Working Group classification of definitive polyomavirus nephropathy: a multicenter validation study in the modern era. Am J Transplant. 2021;21:669–80.

Latus J, Schwab M, Tacconelli E, Pieper FM, Wegener D, Rettenmaier B, et al. Acute kidney injury and tools for risk stratification in 456 patients with hantavirus induced nephropathia epidemica. Nephrol Dial Transplant. 2015;30:245–51.

Lusco MA, Fogo AB, Najafian B, Alpers CE. AJKD atlas of renal pathology: adenovirus infection. Am J Kidney Dis. 2018;71:e1–2.

Outinen T, Makelä S, Clement J, Paakkala A, Pörsti I, Mustonen J. Community acquired severe acute kidney injury caused by hantavirus-induced hemorrhagic fever with renal syndrome has a favorable outcome. Nephron. 2015;130:182–90.

Rane S, Nada M, Minz M, Sakhuja V, Joshi K. Spectrum of cytomegalovirus-induced renal pathology in renal allograft recipients. Transplant Proc. 2012;44:713–7.

Swanepoel CR, Atta MG, D'Agati VD, Estrella MM, Fogo AB, Naicker S, et al. Kidney disease in the setting of HIV infection: conclusions from a kidney disease: improving global outcomes (KDIGO) controversies conference. Kidney Int. 2018;93(3):545–59.

Swanson KJ, Djamali A, Jorgenson MR, Misch EA, Ghaffar A, Zhong W. Cytomegalovirus nephritis in kidney transplant recipients: epidemiology and outcomes of an uncommon diagnosis. Transpl Infect Dis. 2021;23(5):e13702. https://doi.org/10.1111/tid.13702.

Veer M, Abdulmassih R, Como J, Min Z, Bhanot N. Adenoviral nephritis in a renal transplant recipient: case report and literature review. Transpl Infect Dis. 2017;19:e12716.

Wyatt CM, Klotman PE, D'Agati VD. HIV-associated nephropathy: clinical presentation, pathology, and epidemiology in the era of antiretroviral therapy. Semin Nephrol. 2008;28(6):513–22.

Zafrani L, Coppo P, Dettwiler S, Molinier-Frankel V, Agbalika F, Guiard-Schmid JB, et al. Nephropathy associated with the diffuse infiltrative lymphocytosis syndrome. Kidney Int. 2007;72:219–24.

Zaidan M, Lescure FX, Brochériou I, Dettwiler S, Guiard-Schmid JB, Pacanowski J, Rondeau E, Pialoux G, Girard PM, Ronco P, Plaisier E. Tubulointerstitial nephropathies in HIV-infected patients over the past 15 years: a clinico-pathological study. Clin J Am Soc Nephrol. 2013;8:930–8.

Bacterial and Parasitic-Related Tubulointerstitial Nephritis

Nicola Wearne and Bianca Davidson

1 Introduction

Acute tubulointerstitial nephritis [TIN] is an important cause of acute kidney injury [AKI] and can progress to chronic kidney disease [CKD]. In a large, multicenter study, an overall prevalence of 2.7% was reported. However the true incidence is likely underestimated, as many are not referred for kidney biopsy. Drugs are cited as the most common cause of TIN, with infections reported less frequently. In a review of the reported literature, drugs were the leading cause of TIN in approximately 70% of cases with infections resulting in 4.0–15.6%. However, infections remain an important cause and are likely to be region specific.

2 Bacterial Causes of Interstitial Disease

The most common mechanisms by which bacteria cause AKI is from sepsis or systemic inflammatory response syndrome [SIRS]. AKI can be exacerbated by multiorgan failure, hypotension, hemolysis or hepatorenal syndrome. Some bacteria have been specifically associated with acute TIN. These include Staphylococcus *aureus and epidermidis,* Salmonella *typhi and paratyphi,* Legionella *spp*, Yersinia *enterocolitica,* Brucella *spp*, Campylobacter *jejuni,* and Corynebacterium *diphtheriae.* These bacteria directly invade the interstitium of the kidney either through ascending infection or hematogenous spread. Activation of immune responses subsequently result in acute or chronic TIN. Antimicrobial agents used to treat these

N. Wearne (✉) · B. Davidson
Department of Nephrology and Hypertension, Kidney Research Unit, Groote Schuur Hospital, University of Cape Town, Cape Town, Western Cape, South Africa
e-mail: Nicola.wearne@uct.ac.za; Bianca.davidson@uct.ac.za

M. G. Atta, M. A. Perazella (eds.), *Tubulointerstitial Nephritis*,
https://doi.org/10.1007/978-3-030-93438-5_6

infections may also result in TIN. A high level of clinical suspicion, early detection, and management are essential to prevent ongoing kidney injury.

2.1 *Mycobacterium* tuberculosis

Granulomatous interstitial nephritis [GIN] is a variant of TIN where granulomas are seen in the interstitium of the kidney often surrounded by inflammatory cells. The current published literature reports GIN to occur in 0.5–1.37% of patients undergoing kidney biopsy. Although sarcoidosis and drugs are often cited as the commonest cause in developed countries, tuberculosis [TB] is the most common cause in regions endemic with Mycobacterium *tuberculosis*, and heightened where human immunodeficiency virus [HIV]/TB coinfection occurs. In 2019, people living with HIV accounted for 85% (3.5 million) of the total TB infections. Of the 3.5 million, three countries; India, Tanzania, and South Africa accounted for 25%, 17% and 14%, respectively.

Kidney involvement from TB includes localized genitourinary disease, GIN, and GIN occurring from TB immune reconstitution inflammatory syndrome [IRIS]. The impaired CD4 T-cell function seen in untreated HIV with low CD4 counts, alters cytokine secretion leading to poorly formed granulomas. Antiretroviral therapy restores the host's ability to form granulomata which may lead to an intense paradoxical reaction improving granuloma formation resulting in TB-IRIS. A high degree of clinical suspicion is required as a diagnosis to the etiology of GIN can be challenging.

2.2 *Leptospirosis*

Leptospirosis is a zoonotic disease endemic to tropical and temperate regions that is caused by a spirochete; Leptospira *interrogans*. The rat is the major reservoir excreting spirochetes in the urine. The spectrum of kidney injury in humans includes mild proteinuria, urinary sediment abnormalities, tubular dysfunction, and AKI predominantly due to acute TIN. Leptospira enter the host's kidney by penetrating the capillary lumen, adhering to tubular epithelium, and subsequently invading the kidney interstitium. An outer membrane protein of the spirochete actives the immune response via toll-like receptors, ultimately leading to varying degrees of lymphoplasmacytic interstitial nephritis. However, the mechanisms for the tubulointerstitial damage remains multifactorial including hemodynamic instability, hyperbilirubinemia, rhabdomyolysis, immune-mediated inflammation, and direct nephrotoxicity by the spirochete. Kidney involvement usually accompanies pulmonary hemorrhage and liver dysfunction.

2.3 *Leprosy*

Kidney involvement in leprosy is characterized by epithelioid granulomas. The bacilli of Mycobacterium *leprae* may also be seen within the kidney parenchyma. Kidney involvement is characterized by hematuria, mild proteinuria, and renal tubular dysfunction. It can also lead to chronic TIN and amyloidosis progressing to CKD. The mechanism of kidney disease is likely associated with immunological phenomena. Leprosy nephropathy has become a milder disease, which tends to recover after specific treatment.

3 Parasitic Causes of Interstitial Nephritis

Currently there are 342 identified parasites, of which 20 cause disease in humans and may lead to kidney disorders. The four parasites that cause the most significant kidney pathology include malaria, schistosomiasis, filariasis, and leishmaniasis which are classified as neglected tropical disease by the World Health Organization [WHO]. The geographical distribution of these parasites is demonstrated in Fig. 1.

Malaria is the most life-threatening. In 2019, the WHO estimated 229 million cases of malaria worldwide with over 409,000 reported deaths with the African region carrying a high share of the global burden. Malaria-associated AKI has been reported to occur in over 40% of patients with severe malaria. Table 1 outlines how malaria and other major parasites affect the interstitium resulting in kidney dysfunction. Schistosomiasis affects more than 200 million people worldwide and it is endemic in Africa, South America and, the Far East (Fig. 1). Current WHO

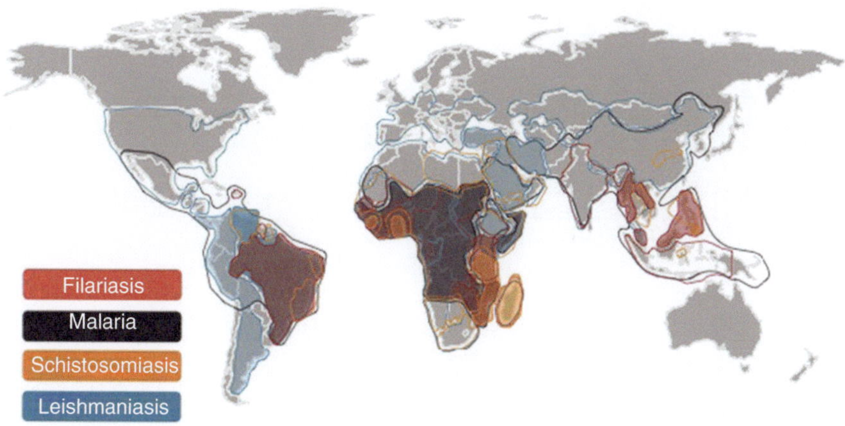

Fig. 1 Geographic distribution of the four commonest parasites that affect the kidney. World map with outlined countries depicting the geographic regions where parasites are found. The highlighted areas demonstrate areas of highest burden

Table 1 Kidney manifestations of parasitic infections

	Clinical syndromes	Kidney involvement	Interstitial disease	gn – ic mediated
Blood and tissue protozoa				
Leishmaniasis (Kala-azar) **Transmission:** insects (sand fly)	**Visceral leishmaniasis:** Low-grade fever, pallor, splenomegaly, hepatomegaly, fatigue, weakness, loss of appetite and weight loss. Laboratory: pancytopenia, hypergammaglobulinemia and hypoalbuminemia.	**Urine abnormalities:** Mild/ moderate proteinuria/ nephrotic syndrome (albuminuria/microalbuminuria and gamma globulins) Microscopic hematuria and leukocyturia. **Interstitial nephritis:** glomerular changes can also be seen. **AKI complicated with:** **Electrolyte disturbances** (in 1/3 patients) due to increased fractional excretion ($\downarrow Na^{2+}$(94.6%), $\downarrow Mg^{2+}$ (41.8%), $\downarrow Ca^{2+}$ (32%), $\downarrow Cl^{-}$(27.2%), and $\downarrow K^{+}$ (26%)). **Tubular defects** (urinary concentration and acidification defects (Type 1 RTA), thought to be due to increased gamma globulins. **Hormone** abnormalities: elevated ACTH, primary adrenal insufficiency, aldosterone excretion abnormalities and SIADH.	*The Leishmania can manipulate the host immune system to evade detection by:* (1) Inducing the production of macrophage-inhibiting cytokines (growth factor β and IL10) and interfering with IFN-**γ** signaling as well as producing polyclonal B-cell activation. (2) Impairing Lymphoid proliferation. (3) Inhibition of natural killer cells.	MesPGN MCGN Collapsing FSGS RPGN Amyloid deposits

Trypanosoma *T. Cruzi* (CHAGAS Disease) **Transmission**: triatomine bug	**Acute presentation:** Fever, inflamed inoculation, lymphadenopathy, hepatosplenomegaly, myocarditis, pericardial effusion, and meningoencephalitis. **Chronic presentation:** cardiac abnormalities, enlargement of the esophagus and colon as well as nerve involvement.	**Urine abnormalities:** Microscopic hematuria. Mild/Moderate proteinuria. **AKI due to:** **Functional reduction in renal blood flow:** cardiac induced hemodynamic instability. **Structural damage** likely by inflammation and renal ischemia resulting in proximal tubular injury and an inflammatory interstitial infiltrate.	*The exact mechanism by which T. cruzi causes kidney disease is still to be elucidated:* Proposed mechanisms: (1) Increased production of pro-inflammatory cytokines and nitric oxide. (2) Renal function loss associated with a high parasitic load (antigen found in the interstitium). (3) Immunological activation and autoantibodies production	MesPGN MCGN
Plasmodium Malaria (1-4) *P. falciparum* *P. vivax greatest human risk.* **Transmission** Anopheles Mosquito	**Acute presentation:** Fever Dark urine (blackwater fever) Jaundice Anemia (hemolytic) Headache/Confusion Hepatomegaly Splenomegaly	**Urinary abnormalities:** +/-Hematuria/ massive hemolysis resulting in hemoglobinuria. **AKI due to**: **Renal hypoperfusion**: increased fluid loss and decreased intake of fluids, hypotension. **Hemolysis:** cytoadherence with adhesion of parasitized RBCs to the vascular endothelial cells resulting in sequestration of RBCs in the circulation of vital organs and hypoxia. **Rhabdomyolysis** and **thrombotic microangiopathy (rare)**	*Mechanism of TIN is multifactorial:* (1) Host immune response to infection. (2) Release of inflammatory cytokines, reactive oxygen species and nitric oxide. (3) Renal hypoperfusion.	Glomerular endothelial damage, Coagulopathy PIGN Mild mesPGN

(continued)

Table 1 (continued)

	Clinical syndromes	Kidney involvement	Interstitial disease	gn – ic mediated
Quartan Malaria *P. Malariae*	**Chronic presentation:** Cyclical fever, flu-like symptoms, and headache.	**Urinary abnormalities:** Proteinuria/ Nephrotic syndrome. **ESKD**		Progressive GN MesPGN MCGN Membranous (rare)
Toxoplasma gondii Toxoplasmosis **Transmission:** Cats	**Acute presentation:** Flu-like illness Lymphadenopathy **Chronic presentation:** Confusion, seizures, meningism, focal neurology, movement disorders, visual changes. Myocarditis Pneumonitis (rare)	**Urinary abnormalities:** Proteinuria/ Nephrotic syndrome. **Interstitial nephritis:** glomerular changes can also be seen. **AKI due to:** Sulfadiazine crystal deposition in the urinary tract.	*Pathogenesis of interstitial renal disease associated with T. gondii infection:* (1) Tubulointerstitial nephritis (Sulfadiazine crystal deposition)	MCGN FSGS

Fluke/Trematode				
Schistosoma 3 **<u>main</u>** species: S. *haematobium* S. *mansoni* S. *japonicum* **Transmission**: larvae released by freshwater snails penetrate the skin during contact with infested water.	**Clinical presentation**: **[S. *haematobium*]** Terminal hematuria. Increased frequency of micturition and dysuria. Bladder and urethral fibrosis and hydronephrosis. Bladder cancer(late). **[S. *japonicum*, S. *mansoni*]** Intestinal manifestations: abdominal pain, diarrhea and bloody stool. Advanced cases: HSM with portal hypertension	**Urinary abnormalities:** Hematuria Proteinuria [if GN: rare cases seen with S. *mansoni*]. **AKI due to:** **Tubular injury:** mainly urinary concentration dysfunction. **Obstruction** from lower urinary fibrosis and strictures. **Further kidney complications:** **Infection:** Secondary bacterial or viral infection are common. **Stone formation**: may occur. **Bladder malignancy** is a late manifestation.	*Urinary Schistosomiasis causes interstitial disease by the following mechanisms:* (1) Cell-mediated disorders [S. *haematobium*] with formation of granulomata along the entire urinary tract (granulomas in interstitium have been reported). (2) Healing results in excessive fibrosis that may lead to strictures, calcifications, and urodynamic abnormalities. (3) Immune-mediated tubulointerstitial nephritis with dense interstitial infiltration and fibrosis can occur [S. *mansoni* and S. *haematobium*]. (4) Host immune evasion and direct parasitic injury.	MesPGN MCGN FSGS Exudative GN Amyloidosis

(continued)

Table 1 (continued)

	Clinical syndromes	Kidney involvement	Interstitial disease	gn – ic mediated
Intestinal roundworm				
Ascaris lumbricoides (round worms) **Transmission:** Fecal oral route	**Acute presentation:** Asymptomatic occasionally fever, dry cough, dyspnea. **Chronic presentation:** Asymptomatic occasionally complicated by bowel or biliary tree obstruction.	**Rare:** AKI in the setting of pancreatitis as a complication of *A. lumbricoides*	*Isolated case reports*: Acute TIN as a form of hypersensitivity reaction in the setting of human parasitosis.	
Tissue roundworms				
Wuchereria bancrofti, (filariasis) ***Brugia malayi*** (filariasis) ***Onchocerca*** *volvulus* (river blind- ness), ***Loa loa*** (African eye worm) **Transmission:** Flies/ mosquito	**Acute presentation:** Asymptomatic Lymphatic filariasis Tropical eosinophilic pneumonia Lymphatic blockade and elephantiasis	**Urine abnormalities:** Chyluria and hematuria Proteinuria Nephrotic syndrome **Kidney failure (rare)**	*Case reports of Interstitial Nephritis:* (1) Direct toxic effect of microfilariae with eosinophilic infiltration and interstitial inflammation. (2) Microfilariae demonstrated in the renal biopsy specimen(rare). (3) Immune complex formation as well as direct toxic effects like tubulointerstitial disease.	Proliferative GN MCGN Amyloidosis

Abbreviations: *Na*$^{2+}$ sodium, *Mg*$^{2+}$ magnesium, *Ca*$^{2+}$ Calcium, *Cl*$^{-}$ Chloride, *K*$^{2+}$ potassium, *Type 1 RTA* type 1 renal tubular acidosis, *AKI* acute kidney injury, *SIADH* syndrome of inappropriate antidiuretic hormone secretion, *IL* interleukin, *IFN* interferon, *GN* glomerulonephritis, *MesPGN* mesangioproliferative glomerulonephritis, *MCGN* mesangiocapillary glomerulonephritis, *RPGN* rapidly progressive glomerulonephritis, *FSGS* focal segmental glomerulonephritis, *PIGN* post-infectious glomerulonephritis, *RBC* red blood cells, *HSM* hepatosplenomegaly, *TIN* tubulointerstitial nephritis, *ESKD* end stage kidney disease estimates state that 112 and 54 million people are infected with Schistosomiasis *haematobium* and *mansoni* respectively. Of the infected subjects, 60% are symptomatic and 10% have kidney dysfunction (Table 1). Leishmaniasis is linked to environmental changes such as deforestation, building of dams, irrigation schemes, and urbanization. An estimated 700,000 to 1 million new cases occur annually. Only a small fraction of those infected by Leishmania parasites develop disease. Finally, worldwide, 893 million people in 49 countries remain threatened by lymphatic filariasis and require preventive chemotherapy to stop the spread of this parasitic infection (Table 1).

3.1 Mechanisms by Which Parasites Affect the Kidney

The mechanisms by which host-parasite interactions cause kidney injury are multifactorial. The interstitial injury from the parasite may occur from three main mechanisms. (1) Direct invasion of the kidneys or urinary tract. For example, Schistosoma ova directly invade the kidney and produce a delayed hypersensitivity reaction leading to granuloma formation. The second mechanism results from acute systemic effects. Malaria demonstrates this as it leads to hemodynamic instability, increased oxidative stress from hemolysis, and cytoadherence leading to microvascular disruption and rarely rhabdomyolysis. The 3rd mechanism is immune mediated inflammation that results from adaptive immune system activation, parasite related injury from host evasion, and antibody production (IgE) with complement activation from alternative and classical pathways. Parasites are also able to evade host immune detection by various mechanisms including the acquisition of host antigens (e.g., schistosomiasis) and down-regulation or suppression of monocytes (e.g., leishmaniasis, schistosomiasis).

4 Conclusion

Drugs are the most common cause of TIN. However, bacteria and parasites may play a more prominent role in endemic areas. Jha et al. emphasizes the differences in environmental risk factors for kidney disease worldwide. With global travel and migration these infections should be considered as part of the diagnosis of kidney dysfunction, in patients who have recently travelled or previously lived in endemic areas. Parasites and bacteria can affect the interstitium by (1) direct invasion (2) systemic effects and (3) by immune mediated inflammation. Importantly antibiotics and antiparasitic treatment can also cause TIN. These may also include over the counter medications, herbal, and local traditional remedies.

Suggested Reading

Andrade L, de Francesco Daher E, Seguro AC, editors. Leptospiral nephropathy. Semin Nephrol. 2008. Elsevier.
Angus DC, van der Poll T. Severe sepsis and septic shock. N Engl J Med. 2013;369(9):840–51.
Arogundade FA, Hassan MO, Omotoso BA, Oguntola SO, Okunola OO, Sanusi AA, et al. Spectrum of kidney diseases in Africa: malaria, schistosomiasis, sickle cell disease, and toxins. Clin Nephrol. 2016;86(7):53.
Baker RJ, Pusey CD. The changing profile of acute tubulointerstitial nephritis. Nephrol Dial Transplant. 2004;19(1):8–11.
Barsoum R. Tropical parasitic nephropathies. Nephrol Dial Transplant. 1999;14(Suppl_3):79–91.
Bharti AR, Nally JE, Ricaldi JN, Matthias MA, Diaz MM, Lovett MA, et al. Leptospirosis: a zoonotic disease of global importance. Lancet Infect Dis. 2003;3(12):757–71.
Bijol V, Mendez GP, Nose V, Rennke HG. Granulomatous interstitial nephritis: a clinicopathologic study of 46 cases from a single institution. Int J Surg Pathol. 2006;14(1):57–63.
Brown DD, Solomon S, Lerner D, Del Rio M. Malaria and acute kidney injury. Pediatr Nephrol. 2020;35(4):603–8.
Costa RS, Monteiro RC, Lehuen A, Joskowicz M, Noël L-H, Droz D. Immune complex-mediated glomerulopathy in experimental Chagas' disease. Clin Immunol Immunopathol. 1991;58(1):102–14.
da Silva Júnior GB, Barbosa OA, de Moura Barros R, Carvalho PDR, de Mendoza TR, Barreto DMS, et al. Amyloidosis and end-stage renal disease associated with leprosy. Rev Soc Bras Med Trop. 2010;43(4):474–6.
da Silva Junior GB, Duarte DB, Barros EJG, Daher EDF. Schistosomiasis-associated kidney disease: a review. Asian Pac J Trop Dis. 2013;3(1):79–84.
da Silva Junior GB, Barros EJG, Daher EDF. Kidney involvement in leishmaniasis—A review. Braz J Infect Dis. 2014;18(4):434–40.
da Silva Junior GB, Antunes VVH, Motta M, Barros EJG, Daher EDF. Chagas disease-associated kidney injury–A review. Nefrol Latinoamericana. 2017a;14(1):22–6.
da Silva Junior GB, Pinto JR, Barros EJG, Farias GMN, Daher EDF. Kidney involvement in malaria: an update. Rev Inst Med Trop Sao Paulo. 2017b;59:e53.
da Silva Junior GB, Jereissati AAR, Neri AKM, da Costa Lino DO, de Oliveira JGR, Daher EDF. Neglected tropical diseases with an impact on kidney function. In: Current topics in tropical emerging diseases and travel medicine. London, United Kingdom: IntechOpen; 2018.
Davidson B, Nel D, Jones E, Manning K, Spies R, Bohmer R, et al. Granulomatous interstitial nephritis on renal biopsy in HIV positive patients: prevalence and causes in Cape Town, South Africa. Nephrology. 2019;24(7):681–8.
De Francesco DE, Martins Dos Santos G. Renal tubular dysfunction in human visceral leishmaniasis (Kala-azar). Clin Nephrol. 2009;71(5):492–500.
Dutra M, Martinelli R, de Carvalho EM, Rodrigues LE, Brito E, Rocha H. Renal involvement in visceral leishmaniasis. Am J Kidney Dis. 1985;6(1):22–7.
Flores-Mireles AL, Walker JN, Caparon M, Hultgren SJ. Urinary tract infections: epidemiology, mechanisms of infection and treatment options. Nat Rev Microbiol. 2015;13(5):269–84.
Goicoechea M, Rivera F, López-Gómez JM, Glomerulonephritis atmotSRo. Increased prevalence of acute tubulointerstitial nephritis. Nephrol Dial Transplant. 2013;28(1):112–5.
Gryseels B, Polman K, Clerinx J, Kestens L. Human schistosomiasis. Lancet. 2006;368(9541):1106–18.
Holaday BJ, Pompeu M, Jeronimo S, Texeira MJ, de Sousa A, Vasconcelos AW, et al. Potential role for interleukin-10 in the immunosuppression associated with kala azar. J Clin Invest. 1993;92(6):2626–32.
https://www.cdc.gov/parasites/malaria/index.html. Accessed 25 May 2021.
https://www.who.int/news-room/fact-sheets/detail/chagas-disease-(american-trypanosomiasis).
https://www.who.int/news-room/fact-sheets/detail/leishmaniasi. Accessed 25 May 2021.

https://www.who.int/news-room/fact-sheets/detail/lymphatic-filariasis. Accessed 25 May 2021.
https://www.who.int/news-room/fact-sheets/detail/malaria. Accessed 25 May 2021.
https://www.who.int/schistosomiasis/epidemiology/table/en/. Accessed 25 May 2021.
https://www.who.int/teams/control-of-neglected-tropical-diseases. Accessed 20 May 2021.
Javaud N, Belenfant X, Stirnemann J, Laederich J, Ziol M, Callard P, et al. Renal granulomatoses: a retrospective study of 40 cases and review of the literature. Medicine. 2007;86(3):170–80.
Jha V, Garcia-Garcia G, Iseki K, Li Z, Naicker S, Plattner B, et al. Chronic kidney disease: global dimension and perspectives. Lancet. 2013;382(9888):260–72.
Joss N, Morris S, Young B, Geddes C. Granulomatous interstitial nephritis. Clin J Am Soc Nephrol. 2007;2(2):222–30.
Jung O, Ditting T, Gröne HJ, Geiger H, Hauser IA. Acute interstitial nephritis in a case of Ascaris lumbricoides infection. Nephrol Dial Transplant. 2004;19(6):1625–8.
Kamath N, Iyengar A. Infections and the kidney: a tale from the tropics. Pediatr Nephrol. 2018;33(8):1317–26.
Langhammer J, Birk HW, Zahner H. Renal disease in lymphatic filariasis: evidence for tubular and glomerular disorders at various stages of the infection. Tropical Med Int Health. 1997;2(9):875–84.
Lawn SD, Bekker L-G, Miller RF. Immune reconstitution disease associated with mycobacterial infections in HIV-infected individuals receiving antiretrovirals. Lancet Infect Dis. 2005;5(6):361–73.
Lemos JRD, Rodrigues WF, Miguel CB, Parreira RC, Miguel RB, de Paula RA, et al. Influence of parasite load on renal function in mice acutely infected with Trypanosoma cruzi. PLoS One. 2013;8(8):e71772.
Lomonte C, Chiarulli G, Cazzato F, Giammaria B, Marchio G, Losurdo N, et al. End-stage renal disease in leprosy. J Nephrol. 2004;17(2):302–5.
Martin-Blondel G, Debard A, Laurent C, Pugnet G, Modesto A, Massip P, et al. Mycobacterial-immune reconstitution inflammatory syndrome: a cause of acute interstitial nephritis during HIV infection. Nephrol Dial Transplant. 2011;26(7):2403–6.
McLaren DJ, Terry R. The protective role of acquired host antigens during schistosome maturation. Parasite Immunol. 1982;4(2):129–48.
Muriithi AK, Leung N, Valeri AM, Cornell LD, Sethi S, Fidler ME, et al. Biopsy-proven acute interstitial nephritis, 1993–2011: a case series. Am J Kidney Dis. 2014;64(4):558–66.
Oliveira GM, Masuda MO, Rocha NN, Schor N, Hooper CS, de Araújo-Jorge TC, et al. Absence of Fas-L aggravates renal injury in acute Trypanosoma cruzi infection. Mem Inst Oswaldo Cruz. 2009;104(8):1063–71.
Plewes K, Turner GD, Dondorp AM. Pathophysiology, clinical presentation, and treatment of coma and acute kidney injury complicating falciparum malaria. Curr Opin Infect Dis. 2018;31(1):69.
Polito MG, Moreira SR, Nishida SK, Mastroianni Kirsztajn G. It is time to review concepts on renal involvement in leprosy: pre-and post-treatment evaluation of 189 patients. Ren Fail. 2015;37(7):1171–4.
Prasad N, Patel MR. Infection-induced kidney diseases. Front Med. 2018;5:327.
Prina E, Lang T, Glaichenhaus N, Antoine J-C. Presentation of the protective parasite antigen LACK by Leishmania-infected macrophages. J Immunol. 1996;156(11):4318–27.
Ray D, Thukral S. Microfilariae in the kidney. Trop J Med Res. 2017;20(1):101.
Rodriguez-Morales AJ. Current topics in tropical emerging diseases and travel medicine: BoD–books on demand. London, United Kingdom: IntechOpen Limited; 2018.
Schistosomiasis. co. Second report of the WHO Expert committee. World Health Organ Tech Rep Ser. 1993;830:1–86.
tbsouthafrica.org.za/resources/who-global-tuberculosis-report-2020. 2020.
Tucker LF. MS. Chapter 3: schistosomiasis. Digenetic trematodes advances in experimental medicine and biology series. 2014;766:47–75.
Van Velthuysen M-L, Florquin S. Glomerulopathy associated with parasitic infections. Clin Microbiol Rev. 2000;13(1):55–66.

Verde FAAL, Verde FAL, Verde IAL, Silva Junior GB, Daher EF, Verde EML. Evaluation of renal function in human visceral leishmaniasis (kala-azar): a prospective study on 50 patients from Brazil. J Nephrol. 2007;20(4):430–6.

Verde FAL, Verde FAAL, Neto AS, Almeida PC, Verde EML. Hormonal disturbances in visceral leishmaniasis (kala-azar). Am J Trop Med Hyg. 2011;84(5):668–73.

Visith S, Kearkiat P. Nephropathy in leptospirosis. J Postgrad Med. 2005;51(3):184.

Yang CW, Wu MS, Pan MJ. Leptospirosis renal disease. Nephrol Dial Transplant. 2001;16(Suppl_5):73–7.

Tubulointerstitial Nephritis Due to Autoimmune Diseases

Maria Prendecki and Charles D. Pusey

1 Introduction

Many systemic autoimmune diseases have been associated with the development of tubulointerstitial nephritis (TIN), including sarcoidosis, Sjogren's syndrome, systemic lupus erythematosus (SLE), tubulointerstitial nephritis and uveitis syndrome (TINU), and ANCA-associated vasculitis (AAV) (Table 1). Underlying autoimmune disease may account for up to 5% of biopsy proven interstitial nephritis. The histopathological findings of TIN due to autoimmune disease are largely in common with those due to other causes such as drug induced or idiopathic. When disease presents acutely, edema, tubular injury, and cellular infiltrate are present; inflammation may be granulomatous. More chronic findings include a persistent cellular infiltrate, tubular atrophy, and interstitial fibrosis. Tubulointerstitial disease may be a secondary phenomenon, occurring in response to glomerular disease, or can occur in isolation. The pathogenesis of interstitial inflammation in the absence of glomerular disease is complex and incompletely understood, although there are several suggested pathogenic mechanisms involving both the innate and adaptive immune systems, which are common to many autoimmune and systemic diseases. These may include direct antibody-mediated damage, or immune complex deposition, with antibodies directed against an antigen located on or secreted by the tubules. Cellular immunity has also been shown to play a role; HLA subtypes are associated with various underlying diseases, and activated T cells are often present in inflammatory infiltrate. Dendritic cells are also likely to be important in pathogenesis by presenting tubular antigens to infiltrating T cells.

M. Prendecki (✉) · C. D. Pusey
Centre for Inflammatory Disease, Department of Immunology and Inflammation, Imperial College London, Hammersmith Campus, London, UK
e-mail: m.prendecki@imperial.ac.uk; c.pusey@imperial.ac.uk

M. G. Atta, M. A. Perazella (eds.), *Tubulointerstitial Nephritis*,
https://doi.org/10.1007/978-3-030-93438-5_7

Table 1 Autoimmune diseases associated with TIN

More common	Less common
Sarcoidosis	Cryoglobulinemia
Systemic lupus erythematosus	Primary biliary cholangitis
TINU	Inflammatory bowel disease
Sjogren's syndrome	Idiopathic hypocomplementemic TIN
ANCA-associated vasculitis	Relapsing polychondritis

2 Sarcoidosis

Sarcoidosis is a multi-system disorder of unknown etiology which is characterized by the presence of non-caseating granulomas. It has been described to occur at any age, but is most common in adults under the age of 50 years. It is slightly more common in females, and more common in certain ethnic groups, such as African-Americans and Scandinavians. The disease has also been described to affect certain ethnic groups more severely, with extra-thoracic manifestations more common in Puerto-Ricans, African-Americans, and Scandinavians.

The pathogenesis of sarcoidosis is incompletely understood; this may be in part due to the heterogeneity of the disease, and historically imprecise definitions used for diagnosis. Despite a large multi-center case-control study carried out by the National Institutes for Health (NIH) in the USA, no defined etiological agent, and no genetic locus for disease susceptibility has been identified. An infectious agent has been implicated as a trigger; presentation is more common in winter and early spring, and there are reports of community outbreaks suggesting disease is either spread person to person or by exposure to a common environmental agent. *Mycobacterium* spp and *Cutibacterium acnes* (formerly *Propionibacterium acnes*) are the most commonly implicated infectious agents. The transmission of sarcoidosis by solid organ transplant, including cardiac and lung, provides further evidence for an infectious etiology. Heavy metals and dust exposure have also been suggested as responsible agents, and exposure to metal dusts such as beryllium or zirconium can result in disease which is clinico-pathologically indistinguishable from sarcoidosis. It is suggested that phagocytosis and presentation of an unknown environmental antigen by macrophages and dendritic cells to CD4+ T cells then leads to T_{H1} cytokine production, such as interleukin-(IL-)2 and interferon (IFN-)γ, and subsequent granuloma formation. Increased circulating IL-17 and T_{H17} positive cellular infiltrates in affected organs have been identified, but the full role of this axis has yet to be identified. Patients with sarcoid have been shown to have a decreased CD4:CD8 T cell ratio in the peripheral blood due to sequestration of CD4+ cells in affected organs, and hypergammaglobulinemia due to generalized B cell hyperactivity is also common.

The respiratory tract is the commonest site of disease in sarcoidosis, with nearly all patients exhibiting pulmonary involvement at some point. Even those with predominantly extra-thoracic disease usually have evidence of subclinical pulmonary features. Outside the lungs, sarcoidosis can involve most organ systems including heart, skin, eyes, nervous system, liver, spleen, lymph nodes, bone marrow, salivary glands, joints, muscles, and genito-urinary tract. Hypercalcemia due to production of calcitriol by activated macrophages in granulomas is common. Sarcoidosis is a diagnosis of exclusion, and is based on suggestive clinical and radiological findings, the presence of non-caseating granulomas on biopsy, and the exclusion of other granulomatous disorders, particularly those due to infectious agents such as TB.

Kidney involvement leading to an impairment of excretory function in sarcoidosis is most commonly due to nephrocalcinosis, nephrolithiasis, and dehydration secondary to hypercalcemia. The presence of interstitial nephritis on kidney biopsy from a single case was first described in 1955 and has been identified in several subsequent small case series. Estimates of incidence vary widely and has been described to be 0.18% in one large biopsy case series. Subclinical disease is likely to be common however, as incidence of up to 40% is reported in post-mortem series. Glomerular involvement in sarcoidosis is rare; focal segmental glomerulosclerosis (FSGS), vasculitis, membranous nephropathy, mesangioproliferative GN (MPGN), and IgA nephropathy have all been described, but disease confined to the tubulointerstitial compartment is more common. Most patients with interstitial nephritis due to sarcoidosis will also have systemic, extra-renal manifestations of disease although there are a few small case series describing patients with kidney limited disease. There are also cases whereby the identification of TIN has led to a subsequent diagnosis of sarcoidosis. As such, a proportion of cases which are diagnosed as idiopathic granulomatous TIN may be in fact due to a first presentation of sarcoidosis.

2.1 Pathology

The inflammatory infiltrate in TIN due to sarcoidosis is classically described to be confined to the kidney cortex but can also occur throughout the kidney parenchyma. In some studies cellular infiltrate is noted to be widespread, affecting >50% of the tissue. Granulomas are present in 70–80% of cases (Fig. 1). Sarcoid is described to be responsible for 28–50% of cases of granulomatous interstitial nephritis (gTIN) with the main differential diagnoses being drugs and TB. In keeping with sarcoid granuloma in other organs, T cells are mainly CD4+. An eosinophilic infiltrate is generally rare. Chronic features of tubular atrophy and fibrosis are common. The clinical features are variable. In one case series of 21 patients with sarcoid biopsied for AKI, only four patients had evidence of gTIN. However, others have reported series of patients with gTIN due to sarcoid in which all patients have derangement of excretory kidney function, including some patients in whom the indication for kidney biopsy was AKI. The most common urinary abnormality is moderate proteinuria; sterile pyuria and microscopic hematuria may also be present. Serum ACE levels may be normal. Gallium scanning has been used to show foci of inflammation in the kidney; however this too may be normal.

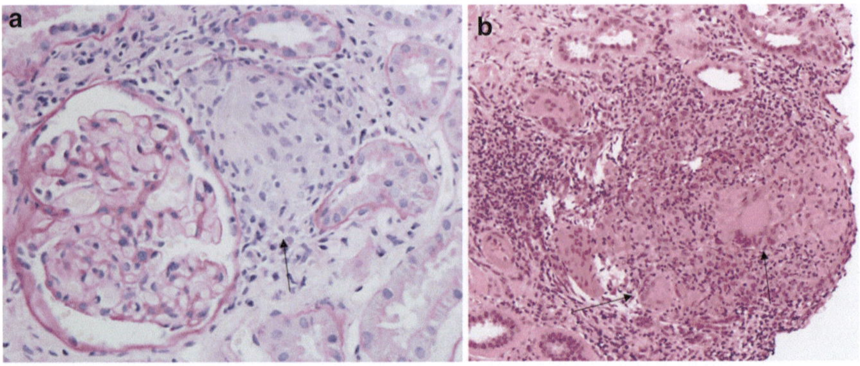

Fig. 1 (**a**) High power and (**b**) Low power photomicrographs of kidney biopsy sections from patients with sarcoidosis showing a granulomatous tubulointerstitial nephritis. Images show mononuclear cell infiltrate and large non-caseating granulomas (black arrows). (Image courtesy of Prof H. T. Cook)

2.2 Treatment and Prognosis

Corticosteroid therapy is the main treatment strategy in patients with TIN and sarcoidosis, with most case series reporting patients showing stabilization or improvement of kidney function. In general, high dose corticosteroids (1 mg/kg up to 60 mg daily) are used followed by corticosteroid taper. Often patients will relapse upon rapid cessation of corticosteroid treatment, although this usually responds to a reintroduction of corticosteroids. Lifelong low dose corticosteroids may be required for patients with frequent relapses. There are isolated case reports of steroid sparing agents such as methotrexate, azathioprine, mycophenolate mofetil, or anti-TNF therapy being used with successful outcomes.

In general, kidney outcomes are good with over 85% of patients responding to corticosteroid treatment, including reports of patients requiring kidney replacement therapy (KRT) recovering independent kidney function. Patients with evidence of significant interstitial fibrosis or tubular atrophy on biopsy often respond less well to treatment. In a case series of native and transplant kidney biopsy findings, only 2 of 2331 patients receiving a kidney transplant (over 10 years) had lost their native kidney function due to confirmed renal sarcoidosis. There is little evidence on the outcomes of kidney transplantation in patients whose native kidney disease was due to sarcoidosis; post-transplant recurrence was detected in one of the two patients in this series. In this case the biopsy was taken incidentally at time of hernia repair, and the patient had stable graft function. Another case series of 18 patients with sarcoidosis who underwent kidney transplant described recurrence of disease in five patients, with kidney involvement in three patients.

3 Systemic Lupus Erythematosus

Systemic lupus erythematosus (SLE) is a multisystem autoimmune disease associated with loss of tolerance to nuclear antigens and production of autoantibodies to them. Immune complex deposition occurs, leading to activation of complement and inflammatory cascades. Around 40% of patients with SLE have kidney disease at the time of diagnosis, and up to 60% may have kidney involvement at some point in their disease course. SLE is more prevalent in women of reproductive age, and in non-white individuals. Among those with SLE, younger age, male gender, and African, Asian or Hispanic ethnicity, are associated with increased likelihood of lupus nephritis (LN).

Lupus nephritis is classified histologically into five main types with differing pathology and clinical features. Tubulointerstitial involvement in LN is common and may be found in 50–70% of patients; however, classifications of LN focus predominantly on glomerular lesions. Tubulointerstitial damage has been associated with more severe glomerular lesions in LN in some but not all studies, and there are also reports of severe TIN occurring in the absence of glomerular disease. It is well recognized that tubulointerstitial damage can play an important role in predicting disease outcomes; in one study, 37% of patients with severe interstitial infiltrate progressed to kidney failure within 2 years.

3.1 *Pathology*

Lupus TIN may be a manifestation of a localized immune process, in contrast to the glomerular lesions which are thought to be dependent on systemic autoimmunity. Tubulointerstitial infiltrates in LN are often composed of B and T lymphocytes, including T follicular helper cells (T_{FH}), and can undergo organization into structures resembling secondary lymphoid organs with a central core of follicular dendritic cells (DCs). There is some evidence that these lymphoid structures are functional, with local proliferation and perpetuation of the immune response occurring in germinal centers. One study suggested that, in a small number of patients in whom repeat biopsy was available, these aggregates showed higher organizational structure over time despite immunosuppressive treatment. Immune complexes are often seen along the tubular basement membrane (TBM) and, in keeping with immune complexes found elsewhere in SLE, they are composed of IgG, IgM, C1q, C3, C5–9 and, rarely IgA. Some studies have suggested that immune complexes in the interstitium are associated with more severe inflammation, although this has not been confirmed in others.

In keeping with the possibility of differing pathogenic mechanisms mediating disease in the glomerulus and tubulointerstitium, there are reports of different antibody isotypes between the two compartments in the same patient. One study has described that B cells in tubulointerstitial infiltrates appear antigenically restricted to cytoplasmic antigens, and identified vimentin, a filament protein secreted by activated macrophages, as the most common target. High serum anti-vimentin antibodies were shown to correlate with severe tubulointerstitial infiltrate and identified a group of patients resistant to conventional treatments. Anti-vimentin antibodies have also been described in a number of other contexts, including autoimmune diseases such as sarcoidosis, and transplantation rejection, suggesting that anti-vimentin antibodies may represent an immune response to chronic kidney inflammation in a number of settings. Other potential autoantibodies which may mediate the development of tubulointerstitial injury in lupus nephritis include dsDNA Ab, which have been shown to directly bind to and activate proximal tubular epithelial cells (PTEC), leading to pro-inflammatory cytokine production. Autoantibodies against acute phase proteins such as C reactive protein (CRP) and pentraxin 3 have also been identified and shown to correlate with tubulointerstitial damage, suggesting a potential role in lupus TIN.

3.2 Treatment and Prognosis

Cases of isolated TIN are too variable and insufficient in number to guide specific treatment strategies. In most cases corticosteroids have been used with improvement in kidney function, although cases are also described where no treatment was used with improvement in kidney function, although not back to previous baseline. Where GN and TIN co-exist, treatment strategy is usually guided by the classification of the glomerular disease. There are several studies showing that the degree of TIN in LN identifies patients at risk of progression to kidney failure to a greater degree than glomerular classification, leading some authors to suggest that patients with both GN and TIN should be treated with the most intensive therapeutic interventions.

4 Tubulointerstitial Nephritis and Uveitis

The syndrome of tubulointerstitial nephritis and uveitis (TINU) was first described by Dobrin in 1975 in two children who presented with acute kidney injury (AKI) due to eosinophilic TIN, together with uveitis, bone marrow granulomas, hypergammaglobulinemia and an acute phase response. No underlying etiological agent was identified, and it was proposed as a new syndrome, termed TINU. Since then, there have been several reported cases and small case series, although granulomas are not always described as present. TINU is a diagnosis of exclusion, as other conditions such as granulomatosis with polyangiitis, sarcoidosis, or toxoplasmosis may also be associated with TIN and uveitis. A recent systematic review identified 592 patients with TINU described in the literature to date. Females were more commonly affected than males, and there were equal numbers of cases described in children and in adults.

The etiology of TINU has not been identified. There is likely genetic susceptibility to developing TINU; cases have been reported in monozygotic twins and sibling pairs. There are reported HLA associations including DRB1*14 and DQA1*01:04 in one series of 31 patients with TIN, 20 of whom had TINU. DRB1*0102, DQA1*01, and DQB1*05 have been identified in another series of 18 patients. It has been suggested there is an infectious trigger to TINU as patients often have prodromal flu-like symptoms, and TINU has been diagnosed in patients with numerous infectious illnesses including TB, EBV, herpes zoster, HTLV, and campylobacter. Drug exposure has also been implicated, including NSAIDs and antibiotics. TINU has also been reported in association with relapsing polychondritis.

Patients with TINU usually have prodromal flu-like symptoms of fever, malaise, arthralgia, and anorexia. Uveitis and ocular symptoms commonly occur after the onset of kidney disease and have been described to relapse. Uveitis is commonly bilateral and anterior, although all of the uveal tract may be affected. Patients with TINU often have evidence of AKI. Moderate proteinuria is common as is evidence of proximal tubular dysfunction. There are several case reports of Fanconi syndrome. Most patients have evidence of hypergammaglobulinemia and an acute phase response.

Diagnosis of TINU is currently a diagnosis of exclusion, although it has been suggested that serum Krebs von den Lunge-6 (KL-6) may be useful as a diagnostic marker; however one study has found it is not specific to TINU and that other causes of TIN may also result in increased levels. Differentiating TINU from sarcoid may be difficult, and some authors suggest that TINU represents an atypical or early presentation of sarcoidosis. Mandeville et al. have developed diagnostic criteria using clinical features from 133 patients identified in 2001.

4.1 Pathology

There is some evidence that TINU is an autoimmune process. Many studies have suggested that an autoantibody against a common antigen in the renal tubular and ciliary epithelium may be responsible, and have demonstrated antibody deposition along the TBM. Other studies, however, have only identified the presence of deposited antibody along the TBM infrequently. Patients with TINU often have autoantibodies including ANCA, Rheumatoid factor, anti-GBM antibody, and ANA. Antibodies against CRP have been identified in TINU and shown to co-localize with modified CRP in kidney and ocular tissue. HLA associations suggest that cellular immunity is important in the pathogenesis of TIN and there may be a skew to a T_{H1}/T_{H17} axis. The interstitial infiltrate in TINU is predominantly CD3+ T

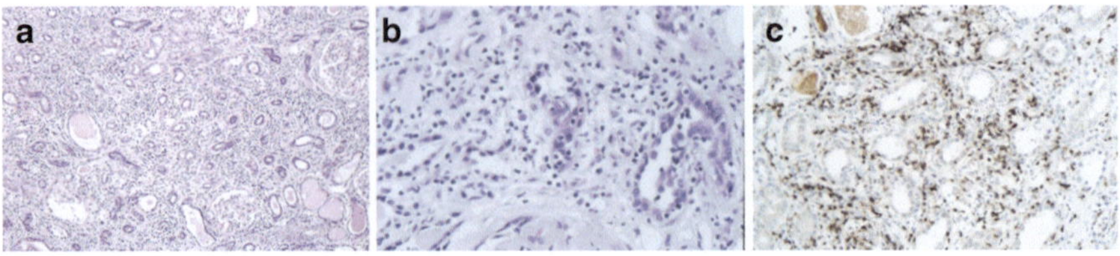

Fig. 2 Photomicrographs of kidney biopsy section from a patient with tubulointerstitial nephritis and uveitis. (**a**) Low power image showing widespread tubulointerstitial mononuclear cell infiltrate with separation of the tubules, tubular atrophy and interstitial edema. Red cell casts can be seen within tubular lumens. (**b**) High power image showing the presence of tubulitis. (**c**) Immunoperoxidase staining for CD3 identifying widespread infiltrate of CD3+ cells (brown staining). (Image courtesy of Prof H. T. Cook)

lymphocytes, with macrophages, plasma cells and eosinophils (Fig. 2). In some studies CD4+ cells have been shown to predominate and in others CD8+ cells. Tubulitis and interstitial edema is often present. Granulomas have been described in around 10% of cases.

4.2 Treatment and Prognosis

In keeping with other rare diseases, there is no evidence based protocol for the treatment of TINU. Most cases are treated with oral glucocorticoids with taper based on response to treatment. Second line, a variety of different immunosuppressive agents have been used including methotrexate, cyclosporine, mycophenolate mofetil and cyclophosphamide. In general, responses to treatment are good, both in terms of the uveitis, and kidney disease. Excretory kidney function has been shown to improve, even in cases where the patient was receiving RRT. There are cases of progression to CKD, and systematic review has identified adult age at onset, and the presence of uveitis beyond the anterior chamber, as risk factors for this. There are reports of patients progressing to develop kidney failure but this is rare. Topical corticosteroids have been described as treatment for isolated uveitis when kidney disease is in remission. Uveitis often follows a relapsing-remitting course, and corticosteroid sparing agents may be required to avoid high cumulative glucocorticoid doses and resultant side effects.

5 Sjogren's Syndrome

Primary Sjogren's syndrome (pSS) is a progressive autoimmune disorder of the exocrine glands, characterized by lymphocytic infiltration, particularly of the salivary and lacrimal glands. Patients typically present with sicca syndrome of dry eyes and dry mouth, which is present in >90% of cases. Extraglandular manifestations are described in around 25% of patients and can occur in multiple organ systems, including TIN, interstitial lung disease, arthritis, cutaneous vasculitis and peripheral neuropathy. Approximately 5% of patients with pSS will develop lymphoma. Sjogren's syndrome has one of the highest female: male imbalances of all autoimmune diseases, with a ratio of up to 15–20:1 in large studies. Those with non-European backgrounds are more commonly affected. Sjogren's syndrome frequently co-exists with other autoimmune diseases, including SLE, rheumatoid arthritis, and systemic sclerosis. The most frequent age of clinical onset of disease is in the sixth decade, although the autoantibodies characteristic of disease are frequently present for many years prior to clinical onset.

The etiology of Sjogren's syndrome is not fully understood but it is thought to be triggered by an environmental factor, likely to be a viral infectious agent, in a susceptible individual. A large GWAS study in patients of European ancestry has identified that HLA-DQB1, and polymorphisms in other loci involved in the innate immune response such as IRF5 and TNIP1, and adaptive immunity such as STAT4, BLK, IL12A and CXCR5, are associated with disease. Although many studies have suggested a role for a viral trigger in disease pathogenesis, no single viral trigger has been identified. Viruses, such as EBV often target salivary glands, and EBV DNA is localized in ectopic lymphoid tissue which is present in some patients with pSS. EBV DNA has been found in the renal tubules of patients with pSS, but also in cases of chronic TIN due to other causes, suggesting it may play a non-specific role in interstitial inflammation.

Sjogren's syndrome is often referred to as an autoimmune epithelitis; epithelial cells are thought not only to be the target of an injurious response but also to perpetuate the autoimmune response by presenting antigen. Epithelial cell activation and injury as a result of viral infection is thought to promote release of pSS associated autoantigens such as Ro and La, and chemokines/chemoattractants. This then leads to an influx of dendritic cells which secrete IFNα and other cytokines leading to influx of lymphocytes and secretion of B cell activating factors. Immune complexes form which lead to a positive feedback loop maintaining production of IFNα. Type 1 interferon pathways have been shown to be implicated in pathogenesis in many studies; IFNα secreting cells are present in biopsy tissue and transcriptional analysis has identified an IFN signature in both biopsy tissue and the peripheral blood. The presence of circulating autoantibodies to the nuclear proteins Ro and La is a key diagnostic feature of pSS. However, these autoantibodies do not seem to play a directly pathogenic role beyond the formation of immune complexes leading to TLR and Fc receptor engagement and an IFNα response.

5.1 Pathology

Estimates of the incidence of kidney involvement vary widely between studies, likely due to differing definitions of disease, and its subclinical presentation in some cases. In some series it has been estimated to be as high as 40%. TIN is the most common kidney lesion seen in pSS and is found in around 75% of patients who undergo kidney biopsy. The cellular infiltrate is predominantly CD4+ T cells with smaller numbers of CD8+ T cells and infrequent B cells. Tubular immune complex deposits are uncommon but when present have been described to co-localize with areas of tubular atrophy and fibrosis. Tubular dysfunction is common in pSS with renal tubular acidosis, Fanconi syndrome and nephrogenic diabetes insipidus all described. These conditions often do not correlate with the histological findings of TIN, and in some studies are more common in younger patients, or in those with CKD. A defect in urinary concentrating ability is the most common abnormality and is present in up to 80% of patients; distal RTA (dRTA) is the second most common abnormality, present in up to 70% in some studies. Patients with dRTA may be asymptomatic or present with hypokalemic symptoms including paralysis. Dynamic testing may be required for diagnosis when the dRTA is incomplete. Patients may also develop nephrocalcinosis or stone disease secondary to dRTA. Proximal tubular dysfunction is estimated to be present in 10–40% of patients, but full Fanconi syndrome is rare. Approximately 25% of patients will have evidence of GN, either in isolation or along with TIN. It is thought to occur later in the disease course than TIN, and GN is predominantly immune complex mediated, with MPGN due to cryoglobulinemia the most common histopathological lesion.

5.2 *Treatment and Prognosis*

A range of immunosuppressive agents have been used in pSS, with some assessed in randomized controlled trials; however none are of proven benefit. In case series of patients with TIN due to pSS, the majority of patients have been treated with corticosteroids, some with additional immunosuppressive agents. Cyclophosphamide, rituximab, azathioprine, and hydroxychloroquine have all been used in small numbers. CKD is common but kidney failure due to pSS is rare. Kidney outcomes are similar in patients with TIN compared to those with GN, but some case series have identified higher mortality in those with GN, possibly due to increased immunosuppression used in these patients. Patients may also need treatment for disorders of tubular function.

6 ANCA-Associated Vasculitis

The anti-neutrophil cytoplasm antibody (ANCA) associated vasculitides (AAV) are a group of rare systemic autoimmune diseases characterized by the presence of circulating ANCA to myeloperoxidase (MPO) or proteinase-3 (PR3) and the presence of necrotizing inflammation of small blood vessels. The three clinical syndromes of AAV are granulomatosis with polyangiitis (GPA), microscopic polyangiitis (MPA) and eosinophilic GPA (EGPA) and there is wide variation in clinical presentation both in organ involvement and disease severity. There are also cases of vasculitis limited to the kidney. There is a slight male preponderance in the incidence of AAV and incidence increases with age. Disease is much less common in non-Caucasian and non-Asian populations and clinical presentation varies between ethnic groups. There are well described genetic and environmental associations with AAV although its etiology is not fully understood. Large GWAS studies have identified HLA associations including HLA-DP (in patients with PR3-ANCA specificity) and HLA-DQ (in patients with MPO-ANCA specificity). Infection has been shown in several studies to precede disease relapse, and in patients with ENT disease nasal carriage of Staphylococci correlates with disease relapse. Molecular mimicry or anti-idiotype antibodies have both been suggested as potential mechanisms.

Anti-neutrophil cytoplasm antibodies have been shown to be directly pathogenic in several clinical and pre-clinical studies and can activate primed neutrophils and monocytes leading to ROS and cytokine production, NETosis and increased endothelial adhesion. NETs in particular have been shown to be mediators of vascular damage but may also play a role in the loss of tolerance to ANCA antigens. There are many studies in preclinical models, and clinical studies, identifying a role for the complement cascade, particularly the alternative pathway.

6.1 Pathology

The main kidney histological lesion in AAV is that of a pauci-immune GN; glomerular disease has been classified into crescentic, focal, mixed, and sclerotic disease, which can be used to predict disease outcomes. Patients will often have interstitial inflammation associated with GN but isolated TIN is rare. Patients with GPA and EGPA may have granulomatous TIN and there is often an eosinophilic infiltrate (Fig. 3). In one case series of 63 patients with EGPA, 28 patients (44%) had evidence of GN accompanied by TIN, and 6 (9.5%) had isolated TIN. Three biopsies had evidence of granuloma formation. The TIN in this cohort was often significant, affecting >25% of the cortical area, and was predominantly eosinophilic. In patients with MPA and GPA interstitial infiltrate has been described to be periglomerular, particularly around glomeruli with severe crescents or sclerosis. Infiltrate is described to be predominantly CD3+ T cells, with a predominance for CD8+ over CD4+ cells. B cells, CD68+ monocytes/macrophages, and neutrophils may also be present. Patients who are MPO-ANCA positive often have greater degree of tubulointerstitial inflammation or scarring.

Isolated TIN in patients with AAV other than EGPA is rare and there are only a small number of cases reported. Most of these cases were in patients with MPO-ANCA specificity, although there is a reported case of a PR3-ANCA positive patient with isolated TIN and granuloma formation. It has been suggested that peritubular capillaritis and tubulitis might lead to the interstitial infiltrate in cases with isolated TIN. Low affinity ANCA recognizing tubular antigens or direct tubular cell injury

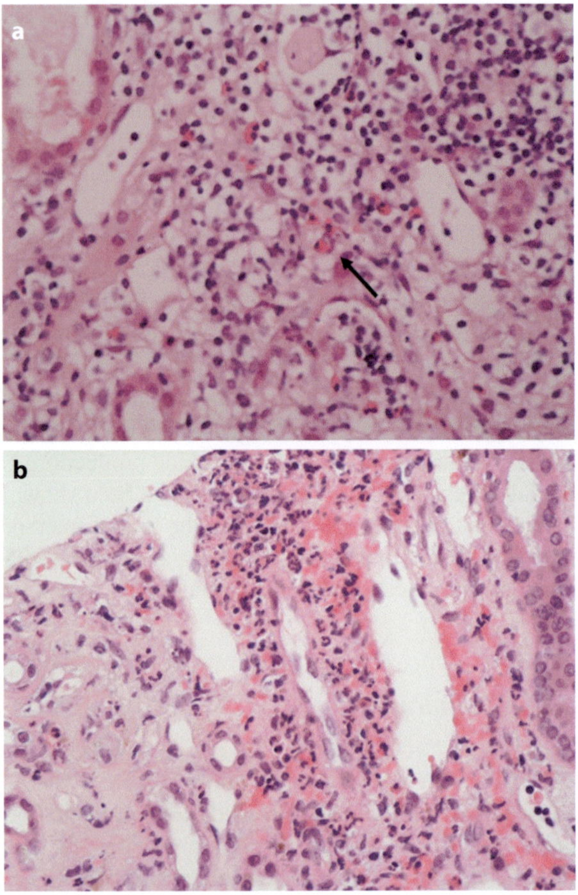

Fig. 3 (**a**) Photomicrograph of kidney biopsy section from a patient with EGPA and eosinophilic tubulointerstitial nephritis. Widespread cellular infiltrate is seen with frequent cells with typical eosinophil morphology (Black arrow). (**b**) Photomicrograph of kidney biopsy section from a patient with MPA showing medullary angiitis with interstitial hemorrhage and polymorphonuclear leucocyte infiltration. (Image courtesy of Prof H. T. Cook)

by ANCA activated leucocytes have been suggested as potential mechanisms by others. There are also several cases described of TIN in AAV which may be of drug induced etiology, but where a role for AAV cannot be ruled out.

6.2 Treatment and Prognosis

In patients with co-existing GN and TIN, patients are treated based on their glomerular disease. Current treatment strategies are supported by the findings of several high quality randomized controlled trials and usual treatment to induce remission is high-dose glucocorticoids and either rituximab or cyclophosphamide. Isolated TIN has in general been treated with less intensive regimens, usually corticosteroid monotherapy, although additional agents have been added in more severe cases. In most cases of TIN there is improvement in excretory kidney function.

7 Other Autoimmune Diseases

Essential mixed cryoglobulinemia (EMC) is characterized by the presence of serum immunoglobulins which are capable of precipitating in the cold. Mixed cryoglobulins are immune complexes formed of either monoclonal and polyclonal (type II) or polyclonal (type III) immunoglobulin. Hepatitis C infection is thought to account for 60–90% of cases in some populations but not all. In some populations Hepatitis C infection is the underlying cause in less than 40% of cases. In non-infectious cases, the predominant kidney lesion is MPGN, seen in over 90% of cases in one series. Over 50% of patients will have evidence of TIN, usually secondary to glomerular lesions, with lymphoid nodules present in some cases. The interstitial infiltrate in EMC is predominantly CD3+ T lymphocytes and monocytes. If hepatitis C infection is present then treatment is with anti-viral therapy. In non-infectious cases, where kidney involvement is serve, treatment is with corticosteroids and cyclophosphamide, or rituximab, sometimes with the addition of plasma exchange.

Primary biliary cholangitis (PBC) is an auto-immune cholestatic liver disease. It predominantly affects women in middle age and over 95% of patients have circulating anti-mitochondrial antibodies. It is characterized by T cell infiltration and destruction of small bile ducts leading to cholestasis, cirrhosis and liver failure. An infectious agent is thought to trigger disease, possibly via a mechanism of molecular mimicry. Distal RTA is common in patients with PBC, and is present in around 30% of patients with advanced liver disease. It is often of no clinical significance. A small number of cases of TIN associated with PBC have been described, sometimes in association with Fanconi syndrome; all cases were in female patients. TIN may be more likely to occur in the early phase of disease prior to the development of hepatic dysfunction or cirrhosis. Interstitial infiltrate is predominantly lymphocytic and can be severe. Some studies have also identified the presence of IgM+ plasma cells. Patients in most reports were treated with corticosteroids with the majority responding to treatment.

Inflammatory bowel disease (IBD) is of complex etiology and there is some debate as to whether it truly represents an autoimmune disease. A likely mechanism for disease is an altered response to the gut microbiome triggering chronic inflammation and involving both the innate and adaptive immune system. Altered T cell function has been implicated in disease pathogenesis. Kidney disease is common in patients with IBD and is present in up to 25% in some case series. TIN in IBD may occur largely due to the use of 5-aminosalicylic acid (5-ASA), with all cases in one recent series demonstrating histological evidence of gTIN and prior exposure to this agent. However there are several reported cases of TIN in patients not receiving 5-ASA, including in those who were treatment naïve and where kidney and bowel disease presented concurrently. In these cases, biopsy showed a predominantly lymphocytic infiltrate, often with granuloma formation. Some studies have suggesting cross-reacting T cell responses with a tubulointerstitial antigen may be mediating disease. Patients are usually treated with corticosteroids, often with an additional agent. Response to treatment is often limited, with several reported cases describing progression to kidney failure.

Idiopathic hypocomplementemic interstitial nephritis is a rare autoimmune cause of isolated TIN. There is thought to be some overlap with IgG4-related disease, particularly in historically described cases, although there are case descriptions which do not fulfil the criteria for IgG4RD. There are limited cases described in the literature, but patients are more likely to be male and in middle to older age groups. Kidney biopsy demonstrates tubular basement membrane IgG, and often C3, deposition with lymphocytic interstitial infiltrates. Treatment is usually with corticosteroids and patients often have significant kidney impairment which progresses despite treatment.

8 Conclusions

Tubulointerstitial nephritis can be found in a diverse range of systemic autoimmune diseases and there may be common immunopathological mechanisms which underlie its development. In patients with autoimmune disease there should be a high index of suspicion for TIN as early disease may be asymptomatic and kidney biopsy is needed to confirm the diagnosis. Most cases are treated with corticosteroids, sometimes with steroid sparing agents. Response to treatment is variable and differs between underlying conditions.

Acknowledgements We are grateful to Prof H. T. Cook for providing the histopathology specimens. MP is supported by a NIHR Clinical Lectureship. We acknowledge support from the NIHR Imperial Biomedical Research Centre.

Suggested Reading

Aasarød K, Haga HJ, Berg KJ, Hammerstrøm J, Jørstad S. Renal involvement in primary Sjögren's syndrome. QJM. 2000;93(5):297–304.

Abed L, Merouani A, Haddad E, Benoit G, Oligny LL, Sartelet H. Presence of autoantibodies against tubular and uveal cells in a patient with tubulointerstitial nephritis and uveitis (TINU) syndrome. Nephrol Dial Transplant. 2008;23(4):1452–5.

Aguilar MC, Lonngi M, de-la-Torre A. Tubulointerstitial nephritis and uveitis syndrome: case report and review of the literature. Ocul Immunol Inflamm. 2016;24(4):415–21.

Ambruzs JM, Walker PD, Larsen CP. The histopathologic spectrum of kidney biopsies in patients with inflammatory bowel disease. Clin J Am Soc Nephrol. 2014;9(2):265–70.

Anders H-J, Saxena R, Zhao M-H, Parodis I, Salmon JE, Mohan C. Lupus nephritis. Nat Rev Dis Primers. 2020;6(1):7.

Aouizerate J, Matignon M, Kamar N, Thervet E, Randoux C, Moulin B, et al. Renal transplantation in patients with sarcoidosis: a French multicenter study. Clin J Am Soc Nephrol. 2010;5(11):2101–8.

Bagnasco SM, Gottipati S, Kraus E, Alachkar N, Montgomery RA, Racusen LC, et al. Sarcoidosis in native and transplanted kidneys: incidence, pathologic findings, and clinical course. PLoS One. 2014;9(10):e110778.

Banerjee A, McKane W, Thiru S, Farrington K. Wegener's granulomatosis presenting as acute suppurative interstitial nephritis. J Clin Pathol. 2001;54(10):787–9.

Baughman RP, Teirstein AS, Judson MA, Rossman MD, Yeager H Jr, Bresnitz EA, et al. Clinical characteristics of patients in a case control study of sarcoidosis. Am J Respir Crit Care Med. 2001;164(10 Pt 1):1885–9.

Båve U, Nordmark G, Lövgren T, Rönnelid J, Cajander S, Eloranta ML, et al. Activation of the type I interferon system in primary Sjögren's syndrome: a possible etiopathogenic mechanism. Arthritis Rheum. 2005;52(4):1185–95.

Berden AE, Ferrario F, Hagen EC, Jayne DR, Jennette JC, Joh K, et al. Histopathologic classification of ANCA-associated glomerulonephritis. J Am Soc Nephrol. 2010;21(10):1628.

Berden AE, Jones RB, Erasmus DD, Walsh M, Noël LH, Ferrario F, et al. Tubular lesions predict renal outcome in antineutrophil cytoplasmic antibody-associated glomerulonephritis after rituximab therapy. J Am Soc Nephrol. 2012;23(2):313–21.

Berger KW, Relman AS. Renal impairment due to sarcoid infiltration of the kidney. N Engl J Med. 1955;252(2):44–9.

Bergner R, Hoffmann M, Waldherr R, Uppenkamp M. Frequency of kidney disease in chronic sarcoidosis. Sarcoidosis Vasc Diffuse Lung Dis. 2003;20(2):126–32.

Berliner AR, Haas M, Choi MJ. Sarcoidosis: the nephrologist's perspective. Am J Kidney Dis. 2006;48(5):856–70.

Boucher A, Droz D, Adafer E, Noël LH. Characterization of mononuclear cell subsets in renal cellular interstitial infiltrates. Kidney Int. 1986;29(5):1043–9.

Brito-Zerón P, Kostov B, Solans R, Fraile G, Suárez-Cuervo C, Casanovas A, et al. Systemic activity and mortality in primary Sjögren syndrome: predicting survival using the EULAR-SS Disease Activity Index (ESSDAI) in 1045 patients. Ann Rheum Dis. 2016;75(2):348–55.

Burke WM, Keogh A, Maloney PJ, Delprado W, Bryant DH, Spratt P. Transmission of sarcoidosis via cardiac transplantation. Lancet (London, England). 1990;336(8730):1579.

Chang A, Henderson SG, Brandt D, Liu N, Guttikonda R, Hsieh C, et al. In situ B cell-mediated immune responses and tubulointerstitial inflammation in human lupus nephritis. J Immunol (Baltimore, Md: 1950). 2011;186(3):1849–60.

Cigni A, Soro G, Faedda R, Caucci F, Amadori F, Manca A, et al. A case of adult-onset tubulointerstitial nephritis and uveitis ("TINU syndrome") associated with sacroileitis and epstein-barr virus infection with good spontaneous outcome. Am J Kidney Dis. 2003;42(3):e11.1–e.7.

Clive DM, Vanguri VK. The syndrome of tubulointerstitial nephritis with uveitis (TINU). Am J Kidney Dis. 2018;72(1):118–28.

Conz PA, Milan M, Bragantini L, La Greca G, Bevilacqua PA. TINU syndrome associated with reduced complement levels. Nephron. 2001;89(3):340–1.

Croia C, Astorri E, Murray-Brown W, Willis A, Brokstad KA, Sutcliffe N, et al. Implication of Epstein-Barr virus infection in disease-specific autoreactive B cell activation in ectopic lymphoid structures of Sjögren's syndrome. Arthritis Rheumatol (Hoboken, NJ). 2014;66(9):2545–57.

de Souza HSP, Fiocchi C. Immunopathogenesis of IBD: current state of the art. Nat Rev Gastroenterol Hepatol. 2016;13(1):13–27.

Deguchi HE, Amemiya T. Two cases of uveitis with tubulointerstitial nephritis in HTLV-1 carriers. Jpn J Ophthalmol. 2003;47(4):372–8.

Dempsey OJ, Paterson EW, Kerr KM, Denison AR. Sarcoidosis. BMJ. 2009;339:b3206.

Dobrin RS, Vernier RL, Fish AL. Acute eosinophilic interstitial nephritis and renal failure with bone marrow-lymph node granulomas and anterior uveitis. A new syndrome. Am J Med. 1975;59(3):325–33.

Du L, Kijlstra A, Yang P. Immune response genes in uveitis. Ocul Immunol Inflamm. 2009;17(4):249–56.

Dubrey S, Shah S, Hardman T, Sharma R. Sarcoidosis: the links between epidemiology and aetiology. Postgrad Med J. 2014;90(1068):582–9.

Dugas M, Wallaert B, Tonnel AB, Voisin C. From subclinical alveolitis to granulomatosis. Sequential evaluation of pulmonary involvement in extrathoracic sarcoidosis. Chest. 1989;96(4):931–3.

Durel CA, Sinico RA, Teixeira V, Jayne D, Belenfant X, Marchand-Adam S, et al. Renal involvement in eosinophilic granulomatosis with polyangiitis (EGPA): a multicentric retrospective study of 63 biopsy-proven cases. Rheumatology (Oxford). 2021;60(1):359–65.

Emamian ES, Leon JM, Lessard CJ, Grandits M, Baechler EC, Gaffney PM, et al. Peripheral blood gene expression profiling in Sjögren's syndrome. Genes Immun. 2009;10(4):285–96.

Evans R, Zdebik A, Ciurtin C, Walsh SB. Renal involvement in primary Sjögren's syndrome. Rheumatology. 2015;54(9):1541–8.

Evans RDR, Laing CM, Ciurtin C, Walsh SB. Tubulointerstitial nephritis in primary Sjögren syndrome: clinical manifestations and response to treatment. BMC Musculoskelet Disord. 2016;17:2.

Facco M, Cabrelle A, Teramo A, Olivieri V, Gnoato M, Teolato S, et al. Sarcoidosis is a Th1/Th17 multisystem disorder. Thorax. 2011;66(2):144–50.

Falk RJ, Terrell RS, Charles LA, Jennette JC. Anti-neutrophil cytoplasmic autoantibodies induce neutrophils to degranulate and produce oxygen radicals in vitro. Proc Natl Acad Sci U S A. 1990;87(11):4115–9.

Fujimoto S, Watts RA, Kobayashi S, Suzuki K, Jayne DR, Scott DG, et al. Comparison of the epidemiology of anti-neutrophil cytoplasmic antibody-associated vasculitis between Japan and the U.K. Rheumatology (Oxford). 2011;50(10):1916–20.

Geetha D, Jin Q, Scott J, Hruskova Z, Hanouneh M, Little MA, et al. Comparisons of guidelines and recommendations on managing antineutrophil cytoplasmic antibody–associated vasculitis. Kidney Int Rep. 2018;3(5):1039–49.

Gorroño-Echebarría MB, Calvo-Arrabal MA, Albarrán F, Alvarez-Mon M. The tubulointerstitial nephritis and uveitis (TINU) syndrome is associated with HLA-DR14 in Spanish patients. Br J Ophthalmol. 2001;85(8):1010–1.

Gottenberg JE, Cagnard N, Lucchesi C, Letourneur F, Mistou S, Lazure T, et al. Activation of IFN pathways and plasmacytoid dendritic cell recruitment in target organs of primary Sjögren's syndrome. Proc Natl Acad Sci U S A. 2006;103(8):2770–5.

Goules AV, Tatouli IP, Moutsopoulos HM, Tzioufas AG. Clinically significant renal involvement in primary Sjögren's syndrome: clinical presentation and outcome. Arthritis Rheum. 2013;65(11):2945–53.

Gulamhusein AF, Hirschfield GM. Primary biliary cholangitis: pathogenesis and therapeutic opportunities. Nat Rev Gastroenterol Hepatol. 2020;17(2):93–110.

Guo W, Woo KT, Choo JCJ, Tan PH, Lim CC. Granulomatosis with polyangiitis and acute tubulointerstitial nephritis in the absence of glomerulonephritis. Am J Med. 2020;133(11):e679–e80.

Gupta A, Jothy S, Somerville P, Zaltzman JS. Hypocomplementaemic immune complex tubulointerstitial nephritis. NDT Plus. 2009;3(1):78–80.

Gur H, Kopolovic Y, Gross DJ. Chronic predominant interstitial nephritis in a patient with systemic lupus erythematosus: a follow up of three years and review of the literature. Ann Rheum Dis. 1987;46(8):617–23.

Hanly JG, O'Keeffe AG, Su L, Urowitz MB, Romero-Diaz J, Gordon C, et al. The frequency and outcome of lupus nephritis: results from an international inception cohort study. Rheumatology (Oxford). 2016;55(2):252–62.

Hannedouche T, Grateau G, Noël LH, Godin M, Fillastre JP, Grünfeld JP, et al. Renal granulomatous sarcoidosis: report of six cases. Nephrol Dial Transplant. 1990;5(1):18–24.

Hilderson I, Van Laecke S, Wauters A, Donck J. Treatment of renal sarcoidosis: is there a guideline? Overview of the different treatment options. Nephrol Dial Transplant. 2013;29(10):1841–7.

Hills SE, Parkes SA, Baker SB. Epidemiology of sarcoidosis in the Isle of ManDOUBLEHYPHEN2: evidence for space-time clustering. Thorax. 1987;42(6):427–30.

Howarth L, Gilbert RD, Bass P, Deshpande PV. Tubulointerstitial nephritis and uveitis in monozygotic twin boys. Pediatr Nephrol (Berlin, Germany). 2004;19(8):917–9.

Hsieh C, Chang A, Brandt D, Guttikonda R, Utset TO, Clark MR. Predicting outcomes of lupus nephritis with tubulointerstitial inflammation and scarring. Arthritis Care Res. 2011;63(6):865–74.

Ishige I, Usui Y, Takemura T, Eishi Y. Quantitative PCR of mycobacterial and propionibacterial DNA in lymph nodes of Japanese patients with sarcoidosis. Lancet (London, England). 1999;354(9173):120–3.

Izzedine H, Simon J, Piette AM, Lucsko M, Baumelou A, Charitanski D, et al. Primary chronic interstitial nephritis in Crohn's disease. Gastroenterology. 2002;123(5):1436–40.

Jonsson R, Theander E, Sjöström B, Brokstad K, Henriksson G. Autoantibodies present before symptom onset in primary Sjögren syndrome. JAMA. 2013;310(17):1854–5.

Joss N, Morris S, Young B, Geddes C. Granulomatous interstitial nephritis. Clin J Am Soc Nephrol. 2007;2(2):222–30.

Kain R, Exner M, Brandes R, Ziebermayr R, Cunningham D, Alderson CA, et al. Molecular mimicry in pauci-immune focal necrotizing glomerulonephritis. Nat Med. 2008;14(10):1088–96.

Kamouchi M, Tsuji H, Hirakata H, Okamura K, Ishitsuka T, Murai K, et al. Tubulointerstitial disorders in the kidney associated with primary biliary cirrhosis (PBC). Clin Nephrol. 1991;35(3):134–5.

Kase S, Kitaichi N, Namba K, Miyazaki A, Yoshida K, Ishikura K, et al. Elevation of serum Krebs von den Lunge-6 levels in patients with tubulointerstitial nephritis and uveitis syndrome. Am J Kidney Dis. 2006;48(6):935–41.

Kessenbrock K, Krumbholz M, Schonermarck U, Back W, Gross WL, Werb Z, et al. Netting neutrophils in autoimmune small-vessel vasculitis. Nat Med. 2009;15(6):623–5.

Kidder D, Rutherford E, Kipgen D, Fleming S, Geddes C, Stewart GA. Kidney biopsy findings in primary Sjögren syndrome. Nephrol Dial Transplant. 2015a;30(8):1363–9.

Kidder D, Stewart GA, Furrie E, Fleming S. The case. Idiopathic hypocomplementemic interstitial nephritis. Diagnosis: idiopathic hypocomplementemic tubulointerstitial nephritis. Kidney Int. 2015b;87(2):485–6.

Kinloch AJ, Cascino MD, Dai J, Bermea RS, Ko K, Vesselits M, et al. Anti-vimentin antibodies: a unique antibody class associated with therapy-resistant lupus nephritis. Lupus. 2020;29(6):569–77.

Kinloch AJ, Chang A, Ko K, Henry Dunand CJ, Henderson S, Maienschein-Cline M, et al. Vimentin is a dominant target of in situ humoral immunity in human lupus tubulointerstitial nephritis. Arthritis Rheumatol (Hoboken, NJ). 2014;66(12):3359–70.

Kitching AR, Anders H-J, Basu N, Brouwer E, Gordon J, Jayne DR, et al. ANCA-associated vasculitis. Nat Rev Dis Primers. 2020;6(1):71.

Knights D, Lassen KG, Xavier RJ. Advances in inflammatory bowel disease pathogenesis: linking host genetics and the microbiome. Gut. 2013;62(10):1505–10.

Kodama T, Imai H, Wakui H, Ohtani H, Komatsuda A, Miura AB. Tubulointerstitial nephritis with renal tubular acidosis and asymptomatic primary biliary cirrhosis accompanied by antibody to a 52-kDa mitochondrial protein alone. Clin Nephrol. 1996;45(6):401–5.

Kolopp-Sarda MN, Miossec P. Contribution of hepatitis C infection to a large cohort of cryoglobulin-positive patients: detection and characteristics. Front Immunol. 2020;11:1183.

Komatsuda A, Wakui H, Ohtani H, Masai R, Okuyama S, Nimura T, et al. Tubulointerstitial nephritis and renal tubular acidosis of different types are rare but important complications of primary biliary cirrhosis. Nephrol Dial Transplant. 2010;25(11):3575–9.

Lee JW, Kim HJ, Sung SH, Lee SJ. A case of tubulointerstitial nephritis and uveitis syndrome with severe immunologic dysregulation. Pediatr Nephrol (Berlin, Germany). 2005;20(12):1805–8.

Lessard CJ, Li H, Adrianto I, Ice JA, Rasmussen A, Grundahl KM, et al. Variants at multiple loci implicated in both innate and adaptive immune responses are associated with Sjögren's syndrome. Nat Genet. 2013;45(11):1284–92.

Levinson RD, Park MS, Rikkers SM, Reed EF, Smith JR, Martin TM, et al. Strong associations between specific HLA-DQ and HLA-DR alleles and the tubulointerstitial nephritis and uveitis syndrome. Invest Ophthalmol Vis Sci. 2003;44(2):653–7.

Li C, Su T, Chu R, Li X, Yang L. Tubulointerstitial nephritis with uveitis in Chinese adults. Clin J Am Soc Nephrol. 2014;9(1):21–8.

Liarski VM, Kaverina N, Chang A, Brandt D, Yanez D, Talasnik L, et al. Cell distance mapping identifies functional T follicular helper cells in inflamed human renal tissue. Sci Transl Med. 2014;6(230):230ra46.

Lin CY, Wu CH, Chen HA, Hsu CY, Wang LH, Su YJ. Long-term renal prognosis among patients with primary Sjögren's syndrome and renal involvement: a nationwide matched cohort study. J Autoimmun. 2020;113:102483.

Lin ZS, Liu XL, Cui Z, Wang SX, Yu F, Zhou FD, et al. Acute tubulointerstitial nephritis with germinal centers in antineutrophil cytoplasmic antibody-associated vasculitis: a case report and literature review. Medicine. 2019;98(48):e18178.

Lino M, Binaut R, Noël L-H, Patey N, Rustin P, Daniel L, et al. Tubulointerstitial nephritis and Fanconi syndrome in primary biliary cirrhosis. Am J Kidney Dis. 2005;46(3):e41–e6.

Liu F, Knight GB, Agnello V. Hepatitis C virus but not GB virus C/hepatitis G virus has a role in type II cryoglobulinemia. Arthritis Rheum. 1999;42(9):1898–901.

Londoño Jimenez A, Mowrey WB, Putterman C, Buyon J, Goilav B, Broder A. Brief report: tubulointerstitial damage in lupus nephritis: a comparison of the factors associated with tubulointerstitial inflammation and renal scarring. Arthritis Rheumatol (Hoboken, NJ). 2018;70(11):1801–6.

Longcope WT, Freiman DG. A study of sarcoidosis; based on a combined investigation of 160 cases including 30 autopsies from The Johns Hopkins Hospital and Massachusetts General Hospital. Medicine. 1952;31(1):1–132.

Lyons PA, Rayner TF, Trivedi S, Holle JU, Watts RA, Jayne DR, et al. Genetically distinct subsets within ANCA-associated vasculitis. N Engl J Med. 2012;367(3):214–23.

Mahévas M, Lescure FX, Boffa JJ, Delastour V, Belenfant X, Chapelon C, et al. Renal sarcoidosis: clinical, laboratory, and histologic presentation and outcome in 47 patients. Medicine. 2009;88(2):98–106.

Maldini C, Seror R, Fain O, Dhote R, Amoura Z, De Bandt M, et al. Epidemiology of primary Sjögren's syndrome in a French multiracial/multiethnic area. Arthritis Care Res. 2014;66(3):454–63.

Mandeville JTH, Levinson RD, Holland GN. The tubulointerstitial nephritis and uveitis syndrome. Surv Ophthalmol. 2001;46(3):195–208.

Mangat P, Jawad AS, Brownlee W. Tubulointerstitial nephritis uveitis syndrome associated with erosive arthropathy of the hip. Rheumatology (Oxford). 2008;47(6):933–6.

Manjón MT, Sánchez-Bursón J, Montero R, Pérez-Requena J, Alonso M, Marenco JL. Two cases of acute tubulointerstitial nephritis associated with panuveitis (TINU syndrome). J Rheumatol. 1999;26(1):234–6.

Maripuri S, Grande JP, Osborn TG, Fervenza FC, Matteson EL, Donadio JV, et al. Renal involvement in primary Sjögren's syndrome: a clinicopathologic study. Clin J Am Soc Nephrol. 2009;4(9):1423–31.

Mayer C, Müller A, Halbritter J, Wirtz H, Stumvoll M. Isolated renal relapse of sarcoidosis under low-dose glucocorticoid therapy. J Gen Intern Med. 2008;23(6):879–82.

Merkel PA, Xie G, Monach PA, Ji X, Ciavatta DJ, Byun J, et al. Identification of functional and expression polymorphisms associated with risk for antineutrophil cytoplasmic autoantibody-associated vasculitis. Arthritis Rheumatol (Hoboken, NJ). 2017;69(5):1054–66.

Milman N, Andersen CB, Burton CM, Iversen M. Recurrent sarcoid granulomas in a transplanted lung derive from recipient immune cells. Eur Respir J. 2005;26(3):549–52.

Mitchell IC, Turk JL, Mitchell DN. Detection of mycobacterial rRNA in sarcoidosis with liquid-phase hybridisation. Lancet (London, England). 1992;339(8800):1015–7.

Mizoguchi S, Katayama K, Murata T, Ishikawa E, Kozuka Y, Honda Y, et al. IgM-positive tubulointerstitial nephritis associated with asymptomatic primary biliary cirrhosis. Kidney Int Rep. 2018;3(4):1004–9.

Musaelyan A, Lapin S, Nazarov V, Tkachenko O, Gilburd B, Mazing A, et al. Vimentin as antigenic target in autoimmunity: a comprehensive review. Autoimmun Rev. 2018;17(9):926–34.

Nakabayashi K, Sumiishi A, Sano K, Fujioka Y, Yamada A, Karube M, et al. Tubulointerstitial nephritis without glomerular lesions in three patients with myeloperoxidase-ANCA-associated vasculitis. Clin Exp Nephrol. 2009;13(6):605–13.

Newman LS, Rose CS, Bresnitz EA, Rossman MD, Barnard J, Frederick M, et al. A case control etiologic study of sarcoidosis: environmental and occupational risk factors. Am J Respir Crit Care Med. 2004;170(12):1324–30.

Newman LS, Rose CS, Maier LA. Sarcoidosis. N Engl J Med. 1997;336(17):1224–34.

Nocturne G, Mariette X. Advances in understanding the pathogenesis of primary Sjögren's syndrome. Nat Rev Rheumatol. 2013;9(9):544–56.

Nussbaum EZ, Perazella MA. Diagnosing acute interstitial nephritis: considerations for clinicians. Clin Kidney J. 2019;12(6):808–13.

O'Dell JR, Hays RC, Guggenheim SJ, Steigerwald JC. Tubulointerstitial renal disease in systemic lupus erythematosus. Arch Intern Med. 1985;145(11):1996–9.

Oliveira B, Jayawardene S, Shah S. Single-centre experience of granulomatous interstitial nephritis-time for a new approach? Clin Kidney J. 2017;10(2):249–54.

Pagni F, Galimberti S, Galbiati E, Rebora P, Pietropaolo V, Pieruzzi F, et al. Tubulointerstitial lesions in lupus nephritis: international multicentre study in a large cohort of patients with repeat biopsy. Nephrology (Carlton). 2016;21(1):35–45.

Pang Y, Tan Y, Li Y, Zhang J, Guo Y, Guo Z, et al. Pentraxin 3 is closely associated with tubulointerstitial injury in lupus nephritis: a large multicenter cross-sectional study. Medicine. 2016;95(3):e2520.

Pardi DS, Tremaine WJ, Sandborn WJ, McCarthy JT. Renal and urologic complications of inflammatory bowel disease. Am J Gastroenterol. 1998;93(4):504–14.

Peräsaari J, Saarela V, Nikkilä J, Ala-Houhala M, Arikoski P, Kataja J, et al. HLA associations with tubulointerstitial nephritis with or without uveitis in Finnish pediatric population: a nation-wide study. Tissue Antigens. 2013;81(6):435–41.

Plafkin C, Zhong W, Singh T. ANCA vasculitis presenting with acute interstitial nephritis without glomerular involvement. Clin Nephrol Case Stud. 2019;7:46–50.

Polci R, Mangeri M, Faggiani R, Cristi E, Ranalli TV, Feriozzi S. Granulomatous interstitial nephritis in a patient with Crohn's disease. Ren Fail. 2012;34(9):1156–9.

Prendecki M, Tanna A, Salama AD, Tam FW, Cairns T, Taube D, et al. Long-term outcome in biopsy-proven acute interstitial nephritis treated with steroids. Clin Kidney J. 2017;10(2):233–9.

Prezant DJ, Dhala A, Goldstein A, Janus D, Ortiz F, Aldrich TK, et al. The incidence, prevalence, and severity of sarcoidosis in New York City firefighters. Chest. 1999;116(5):1183–93.

Radford DJ, Luu NT, Hewins P, Nash GB, Savage CO. Antineutrophil cytoplasmic antibodies stabilize adhesion and promote migration of flowing neutrophils on endothelial cells. Arthritis Rheum. 2001;44(12):2851–61.

Rajakariar R, Sharples EJ, Raftery MJ, Sheaff M, Yaqoob MM. Sarcoid tubulo-interstitial nephritis: long-term outcome and response to corticosteroid therapy. Kidney Int. 2006;70(1):165–9.

Ramos-Casals M, Brito-Zerón P, Seror R, Bootsma H, Bowman SJ, Dörner T, et al. Characterization of systemic disease in primary Sjögren's syndrome: EULAR-SS Task Force recommendations for articular, cutaneous, pulmonary and renal involvements. Rheumatology. 2015;54(12):2230–8.

Regusci A, Lava SAG, Milani GP, Bianchetti MG, Simonetti GD, Vanoni F. Tubulointerstitial nephritis and uveitis syndrome: a systematic review. Nephrol Dial Transplant. 2021;9:gfab030. https://doi.org/10.1093/ndt/gfab030. Epub ahead of print.

Ren H, Wang WM, Chen XN, Zhang W, Pan XX, Wang XL, et al. Renal involvement and followup of 130 patients with primary Sjögren's syndrome. J Rheumatol. 2008;35(2):278–84.

Robson MG, Banerjee D, Hopster D, Cairns HS. Seven cases of granulomatous interstitial nephritis in the absence of extrarenal sarcoid. Nephrol Dial Transplant. 2003;18(2):280–4.

Roth AJ, Brown MC, Smith RN, Badhwar AK, Parente O, Chung H, et al. Anti-LAMP-2 antibodies are not prevalent in patients with antineutrophil cytoplasmic autoantibody glomerulonephritis. J Am Soc Nephrol. 2012;23(3):545–55.

Saha MK, Tarek H, Sagar V, Abraham P. Role of tumor necrosis factor inhibitor in granulomatous interstitial nephritis secondary to Crohn's disease. Int Urol Nephrol. 2014;46(1):229–33.

Saito I, Servenius B, Compton T, Fox RI. Detection of Epstein-Barr virus DNA by polymerase chain reaction in blood and tissue biopsies from patients with Sjogren's syndrome. J Exp Med. 1989;169(6):2191–8.

Sakai N, Wada T, Shimizu M, Segawa C, Furuichi K, Kobayashi K-I, et al. Tubulointerstitial nephritis with anti-neutrophil cytoplasmic antibody following indomethacin treatment. Nephrol Dial Transplant. 1999;14(11):2774.

Sakthivel P, Bruder D. Mechanism of granuloma formation in sarcoidosis. Curr Opin Hematol. 2017;24(1):59–65.

Sangaletti S, Tripodo C, Chiodoni C, Guarnotta C, Cappetti B, Casalini P, et al. Neutrophil extracellular traps mediate transfer of cytoplasmic neutrophil antigens to myeloid dendritic cells toward ANCA induction and associated autoimmunity. Blood. 2012;120(15):3007–18.

Santoro D, Vita G, Rovito S, Venuto L, Cavallari V, Vita R, et al. Drug-induced TINU syndrome and genetic characterization. Clin Nephrol. 2012;78(3):230–6.

Satoskar AA, Brodsky SV, Nadasdy G, Bott C, Rovin B, Hebert L, et al. Discrepancies in glomerular and tubulointerstitial/vascular immune complex IgG subclasses in lupus nephritis. Lupus. 2011;20(13):1396–403.

Shah S, Carter-Monroe N, Atta MG. Granulomatous interstitial nephritis. Clin Kidney J. 2015;8(5):516–23.

Shimazaki K, Jirawuthiworavong GV, Nguyen EV, Awazu M, Levinson RD, Gordon LK. Tubulointerstitial nephritis and uveitis syndrome: a case with an autoimmune reactivity against retinal and renal antigens. Ocul Immunol Inflamm. 2008;16(1):51–3.

Shiozawa S, Shiozawa K, Shimizu S, Nakada M, Isobe T, Fujita T. Clinical studies of renal disease in Sjögren's syndrome. Ann Rheum Dis. 1987;46(10):768–72.

Simon AH, Alves-Filho G, Ribeiro-Alves MA. Acute tubulointerstitial nephritis and uveitis with antineutrophil cytoplasmic antibody. Am J Kidney Dis. 1996;28(1):124–7.

Singer DR, Evans DJ. Renal impairment in sarcoidosis: granulomatous nephritis as an isolated cause (two case reports and review of the literature). Clin Nephrol. 1986;26(5):250–6.

Singh AK, Ucci A, Madias NE. Predominant tubulointerstitial lupus nephritis. Am J Kidney Dis. 1996;27(2):273–8.

Steinmetz OM, Velden J, Kneissler U, Marx M, Klein A, Helmchen U, et al. Analysis and classification of B-cell infiltrates in lupus and ANCA-associated nephritis. Kidney Int. 2008;74(4):448–57.

Taheri S, Taheri D. Short course of cyclophosphamide therapy may reduce recurrence in patients with tubulointerstitial nephritis and uveitis syndrome. Saudi J Kidney Dis Transpl. 2009;20(4):655–7.

Takahashi N, Kimura H, Kawajiri Y, Mikami D, Yamamoto C, Kasuno K, et al. Tubulointerstitial nephritis with IgM-positive plasmacytoid large lymphocyte infiltration in a patient with primary biliary cirrhosis and Sjögren's syndrome. Clin Nephrol. 2010;74(1):74–80.

Tan Y, Yu F, Qu Z, Su T, Xing GQ, Wu LH, et al. Modified C-reactive protein might be a target autoantigen of TINU syndrome. Clin J Am Soc Nephrol. 2011;6(1):93–100.

Tan Y, Yu F, Yang H, Chen M, Fang Q, Zhao MH. Autoantibodies against monomeric C-reactive protein in sera from patients with lupus nephritis are associated with disease activity and renal tubulointerstitial lesions. Hum Immunol. 2008;69(12):840–4.

Taylor RG, Fisher C, Hoffbrand BI. Sarcoidosis and membranous glomerulonephritis: a significant association. Br Med J (Clin Res Ed). 1982;284(6325):1297–8.

Tengnér P, Halse AK, Haga HJ, Jonsson R, Wahren-Herlenius M. Detection of anti-Ro/SSA and anti-La/SSB autoantibody-producing cells in salivary glands from patients with Sjögren's syndrome. Arthritis Rheum. 1998;41(12):2238–48.

Terrier B, Carrat F, Krastinova E, Marie I, Launay D, Lacraz A, et al. Prognostic factors of survival in patients with non-infectious mixed cryoglobulinaemia vasculitis: data from 242 cases included in the CryoVas survey. Ann Rheum Dis. 2013;72(3):374–80.

Thumfart J, Müller D, Rudolph B, Zimmering M, Querfeld U, Haffner D. Isolated sarcoid granulomatous interstitial nephritis responding to infliximab therapy. Am J Kidney Dis. 2005;45(2):411–4.

Timmermans SAMEG, Christiaans MHL, Abdul-Hamid MA, Stifft F, Damoiseaux JGMC, van Paassen P. Granulomatous interstitial nephritis and Crohn's disease. Clin Kidney J. 2016;9(4):556–9.

Vanhaesebrouck P, Carton D, De Bel C, Praet M, Proesmans W. Acute tubulo-interstitial nephritis and uveitis syndrome (TINU syndrome). Nephron. 1985;40(4):418–22.
Vidal E, Rogues AM, Aldigier JC. The Tinu syndrome or the Sjögren syndrome? Ann Intern Med. 1992;116(1):93.
Vokurka M, Lecossier D, du Bois RM, Wallaert B, Kambouchner M, Tazi A, et al. Absence of DNA from mycobacteria of the M. tuberculosis complex in sarcoidosis. Am J Respir Crit Care Med. 1997;156(3 Pt 1):1000–3.
Wakaki H, Sakamoto H, Awazu M. Tubulointerstitial nephritis and uveitis syndrome with autoantibody directed to renal tubular cells. Pediatrics. 2001;107(6):1443–6.
Waters AM, Zachos M, Herzenberg AM, Harvey E, Rosenblum ND. Tubulointerstitial nephritis as an extraintestinal manifestation of Crohn's disease. Nat Clin Pract Nephrol. 2008;4(12):693–7.
Watts RA, Mahr A, Mohammad AJ, Gatenby P, Basu N, Flores-Suarez LF. Classification, epidemiology and clinical subgrouping of antineutrophil cytoplasmic antibody (ANCA)-associated vasculitis. Nephrol Dial Transplant. 2015;30(Suppl 1):i14–22.
Weening JJ, D'Agati VD, Schwartz MM, Seshan SV, Alpers CE, Appel GB, et al. The classification of glomerulonephritis in systemic lupus erythematosus revisited. J Am Soc Nephrol. 2004;15(2):241.
Weidner S, Carl M, Riess R, Rupprecht HD. Histologic analysis of renal leukocyte infiltration in antineutrophil cytoplasmic antibody-associated vasculitis: importance of monocyte and neutrophil infiltration in tissue damage. Arthritis Rheum. 2004;50(11):3651–7.
Wen YK, Chen ML. Transformation from tubulointerstitial nephritis to crescentic glomerulonephritis: an unusual presentation of ANCA-associated renal vasculitis. Ren Fail. 2006;28(2):189–91.
Werfel U, Schneider J, Rödelsperger K, Kotter J, Popp W, Woitowitz HJ, et al. Sarcoid granulomatosis after zirconium exposure with multiple organ involvement. Eur Respir J. 1998;12(3):750.
Wilson PC, Kashgarian M, Moeckel G. Interstitial inflammation and interstitial fibrosis and tubular atrophy predict renal survival in lupus nephritis. Clin Kidney J. 2018;11(2):207–18.
Winchester R, Wiesendanger M, Zhang HZ, Steshenko V, Peterson K, Geraldino-Pardilla L, et al. Immunologic characteristics of intrarenal T cells: trafficking of expanded CD8+ T cell β-chain clonotypes in progressive lupus nephritis. Arthritis Rheum. 2012;64(5):1589–600.
Winer RL, Cohen AH, Sawhney AS, Gorman JT. Sjögren's syndrome with immune-complex tubulointerstitial renal disease. Clin Immunol Immunopathol. 1977;8(3):494–503.
Xiao H, Schreiber A, Heeringa P, Falk RJ, Jennette JC. Alternative complement pathway in the pathogenesis of disease mediated by anti-neutrophil cytoplasmic autoantibodies. Am J Pathol. 2007;170(1):52–64.
Yao YH, Lin CC, Chung YM, Yang AH, Li SY, Lin CC, et al. Tubulointerstitial nephritis and uveitis syndrome (TINU) with Fanconi's syndrome. Clin Nephrol. 2011;75(Suppl 1):75–8.
Yılmaz H, Kaya M, Özbek M, ÜUreten K, Safa Yİ. Hypokalemic periodic paralysis in Sjogren's syndrome secondary to distal renal tubular acidosis. Rheumatol Int. 2013;33(7):1879–82.
Yu F, Haas M, Glassock R, Zhao M-H. Redefining lupus nephritis: clinical implications of pathophysiologic subtypes. Nat Rev Nephrol. 2017;13(8):483–95.
Yung S, Ng CY, Au KY, Cheung KF, Zhang Q, Zhang C, et al. Binding of anti-dsDNA antibodies to proximal tubular epithelial cells contributes to renal tubulointerstitial inflammation. Clin Sci (London, England: 1979). 2017;131(1):49–67.
Yung S, Tsang RC, Sun Y, Leung JK, Chan TM. Effect of human anti-DNA antibodies on proximal renal tubular epithelial cell cytokine expression: implications on tubulointerstitial inflammation in lupus nephritis. J Am Soc Nephrol. 2005;16(11):3281–94.
Zaidan M, Terrier B, Pozdzik A, Frouget T, Rioux-Leclercq N, Combe C, et al. Spectrum and prognosis of noninfectious renal mixed cryoglobulinemic GN. J Am Soc Nephrol. 2016;27(4):1213–24.
Zeier M, Schmidt R, Andrassy K, Waldherr R, Ritz E. Idiopathic interstitial nephritis complicating ulcerative colitis. Nephrol Dial Transplant. 1990;5(10):901.

IgG4-Related Tubulointerstitial Kidney Disease

Alessia Buglioni, Sanjeev Sethi, and Lynn D. Cornell

1 Overview of IgG4-Related Disease (IgG4-RD)

IgG4-related disease (IgG4-RD) is a systemic immune-mediated process that was first recognized as an IgG4-associated process in the pancreas (autoimmune pancreatitis). The inflammation can cause a variety of signs and symptoms also depending upon which organ system is involved. Most patients have a multi-organ disease process. Wallace et al. have recently described and proposed four disease phenotypes: those affected by (1) pancreato-hepato-biliary disease, (2) retroperitoneal fibrosis and/or aortitis, (3) head and neck-limited disease, and (4) classic Mikulicz syndrome (i.e., symmetric enlargement of the lacrimal and major salivary glands) with systemic involvement. Kidney involvement occurred most commonly (36%) as part of the Mikulicz syndrome phenotype, and least commonly (7%) in the head and neck-limited disease phenotype. The stereotypical patient is a middle-age to older man. Wallace et al. are also the authors of the most recent guidelines for the diagnosis of IgG4-RD: "The 2019 American College of Rheumatology/European League Against Rheumatism Classification Criteria for IgG4-Related Disease". In addition to inclusion criteria, this classification includes absolute clinical, serologic, radiologic, and pathologic exclusion criteria, with the goal of reducing misdiagnosis.

The histology of IgG4-RD encompasses the different organs possibly involved. There are three major histologic features recognized as characteristic of IgG4-RD, regardless of the location, and those are (1) a dense lymphoplasmacytic infiltrate, (2) a background of "storiform" fibrosis, and (3) obliterative phlebitis in organs where large veins are present within the parenchyma. In the right clinical context,

A. Buglioni (✉) · S. Sethi · L. D. Cornell
Division of Anatomic Pathology, Department of Laboratory Medicine and Pathology, Mayo Clinic, Rochester, MN, USA
e-mail: buglioni.alessia@mayo.edu; Sethi.Sanjeev@mayo.edu; Cornell.Lynn@mayo.edu

M. G. Atta, M. A. Perazella (eds.), *Tubulointerstitial Nephritis*,
https://doi.org/10.1007/978-3-030-93438-5_8

the presence of at least two of these three findings would support IgG4-RD. However, there is variability among solid organs and in some, such as lungs, and lacrimal and minor salivary glands, this typical histology may not be present.

The prevalence of IgG4-RD is still difficult to assess and is probably underestimated due to the challenge of recognizing it; however, awareness among health care providers and suspicion and identification of the condition are increasing, likely allowing a more realistic epidemiologic assessment in the future.

2 IgG4-Related Kidney Disease (IgG4-RKD)

The kidney is a frequently involved organ (IgG4-related kidney disease, IgG4-RKD), reported in approximately 25% of the cases, in a context of a systemic disease as well as a single-organ condition. The most common pattern of injury seen in IgG4-RKD is a plasma cell-rich tubulointerstitial nephritis (IgG4-TIN). The process can cause mass-like foci of inflammation and fibrosis. Normal kidney parenchyma may be present between the single foci. Primary glomerular involvement has been reported, particularly in the form of IgG4-related membranous glomerulonephritis. Although the main topic of this chapter will be IgG4-TIN, membranous glomerulonephritis will be briefly discussed. Occasionally, retroperitoneal fibrosis and/or aortitis at the level of the kidney/ureters can also be associated with obstructive uropathy with associated acute kidney injury (AKI).

3 Clinical Manifestations of IgG4-RKD

A variety of clinical signs and symptoms can characterize IgG4-RKD. Most commonly, kidney dysfunction is the initial manifestation; this may be acute or chronic. Patients may present with kidney mass lesion(s) with or without accompanying kidney dysfunction. Less commonly, proteinuria (due to membranous glomerulonephritis) prompts further clinical evaluation. Depending upon which kidney compartment is mostly affected, clinical findings may be different.

3.1 IgG4-Tubulointerstitial Nephritis

IgG4-RKD more often involves the tubulointerstitial compartment and patients can present with electrolyte imbalances and metabolic acidosis, which can all be part of the spectrum of signs and symptoms of IgG4-TIN. Hypocomplementemia can also be detected, and occurs more commonly with IgG4-TIN than when other organs are involved by IgG4-RD.

3.2 *IgG4-Related Membranous Glomerulonephritis*

When primary glomerular involvement is present (as the only finding or with concurrent IgG4-TIN), the most common pattern of injury is membranous glomerulonephritis, which in this disease is termed IgG4-related membranous glomerulonephritis (IgG4-MGN). Patients will likely present with increased serum creatinine and nephrotic range proteinuria with or without nephrotic syndrome. Importantly, PLA2R antibodies, positive in many cases of primary membranous glomerulonephritis, are generally not detected in IgG4-related MGN. In both conditions, a kidney biopsy is warranted to establish the diagnosis. Although often detected, increased serum IgG4 may not be present at the time of clinical presentation or kidney biopsy, and increased IgG4 is not specific for IgG4-related disease. Approximately 30% of patients with IgG4-RKD have a positive ANA, but this is usually low titer. ANCA (anti-MPO or anti-PR3) positivity is an exclusion criterion for IgG4-RD.

Kidney dysfunction may not be the initially observed abnormality bringing the patient to the clinician's attention. Occasionally, imaging studies performed for other reasons could reveal a mass-forming lesion in the kidney. In these instances, the suspicion of a malignancy leads to the kidney biopsy. Impaired kidney function may or not be present when kidney lesions/abnormalities due to IgG4-TIN are detected by imaging. For a more detailed description of possible radiological findings in the setting of IgG4-TIN, we refer the reader to the following section entitled "Radiologic findings in IgG4-TIN". Note that, the classical radiological features discussed here are due to the expansile nature of the abundant interstitial fibrosis characterizing IgG4-TIN; thus, if IgG4-RKD is limited to the glomerulus (i.e. IgG4-related MGN), imaging might not be contributory. Also, the ability to appreciate renal parenchyma lesions by imaging studies implies a more florid and extended interstitial process. The absence of radiologic abnormalities does not exclude a diagnosis of IgG4-TIN.

As already mentioned, many patients (approximately 80%) with kidney involvement will likely have additional organ(s) affected and possibly symptomatic. At the time of kidney biopsy, having up to 2–3 additional organs involved is very possible. Pancreas, liver/biliary tracts, and retroperitoneal region are common other sites affected.

4 Radiologic Findings in IgG4-TIN

More than half of patients with IgG4-RKD have kidney abnormalities on imaging studies. Of the cases that show radiographic abnormalities, contrast-enhanced computed tomography and magnetic resonance are about equal in detecting the characteristic features of IgG4-TIN. Recognized findings include multiple and bilateral low-density lesions, mostly localized superficially in the renal cortex. These lesions have been further classified according to four patterns: small nodules (<1 cm), well-defined or ill-defined round lesions (Fig. 1), well-defined wedge-shaped lesions (Fig. 2) or diffuse patchy distribution. Sometimes, one of the lesions dominates over the others causing a mass effect and distorting the renal contour. Besides direct kidney involvement, "pararenal" signs have also been observed, such as a rim of soft tissue surrounding the kidney, bilateral renal sinuses nodules and diffuse thickening of the renal pelvic wall.

5 The Spectrum of the Pathology of IgG4-RKD

Based upon the compartment/s affected, IgG4-RKD can have multiple different histological findings.

5.1 Tubulointerstitial and Vascular Involvement

IgG4-TIN is a plasma cell-rich TIN characterized by variable degrees of interstitial inflammation associated with an expansile fibrotic process. Figure 3(a–c) shows these peculiar features that can be appreciated on light microscopy. The inflammation is usually composed of mononuclear cells, some eosinophils and abundant polytypic plasma cells. The fibrosis, sometimes so-called "storiform" for its peculiar pattern of growth, pushes the atrophic tubules apart from each other and destroys some of them while expanding. The interstitial stromal cells are spindled cells that can form fascicles and on high-power may show mild nuclear atypia. For these reasons, it may be hard to distinguish IgG4-TIN from a heavily inflamed inflammatory

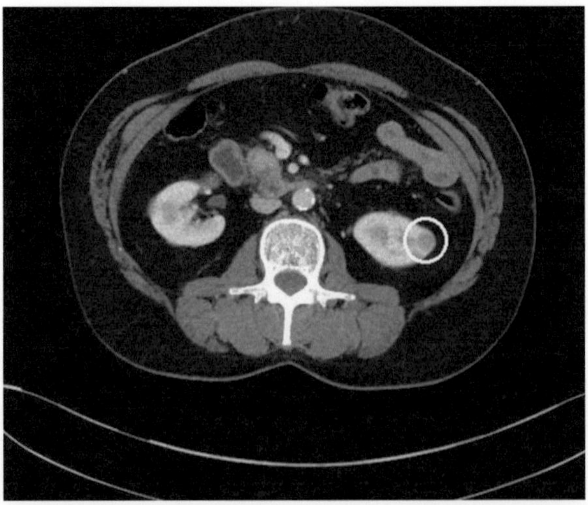

Fig. 1 This CT abdomen with contrast shows a round low density in the left kidney (within the circle). (Courtesy of Dr. Naoki Takahashi, Mayo Clinic)

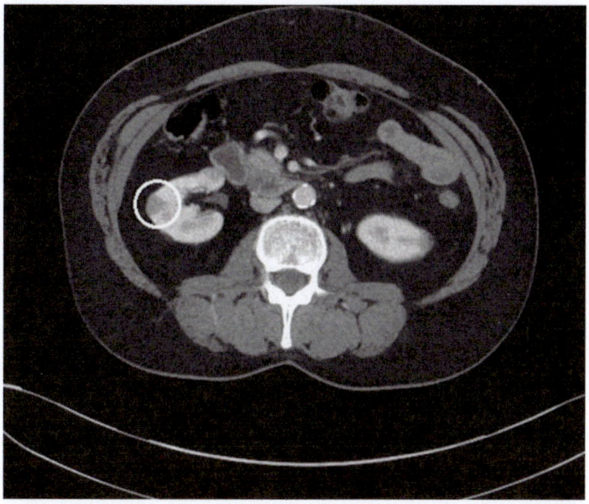

Fig. 2 This CT abdomen with contrast shows a wedge-shaped low density in the right kidney (within the circle). (Courtesy of Dr. Naoki Takahashi, Mayo Clinic)

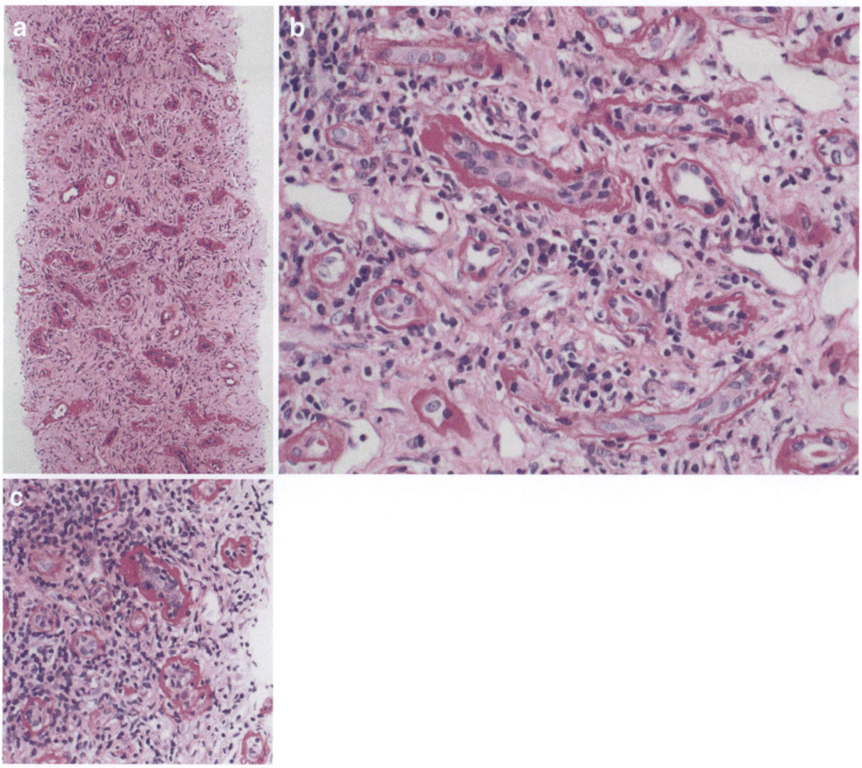

Fig. 3 Classic histological features of IgG4-TIN. Part **a** shows the expansile interstitial fibrosis admixed with inflammation and associated with atrophic tubules with thickened basement membrane. Appreciable is the spindly appearance of this interstitial process. Part **b** is a high-power view that highlights the plasma cell component of the interstitial inflammatory process. Part **c** shows foci of mononuclear cell tubulitis (all pictures are PAS stain)

myofibroblastic tumor (IMT), particularly in a needle core biopsy. IMTs will not have abundant IgG4-positive plasma cells within their inflammatory infiltrate and many will show positive cytoplasmic/membranous staining with anaplastic lymphoma kinase (ALK) immunostain (reflecting an ALK-1 rearrangement). This differential diagnosis is important to keep in mind, also to recall how exuberant the tumor-like growth pattern of the interstitial fibrosis can be in IgG4-TIN. Imaging might also be helpful in distinguishing between IgG4-TIN and IMT (multiple versus single lesion, respectively).

In addition to the variable degree of interstitial inflammation, lymphocytes and/or plasma cells have been observed infiltrating the tubular epithelium (lymphocytic and plasma cell tubulitis, respectively), in most cases.

Vascular involvement is present in IgG4-RD. Obliterative phlebitis has been described in kidney specimens that contain larger veins, although phlebitis is very uncommon in IgG4-TIN. The kidney is an exception in that, within the parenchyma, there are no large veins. However, a few arteries are usually sampled even within a needle core biopsy and arteritis may be identified. Indeed, Sharma et al. reported a case of IgG4-TIN with severe plasma cell-rich arteritis. As distinct from ANCA-associated vasculitis, fibrinoid necrosis/karyorrhectic debris of the arterial wall is not present in IgG4-plasma cell arteritis.

To support the diagnosis of IgG4-TIN, immunohistochemical studies with IgG and IgG4 stains are essential (Fig. 4a, b). The proposed diagnostic criteria from Raissian in 2011 include a moderate increase number of IgG4-positive plasma cells, greater than 10/high-power field, in the most concentrated field. This may translate into an increased IgG4/IgG plasma cell ratio (>40%); however, there is yet no established cut off for the IgG4/IgG ratio in the kidney as has been proposed in other organs. The final diagnosis should be based on the constellation of histological, radiological, laboratory, and clinical findings. Other inflammatory conditions that

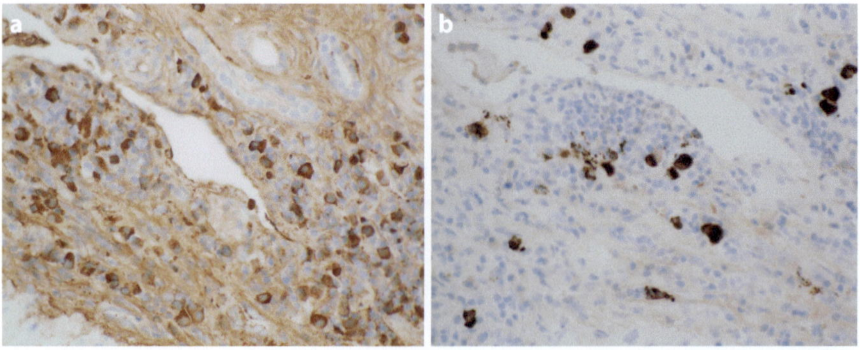

Fig. 4 IgG and IgG4 immunohistochemistry in a case of IgG4-TIN. Part **a** shows a high-power view of a field rich in IgG-positive plasma cells (approximately 70–80/HPF). The same field is represented in part **b** and stained with IgG4. The number of IgG4-positive plasma cells is greater than 10/HPF; the IgG4/IgG ratio is approximately 20%. This finding should be interpreted in conjunction with histological, radiological, clinical and/or laboratory data

can cause increased IgG4+ plasma cells– in particular ANCA associated interstitial inflammation – need to be excluded before making a diagnosis of IgG4-TIN.

On immunofluorescence, there are numerous immune complex deposits (manifest as granular staining) along the tubular basement membranes that stain for IgG, kappa and lambda, usually with lesser staining for C3 (Fig. 5). Trace/weak granular staining with C1q, IgM and IgA can also be occasionally appreciated. After performing IgG subclasses, the deposits show dominant staining with IgG4 with variable intensity of the remaining subclasses. Immune complex deposits may be seen in the interstitium and Bowman's capsule, but usually in IgG4-TIN the glomeruli have no deposits. Electron microscopy will confirm the presence of amorphous electron-dense immune deposits in the thickened tubular basement membranes and interstitium (Fig. 6).

The differential diagnosis of IgG4-TIN is broad and includes IMT, as previously discussed. There are other histological entities that can show increased IgG4-positive plasma cells in the interstitium. ANCA-associated granulomatosis with polyangiitis (GPA) can be mass-forming and can have an increased number of IgG4-positive plasma cells as well as dense interstitial fibrosis. However, different from IgG4-TIN, necrosis and karyorrhectic debris are often seen in GPA (in the interstitium and/or arterial walls) and there are no tubulointerstitial immune complex deposits. Multicentric Castleman disease is often seen in immunocompromised patients (HIV-positive) and it is associated with HHV-8 infection; it can have an increased number of IgG4-positive plasma cells but the expansile fibrosis and the tubulointerstitial immune deposits would not be present. The entity known as

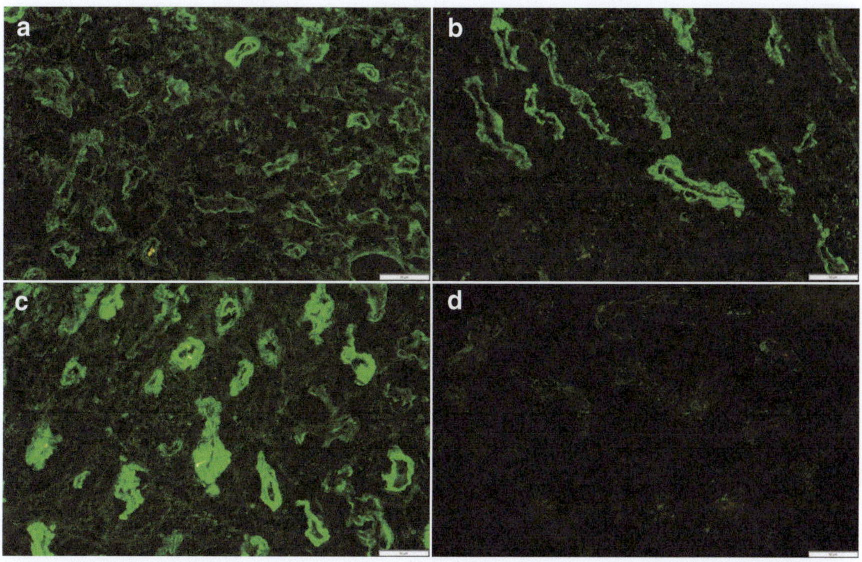

Fig. 5 Immunofluorescence findings in IgG4-TIN. Parts **a–d** illustrate granular immune deposits along the thickened tubular basement membranes. In the background, interstitial immune deposits can also be appreciated. (All pictures taken at 40×)

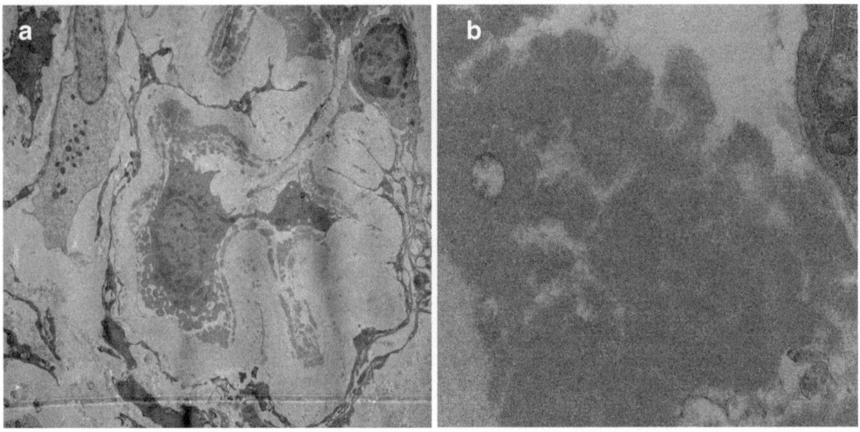

Fig. 6 Electron-dense amorphous tubular basement membrane deposits. Part **a** shows lower power view of the electron-dense deposits along the thickened tubular basement membrane. Part **b** is a high-power view that highlights no substructure

idiopathic hypocomplementemic interstitial nephritis, described before IgG4-TIN was recognized, likely represents IgG4-TIN. Other disease processes in the differential diagnosis of IgG4-TIN are: Sjogren syndrome-associated TIN, which does not usually show increased IgG4-positive plasma cells but will sometimes have tubular basement membrane immune deposits; lupus nephritis may present with tubular basement membrane immune deposits but is usually associated with glomerular (mesangial and/or capillary wall) deposits as well, and is not characterized by the expansile fibrosis; chronic pyelonephritis can present as a mass on imaging studies but histologically will likely show many neutrophils within the interstitial inflammatory infiltrate as well as possible neutrophilic casts; lymphoma could also present as a mass, however, monoclonality by immunohistochemistry and/or molecular testing will support such a diagnosis over IgG4-TIN. Although rare, syphilitic infection of the kidney could also be considered in the differential, as it may be associate with a plasma cell-rich mononuclear cell interstitial nephritis, interstitial fibrosis and membranous nephritis. However, there should be very few IgG4-positive interstitial plasma cells and no tubulointerstitial immune deposits. Other infectious processes, such as HIV, and drugs should also be in the differential of IgG4-interstitial nephritis.

5.2 Glomerular Involvement

The most common glomerular disease in IgG4-RD is IgG4-related MGN. On light microscopy, findings overlap with primary membranous nephropathy and are those of thickened glomerular basement membranes with subepithelial immune deposits seen with special stains (negative on silver, “pinholes”, and fuchsinophilic on trichrome). On immunofluorescence studies the subepithelial deposits stain for IgG, C3, kappa, and lambda, and can be IgG4-dominant, identical to primary (idiopathic) membranous nephropathy. IgG4-related MGN may or may not occur in conjunction with IgG4-TIN. The differential diagnosis includes primary or other forms of secondary MGN; clinical correlation becomes extremely important.

6 Treatment and Prognosis of IgG4-RKD

All symptomatic patients should undergo treatment. If not contraindicated, steroids (prednisone) alone are generally the first approach to induce remission. The vast majority of patients show a brisk response with improvement of symptoms, radiographic features, and laboratory findings. If a multi-drug approach is needed, immunosuppressants and/or biologic agents (i.e. azathioprine, mycophenolate mofetil, and rituximab) should be added. The duration of the treatment depends upon the clinical response, and remission is obtained when there are resolution of symptoms and improvement/normalization of the laboratory and radiologic alterations. Maintenance therapy could be adopted (with glucocorticoid or with a steroids-free protocol), as relapsing disease is a well-known complication after discontinuation of treatment. However, there is no consensus in this regard. If a patient is or becomes refractory to the therapeutic approach chosen, different immunosuppressants and combinations can be attempted.

The prognosis of IgG4-RKD is variable. The severity of the fibrosis has been proposed to play a role, as it has been shown in the salivary glands and an earlier intervention can improve the outcome. Still, even in patients with IgG4-TIN and severe interstitial fibrosis and tubular atrophy on kidney biopsy show a response to steroid or other immunosuppressive treatment. Transplant is a consideration in end-stage kidney disease due to IgG4-RKD. Recurrence of IgG4-TIN post-transplant is rare: there has been only one observed and reported case of recurrent IgG4-TIN in the kidney transplant, and this occurred in the setting of chronic antibody-mediated rejection, and so this may have been the result of under-immunosuppression.

7 The Pathogenesis of IgG4-RD

The immunopathogenesis of IgG4-RD includes the important role played by the B-cells. It has been shown that there is an oligoclonal expansion of a subset of circulating plasmablasts with an activated phenotype, along with production, expression, and secretion of IgG4. These cells are generated in a T-cell-dependent manner and show enhanced somatic hypermutation within heavy chain variable and framework regions. Pillai et al. illustrated a possible model of pathogenesis. The hypothesis is that after exposure to some still-to-be-identified antigen, cytotoxic CD4+ and CD8+ T-cells and activated B-cells/plasma cells infiltrate the tissue, perpetuating an exaggerated inflammatory response. In this context of tissue damage, the B-cells may start presenting self-antigens on specific HLA class II molecules to the cytotoxic CD4+ and CD8+ T-cells which would be reactivated at tissue site. Finally, the polarized T-cells would induce apoptotic cellular death, and the secretion of cytokines by these immune cells would induce healing fibrosis. Circulating T follicular helper-2 cells seem to be involved in IgG4 class-switching of the B-cells through the production of interleukin-4. Interestingly, the IgG4 molecules are thought to be recruited to downregulate the inflammation; they weakly activate the complement cascade and do not participate to antibody-dependent cell-mediated cytotoxicity. The specificity of the HLA class II molecule would explain the propensity of only some subjects to develop IgG4-RD. The inflammation and autoimmunity speculated could explain the well-documented response of IgG4-RD to steroids and other immunosuppressant drugs, as well as the relapse once the therapy is withdrawn. Also, this disarray of immunity could explain some propensity to develop other autoimmune or chronic allergic processes. Many questions remain and deserve further investigation, including why and how this disease forms inflammatory mass lesions with peculiar fibrosis, what are the antigens involved in disease pathogenesis, and what is the role of tissue immune complex deposits and IgG4 in this disease.

Suggested Reading

Alexander MP, Larsen CP, Gibson IW, Nasr SH, Sethi S, Fidler ME, Raissian Y, Takahashi N, Chari S, Smyrk TC, Cornell LD. Membranous glomerulonephritis is a manifestation of IgG4-related disease. Kidney Int. 2013;83(3):455–62. https://doi.org/10.1038/ki.2012.382. Epub 2012 Dec 19. PMID: 23254897.

Chen YC, Lee N, Chang CT, Wu MS. Salt loss and hyponatraemia in a patient with syphilitic nephritis. Nephrol Dial Transplant. 2005;20(6):1248–50. https://doi.org/10.1093/ndt/gfh778. Epub 2005 Apr 26. PMID: 15855196.

Cheuk W, Yuen HKL, Chan JKC. Chronic sclerosing dacryoadenitis: part of the spectrum of IgG4-related Sclerosing disease? Am J Surg Pathol. 2007;31(4):643–5. https://doi.org/10.1097/01.pas.0000213445.08902.11.

Chibbar R, Wright GR, Dokouhaki P, Dumanski S, Prasad B, Mengel M, Cornell LD, Shoker A. Recurrent IgG4-related tubulointerstitial nephritis concurrent with chronic active antibody mediated rejection: a case report. Am J Transplant. 2018;18(7):1799–803. https://doi.org/10.1111/ajt.14758. Epub 2018 Apr 24. PMID: 29607610.

Cornell LD, Chicano SL, Deshpande V, Collins AB, Selig MK, Lauwers GY, Barisoni L, Colvin RB. Pseudotumors due to IgG4 immune-complex tubulointerstitial nephritis associated with autoimmune pancreatocentric disease. Am J Surg Pathol. 2007;31(10):1586–97. https://doi.org/10.1097/PAS.0b013e318059b87c.

Cortazar FB, Stone JH. IgG4-related disease and the kidney. Nat Rev Nephrol. 2015;11(10):599–609. https://doi.org/10.1038/nrneph.2015.95. Epub 2015 Jun 30. PMID: 26122730.

Deshpande V, Zen Y, Chan JK, Yi EE, Sato Y, Yoshino T, Klöppel G, Heathcote JG, Khosroshahi A, Ferry JA, Aalberse RC, Bloch DB, Brugge WR, Bateman AC, Carruthers MN, Chari ST, Cheuk W, Cornell LD, Fernandez-Del Castillo C, Forcione DG, Hamilos DL, Kamisawa T, Kasashima S, Kawa S, Kawano M, Lauwers GY, Masaki Y, Nakanuma Y, Notohara K, Okazaki K, Ryu JK, Saeki T, Sahani DV, Smyrk TC, Stone JR, Takahira M, Webster GJ, Yamamoto M, Zamboni G, Umehara H, Stone JH. Consensus statement on the pathology of IgG4-related disease. Mod Pathol. 2012;25(9):1181–92. https://doi.org/10.1038/modpathol.2012.72. Epub 2012 May 18. PMID: 22596100.

Imai H, Hamai K, Komatsuda A, Ohtani H, Miura AB. IgG subclasses in patients with membranoproliferative glomerulonephritis, membranous nephropathy, and lupus nephritis. Kidney Int. 1997;51(1):270–6. https://doi.org/10.1038/ki.1997.32. PMID: 8995742.

Jo JH, Park YS, Jeon YK, Nam SJ, Huh J. Comparison of plasma cell type of Castleman's disease and IgG4-related sclerosing disease: a histopathological and immunohistochemical study. Pathobiology. 2011;78(4):227–32. https://doi.org/10.1159/000327357. Epub 2011 Jul 19. PMID: 21778790.

Kamisawa T, Zen Y, Pillai S, Stone JH. IgG4-related disease. Lancet. 2015;385(9976):1460–71. https://doi.org/10.1016/S0140-6736(14)60720-0. Epub 2014 Dec 4. PMID: 25481618.

Kawano M, Saeki T, Nakashima H. IgG4-related kidney disease and retroperitoneal fibrosis: an update. Mod Rheumatol. 2019;29(2):231–9. https://doi.org/10.1080/14397595.2018.1554321. Epub 2019 Jan 8. PMID: 30499730.

Khosroshahi A, Wallace ZS, Crowe JL, Akamizu T, Azumi A, Carruthers MN, Chari ST, Della-Torre E, Frulloni L, Goto H, Hart PA, Kamisawa T, Kawa S, Kawano M, Kim MH, Kodama Y, Kubota K, Lerch MM, Löhr M, Masaki Y, Matsui S, Mimori T, Nakamura S, Nakazawa T, Ohara H, Okazaki K, Ryu JH, Saeki T, Schleinitz N, Shimatsu A, Shimosegawa T, Takahashi H, Takahira M, Tanaka A, Topazian M, Umehara H, Webster GJ, Witzig TE, Yamamoto M, Zhang W, Chiba T, Stone JH, Second International Symposium on IgG4-Related Disease. International consensus guidance statement on the management and treatment of IgG4-related disease. Arthritis Rheumatol. 2015;67(7):1688–99. https://doi.org/10.1002/art.39132. PMID: 25809420.

Leung N, Ytterberg SR, Blute ML, Lager DJ, Specks U, Fervenza FC. Wegener's granulomatosis presenting as multiple bilateral renal masses. Nephrol Dial Transplant. 2004;19(4):984–7. https://doi.org/10.1093/ndt/gfh058. PMID: 15031361.

Martínez-de-Alegría A, Baleato-González S, García-Figueiras R, Bermúdez-Naveira A, Abdulkader-Nallib I, Díaz-Peromingo JA, Villalba-Martín C. IgG4-related disease from head to toe. Radiographics. 2015;35(7):2007–25. https://doi.org/10.1148/rg.357150066. Epub 2015 Oct 16. PMID: 26473450.

Mattoo H, Mahajan VS, Della-Torre E, Sekigami Y, Carruthers M, Wallace ZS, Deshpande V, Stone JH, Pillai S. De novo oligoclonal expansions of circulating plasmablasts in active and relapsing IgG4-related disease. J Allergy Clin Immunol. 2014;134(3):679–87. https://doi.org/10.1016/j.jaci.2014.03.034. Epub 2014 May 6. PMID: 24815737; PMCID: PMC4149918.

Miyabe K, Zen Y, Cornell LD, Rajagopalan G, Chowdhary VR, Roberts LR, Chari ST. Gastrointestinal and extra-intestinal manifestations of IgG4-related disease. Gastroenterology. 2018;155(4):990–1003.e1. https://doi.org/10.1053/j.gastro.2018.06.082. Epub 2018 Sep 12. PMID: 30012334.

Muraki T, Hamano H, Ochi Y, Komatsu K, Komiyama Y, Arakura N, Yoshizawa K, Ota M, Kawa S, Kiyosawa K. Autoimmune pancreatitis and complement activation system. Pancreas. 2006;32(1):16–21. https://doi.org/10.1097/01.mpa.0000188308.75043.e4. PMID: 16340739.

Perugino CA, Stone JH. IgG4-related disease: an update on pathophysiology and implications for clinical care. Nat Rev Rheumatol. 2020;16(12):702–14. https://doi.org/10.1038/s41584-020-0500-7. Epub 2020 Sep 16. PMID: 32939060.

Pillai S, Perugino C, Kaneko N. Immune mechanisms of fibrosis and inflammation in IgG4-related disease. Curr Opin Rheumatol. 2020;32(2):146–51. https://doi.org/10.1097/BOR.0000000000000686. PMID: 31842033.

Raissian Y, Nasr SH, Larsen CP, Colvin RB, Smyrk TC, Takahashi N, Bhalodia A, Sohani AR, Zhang L, Chari S, Sethi S, Fidler ME, Cornell LD. Diagnosis of IgG4-related tubulointerstitial nephritis. J Am Soc Nephrol. 2011;22(7):1343–52. https://doi.org/10.1681/ASN.2011010062. Epub 2011 Jun 30. PMID: 21719792; PMCID: PMC3137582.

Qi A, Fiset PO, Pilozzi-Edmonds L. Syphilis-related rapidly progressive glomerulonephritis: a case presentation. BMC Nephrol. 2021;22(1):196. https://doi.org/10.1186/s12882-021-02404-z. PMID: 34034668; PMCID: PMC8146206.

Saeki T, Nishi S, Imai N, Ito T, Yamazaki H, Kawano M, Yamamoto M, Takahashi H, Matsui S, Nakada S, Origuchi T, Hirabayashi A, Homma N, Tsubata Y, Takata T, Wada Y, Saito A, Fukase S, Ishioka K, Miyazaki K, Masaki Y, Umehara H, Sugai S, Narita I. Clinicopathological characteristics of patients with IgG4-related tubulointerstitial nephritis. Kidney Int. 2010;78(10):1016–23. https://doi.org/10.1038/ki.2010.271. Epub 2010 Aug 18. PMID: 20720530.

Salvadori M, Tsalouchos A. Immunoglobulin G4-related kidney diseases: an updated review. World J Nephrol. 2018;7(1):29–40. https://doi.org/10.5527/wjn.v7.i1.29. PMID: 29359118; PMCID: PMC5760510.

Satoskar AA, Kovach P, O'Reilly K, Nadasdy T. An uncommon cause of membranous glomerulonephritis. Am J Kidney Dis. 2010;55(2):386–90. https://doi.org/10.1053/j.ajkd.2009.06.015. Epub 2009 Jul 30. PMID: 19643521.

Sharma SG, Vlase HL, D'Agati VD. IgG4-related tubulointerstitial nephritis with plasma cell-rich renal arteritis. Am J Kidney Dis. 2013;61(4):638–43. https://doi.org/10.1053/j.ajkd.2012.07.031. Epub 2012 Dec 1. PMID: 23206533.

Shimizu Y, Yamamoto M, Naishiro Y, Sudoh G, Ishigami K, Yajima H, Tabeya T, Matsui M, Suzuki C, Takahashi H, Seki N, Himi T, Yamashita K, Noguchi H, Hasegawa T, Suzuki Y, Honda S, Abe T, Imai K, Shinomura Y. Necessity of early intervention for IgG4-related diseaseDOUBLEHYPHENdelayed treatment induces fibrosis progression. Rheumatology (Oxford). 2013;52(4):679–83. https://doi.org/10.1093/rheumatology/kes358. Epub 2012 Dec 19. PMID: 23258649.

Soulier J, Grollet L, Oksenhendler E, Cacoub P, Cazals-Hatem D, Babinet P, d'Agay MF, Clauvel JP, Raphael M, Degos L, et al. Kaposi's sarcoma-associated herpesvirus-like DNA sequences in multicentric Castleman's disease. Blood. 1995;86(4):1276–80. PMID: 7632932.

Takahashi N, Kawashima A, Fletcher JG, Chari ST. Renal involvement in patients with autoimmune pancreatitis: CT and MR imaging findings. Radiology. 2007;242(3):791–801. https://doi.org/10.1148/radiol.2423060003. Epub 2007 Jan 17. PMID: 17229877.

Taylor MS, Chougule A, MacLeay AR, Kurzawa P, Chebib I, Le L, Deshpande V. Morphologic overlap between inflammatory myofibroblastic tumor and IgG4-related disease: lessons from next-generation sequencing. Am J Surg Pathol. 2019;43(3):314–24. https://doi.org/10.1097/PAS.0000000000001167. PMID: 30451733; PMCID: PMC6637760.

Wallace ZS, Deshpande V, Mattoo H, Mahajan VS, Kulikova M, Pillai S, Stone JH. IgG4-related disease: clinical and laboratory features in one hundred twenty-five patients. Arthritis Rheumatol. 2015;67(9):2466–75. https://doi.org/10.1002/art.39205. PMID: 25988916; PMCID: PMC4621270.

Wallace ZS, Naden RP, Chari S, Choi HK, Della-Torre E, Dicaire JF, Hart PA, Inoue D, Kawano M, Khosroshahi A, Lanzillotta M, Okazaki K, Perugino CA, Sharma A, Saeki T, Schleinitz N, Takahashi N, Umehara H, Zen Y, Stone JH, Members of the ACR/EULAR IgG4-RD Classification Criteria Working Group. The 2019 American College of Rheumatology/European League against rheumatism classification criteria for IgG4-related disease. Ann Rheum Dis. 2020;79(1):77–87. https://doi.org/10.1136/annrheumdis-2019-216561. Epub 2019 Dec 3. PMID: 31796497.

Wang L, Zhang P, Wang M, Feng R, Lai Y, Peng L, Fei Y, Zhang X, Zhao Y, Zeng X, Zhang F, Zhang W. Failure of remission induction by glucocorticoids alone or in combination with immunosuppressive agents in IgG4-related disease: a prospective study of 215 patients. Arthritis Res Ther. 2018;20(1):65. https://doi.org/10.1186/s13075-018-1567-2. PMID: 29636109; PMCID: PMC5894179.

Wu C, Zeng YP. Mikulicz disease. JAMA Dermatol. 2020;156(4):451. https://doi.org/10.1001/jamadermatol.2019.4260. PMID: 31913425.

Yamamoto H, Yamaguchi H, Aishima S, Oda Y, Kohashi K, Oshiro Y, Tsuneyoshi M. Inflammatory myofibroblastic tumor versus IgG4-related sclerosing disease and inflammatory pseudotumor: a comparative clinicopathologic study. Am J Surg Pathol. 2009;33(9):1330–40. https://doi.org/10.1097/pas.0b013e3181a5a207. PMID: 19718789.

Yoshida K, Toki F, Takeuchi T, Watanabe S, Shiratori K, Hayashi N. Chronic pancreatitis caused by an autoimmune abnormality. Proposal of the concept of autoimmune pancreatitis. Dig Dis Sci. 1995;40(7):1561–8. https://doi.org/10.1007/BF02285209. PMID: 7628283.

Yunyun F, Yu P, Panpan Z, Xia Z, Linyi P, Jiaxin Z, Li Z, Shangzhu Z, Jinjing L, Di W, Yamin L, Xiaowei L, Huadan X, Xuan Z, Xiaofeng Z, Fengchun Z, Yan Z, Wen Z. Efficacy and safety of low dose Mycophenolate mofetil treatment for immunoglobulin G4-related disease: a randomized clinical trial. Rheumatology (Oxford). 2019;58(1):52–60. https://doi.org/10.1093/rheumatology/key227. PMID: 30124952.

Zen Y, Nakanuma Y. IgG4-related disease. Am J Surg Pathol. 2010;34(12):1812–9. https://doi.org/10.1097/PAS.0b013e3181f7266b.

Anti-Brush Border Antibody (ABBA)-Associated Tubulointerstitial Disease

Laurence Beck and Tiffany Caza

Antibodies against components of the proximal tubular brush border have played a major role in experimental models of immune-complex mediated kidney disease. In particular, the Heymann nephritis model of membranous nephropathy was generated by immunizing Lewis rats against homogenates of brush border extract. The antibodies produced after immunization against brush border, in particular to a subfraction known as Fx1a, were found to primarily target the brush border antigen gp330, now better known as megalin. In the rat, megalin is expressed by the glomerular podocyte as well as by proximal tubular brush border, presenting a target for circulating antibodies within the glomerulus that led to the subepithelial deposits characteristic of membranous nephropathy. Although these anti-megalin antibodies also targeted proximal tubule, this experimental model proved most useful for the understanding of the glomerular mechanisms leading to the nephrotic syndrome.

Megalin, more formally known as low-density lipoprotein (LDL)-related protein 2 (LRP2), is a transmembrane receptor that, in a complex with cubilin (CUBN), is responsible for the endocytic uptake of multiple ligands by the proximal tubule. This 517 kDa glycoprotein has a very large extracellular domain that can bind diverse proteins such as albumin, lipoproteins, and vitamin-binding proteins. Dysfunction of the megalin-cubilin complex results of loss of albumin and other proteins into the urine due to deficient proximal tubular resorption. Mice genetically deficient for megalin exhibit defective tubular function and proteinuria. Human genetic mutation involving LRP2 causes the Donnai-Barrow or

L. Beck (✉)
Department of Medicine, Nephrology Section, Boston Medical Center and Boston University School of Medicine, Boston, MA, USA
e-mail: Laurence.Beck@bmc.org

T. Caza
Arkana Laboratories, Little Rock, AR, USA
e-mail: tiffany.caza@arkanalabs.com

M. G. Atta, M. A. Perazella (eds.), *Tubulointerstitial Nephritis*,
https://doi.org/10.1007/978-3-030-93438-5_9

facio-oculo-acoustico-renal (DB/FOAR) syndrome associated with proteinuric disease and developmental abnormalities while genetic mutation involving CUBN causes Imerslund-Gräsbeck syndrome (IGS) or selective vitamin B(12) (cobalamin) malabsorption with proteinuria.

Once megalin was identified as the antigenic target in the experimental model of membranous nephropathy, focus shifted to humans to see if there was any evidence for anti-megalin or anti-brush border antibodies. Two case reports from this period documented evidence of kidney disease associated with antibodies reactive with proximal tubular brush border, in a 34-year-old male with proteinuria and a 59-year-old male with kidney failure and a thymic tumor. Of note, both revealed segmental glomerular deposits as well as more uniform IgG- and C3-containing deposits in Bowman's capsule. Despite these intriguing cases, it was quickly determined that the majority of human membranous nephropathy could not be explained by antibodies to megalin, and there were no further descriptions of similar cases.

Decades later, and after the major target of human membranous nephropathy was found to be the phospholipase A2 receptor, Rosales and colleagues described a 73-year-old male with rapidly-progressive kidney disease who was found to have tubulointerstitial nephritis with acute tubular injury, loss of proximal tubular brush border, and TBM deposits. Similar to the 1981 cases, this patient had some features of membranous nephropathy with segmental subepithelial deposits along glomerular capillary loops. The patient required hemodialysis and never recovered kidney function despite corticosteroid treatment. Four years later, the patient received a kidney transplant. Remarkably, within 7 weeks of transplantation, the same pathologic process occurred with the same features on biopsy. Pre- and post-transplant serum specimens reacted strongly with brush border by indirect immunofluorescence for IgG, suggesting the presence of circulating antibodies to a component of tubular brush border. Preliminary investigations did not identify the target antigen.

It was not until a detailed analysis of a cohort of similar cases was performed that the target antigen in anti-brush border antibody disease was identified to be LRP2. In this study, serum from several representative cases revealed IgG4 reactivity with a large protein present in extracts from human kidney cortex. Mass spectrometric analysis of candidate bands immunoprecipitated by human IgG suggested LRP2 as a likely target. Autoantibodies to LRP2, particularly to the N-terminal region of the protein, were found in the majority of cases. Co-localization of IgG and LRP2 by confocal immunofluorescence imaging showed that the IgG within TBM deposits co-localized with LRP2 only in this particular disorder and not in other pathological entities that can also show IgG-containing TBM deposits such as lupus nephritis, IgG4-related systemic disease, or BK polyomavirus nephropathy.

Common clinical and histopathologic features became evident from this case series. The ten patients were elderly with a mean age of 73 and the majority were male. They presented with acute kidney injury and sub-nephrotic levels of proteinuria. Fifty percent progressed to end-stage kidney disease.

There is a spectrum of histopathologic severity in anti-brush border antibody disease, with the predominant finding being acute (Fig. 1a) or protracted tubular injury (Fig. 1b) without significant associated inflammation. Immunofluorescence

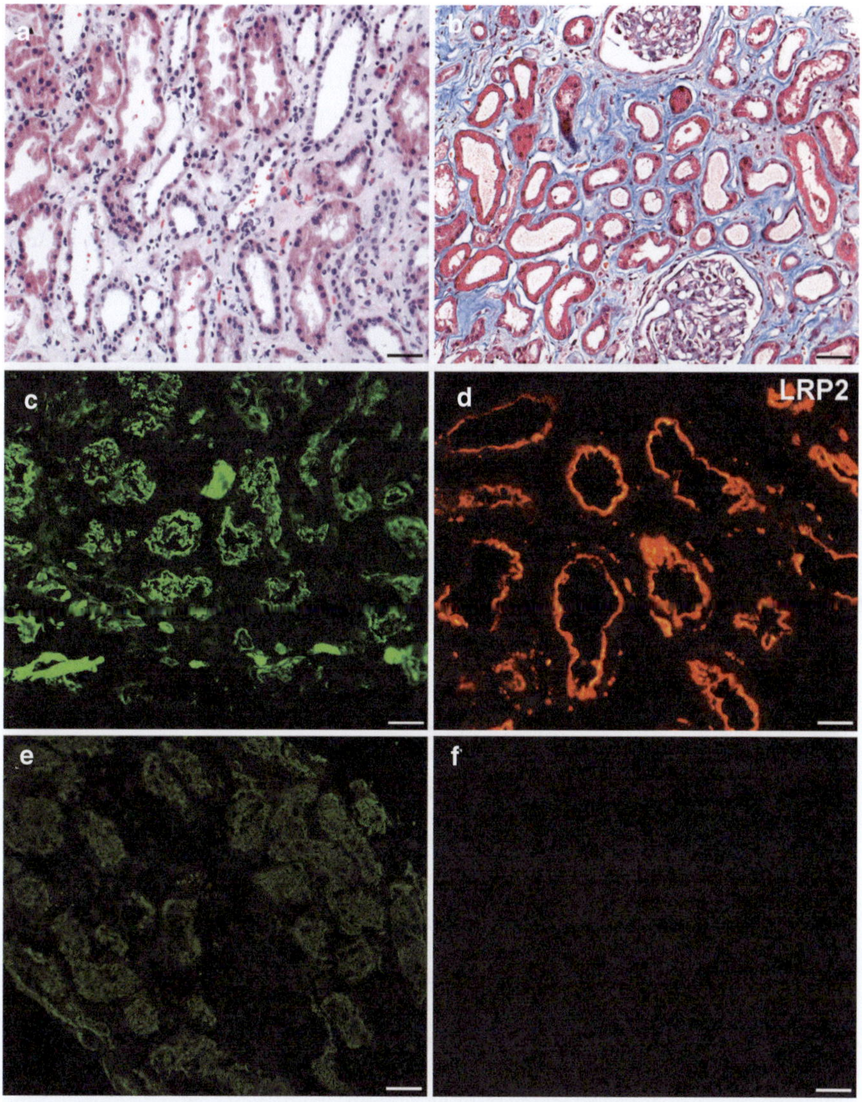

Fig. 1 Histopathology of tubular injury in anti-brush border antibody disease. (**a**) Acute tubular injury and interstitial edema, H & E, scale bar = 50 μm (**b**) Protracted pattern of tubular injury showing interstitial fibrosis separating simplified tubular profiles, Masson-Trichrome, scale bar = 100 μm (**c**) Immunoglobulin staining of the proximal tubular brush borders and tubular basement membranes, scale bar = 50 μm (**d**) LRP2 immunofluorescence within tubular basement membrane deposits, scale bar = 20 μm (**e**) IgG seroreactivity against proximal tubular brush borders by indirect immunofluorescence, scale bar = 50 μm (**f**) Normal human serum lacks IgG reactivity against proximal tubular brush borders, scale bar = 50 μm

for IgG, kappa light chain, and lambda light chain shows granular TBM deposits and is positive along the proximal tubular brush borders (Fig. 1c). LRP2 staining is positive within TBM deposits along the same distribution as IgG (Fig. 1d). Patient sera shows reactivity against the proximal tubular brush borders in the same distribution as IgG on biopsy (Fig. 1e), while normal human serum does not highlight brush borders (Fig. 1f).

In addition to tubulointerstitial injury, a majority of patients have glomerular involvement with deposition of IgG immune complexes along the glomerular basement membranes (Fig. 2a) and along Bowman's capsule (Fig. 2b). A segmental membranous glomerulopathy is frequently present with subepithelial IgG immune deposits within some capillary loops (Fig. 2c, d, f). LRP2 is seen only rarely within the glomerular capillary loop deposits (Fig. 2e), with negative staining along glomerular capillaries in the majority of cases. It is plausible that a lack of staining could result from steric hindrance of existing autoantibodies and commercial anti-LRP2 antibodies or owing to the low expression level of LRP2 in podocytes.

A number of additional cases have been reported in the literature since this initial series, which have often shown disparate clinical presentations and collisions with other concurrent kidney diseases. While a majority of biopsies in the initial series demonstrated acute or protracted tubular injury without significant interstitial inflammation, cases of anti-LRP2 nephropathy have now been reported in the setting of acute interstitial nephritis (AIN), including plasma cell rich AIN mimicking IgG4-associated kidney disease. There are two reported cases of anti-LRP2 nephropathy in association with low-grade B-cell lymphomas (small lymphocytic lymphoma and lymphoplasmacytic lymphoma). Anti-LRP2 nephropathy has also been observed in the setting of lupus nephritis and minimal change disease. It is plausible that proteinuria may be necessary for autoantibodies to access the luminal brush border, which might explain collisions of ABBA with other proteinuric kidney diseases.

The optimal treatment for anti-LRP2 nephropathy has not been defined and we are limited to anecdotal reports as to the success or failure of immunosuppressive therapy. Since it is assumed that the autoantibodies are directly pathogenic and lead to acute tubular injury and rapid loss of kidney function, treatments that can most quickly lead to autoantibody depletion should be considered. Corticosteroids alone do not seem to slow the disease process. Regimens with anti-B cell agents such as rituximab or pulse corticosteroids with alkylating agents have shown some limited success. A decline and disappearance of anti-LRP2 antibody titer (immunologic remission) was associated with stabilization of kidney function after treatment with corticosteroids and cyclophosphamide. Treatment with rituximab in the case associated with chronic lymphocytic leukemia resulted in stabilization of kidney function and a drop in ABBA titer.

Antibodies to other tubular elements can also rarely cause a tubulointerstitial nephritis. A 2016 report describes antibodies to the collecting-duct specific aquaporin 2 that led to tubulointerstitial nephritis. The prevalence of this type of anti-tubular disease is unknown. Another entity is anti-TBM disease, of which the target is the 'tubulointerstitial nephritis antigen'. It is identified by linear IgG, kappa, and

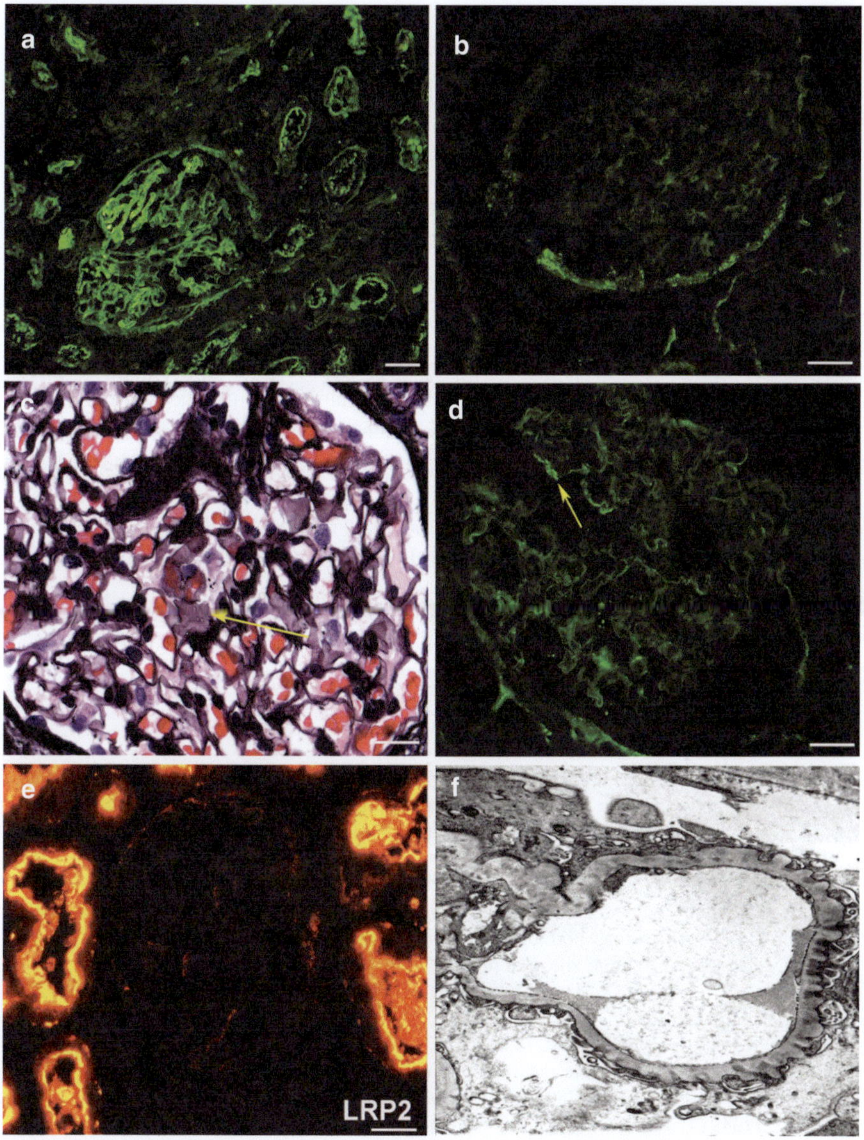

Fig. 2 Histopathologic characteristics of glomerular involvement in anti-brush border antibody disease. (**a**) IgG highlighting glomerular and tubulointerstitial deposits, scale bar = 50 μm. (**b**) Granular IgG staining along Bowman's capsule, scale bar = 20 μm. (**c**) Capillary loop 'holes', Jones methenamine silver, scale bar = 20 μm. (**d**) Segmental distribution of IgG staining along glomerular capillary loops, scale bar = 20 μm. (**e**) LRP2 immunostaining segmentally present along the glomerular basement membranes, Bowman's capsule, and along tubular basement membranes, scale bar = 20 μm. (**f**) Electron photomicrograph displaying subepithelial electron-dense deposits

lambda light chain staining is along the TBM of the proximal tubules. This disease is rare but has been reported in both adults and children and can have concurrent glomerular deposits (Bowman's capsule and subepithelial), similar to ABBA. There are additional autoimmune tubulointerstitial kidney diseases with TBM deposits, including idiopathic hypocomplementemic tubulointerstitial nephritis, tubulointerstitial nephritis in graft-versus-host disease, IgG4-related kidney disease, and lupus nephritis, for which the antigenic targets are largely unknown.

In summary, anti-brush border antibody disease or anti-LRP2 nephropathy is a disease of unclear prevalence that can be associated with rapid progression to end-stage kidney disease. As it more commonly occurs in the elderly, who may be less likely to undergo kidney biopsy, it may be underdiagnosed. Biopsy features that should raise suspicion for anti-LRP2 nephropathy include the presence of TBM immune deposits in association with both Bowman's capsule and segmental glomerular subepithelial deposits, especially when accompanied by proximal tubule brush border IgG positivity. Serum reactivity to proximal tubule brush border on normal kidney sections is typically present, and the finding of circulating anti-LRP2 or the presence of LRP2 within tubular deposits is diagnostic. When feasible, treatment should be directed at reducing antibody levels through the use of immunosuppressive agents that can target B cells.

Suggested Reading

Beck LH Jr, Bonegio RG, Lambeau G, Beck DM, Powell DW, Cummins TD, Klein JB, Salant DJ. M-type phospholipase A2 receptor as target antigen in idiopathic membranous nephropathy. N Engl J Med. 2009;361(1):11–21. https://doi.org/10.1056/NEJMoa0810457. PMID: 19571279; PMCID: PMC2762083.

Caliskan Y, Caza T, Mosman A, Elawa U, Philipneri M, Martin K, Bastani B. A case of immune complex mediated tubulointerstitial disease and nephrotic syndrome: anti LRP-2 Nephropathy with diffuse podocyte effacement. J Nephrol. 2020. https://doi.org/10.1007/s40620-020-00762-9. Epub ahead of print. PMID: 32472527.

Campbell RE, Uhlenhopp D, Shaw M, Dai DF, Sekar A. Anti-brush border antibody (ABBA)-associated renal disease. QJM. 2020;113(8):561–2. https://doi.org/10.1093/qjmed/hcaa015. PMID: 31995201; PMCID: PMC7825481.

Christensen EI, Birn H. Megalin and cubulin: synergistic endocytic receptors in renal proximal tubule. Am J Phys. 2001;280:F562–73. https://doi.org/10.1152/ajprenal.2001.280.4.F562. PMID: 11249847.

Dinesh KP, Raniele D, Michels K, Avasare RS, Larsen CP, Kayton R, Khalighi MA, Andeen NK. Anti-LRP2 nephropathy with abundant IgG4-positive plasma cells: a case report. Am J Kidney Dis. 2019;74(1):132–7. https://doi.org/10.1053/j.ajkd.2018.12.039. Epub 2019 Mar 12. PMID: 30876746.

Douglas MF, Rabideau DP, Schwartz MM, Lewis EJ. Evidence of autologous immune-complex nephritis. N Engl J Med. 1981;305(22):1326–9. https://doi.org/10.1056/NEJM198111263052206. PMID: 6457246.

Dvanajscak Z, Murphy JD, Larsen CP, Padala SA. Anti-brush border antibody disease (anti-LRP2 nephropathy) associated with lupus nephritis. Kidney Int Rep. 2020;5(9):1590–4. https://doi.org/10.1016/j.ekir.2020.06.025. PMID: 32954086; PMCID: PMC7486196.

Gallan AJ, Garg A, Collins AB, Beck LH Jr, Trivin-Avillach C, Henriksen KJ, Chang A. Anti-LRP2 nephropathy. Kidney Int Rep. 2020;5(12):2365–70. https://doi.org/10.1016/j.ekir.2020.09.011. PMID: 33305133; PMCID: PMC7710829.

Gamayo A, Hecox D, Dicker L, Vecchiarelli L, Raess PW, Khalighi M, Andeen NK. Anti-LRP2 nephropathy with concurrent kidney infiltration by lymphoma. Clin Kidney J. 2019;13(3):468–72. https://doi.org/10.1093/ckj/sfz166. PMID: 32701074; PMCID: PMC7367117.

Iványi B, Haszon I, Endreffy E, Szenohradszky P, Petri IB, Kalmár T, Butkowski RJ, Charonis AS, Túri S. Childhood membranous nephropathy, circulating antibodies to the 58-kD TIN antigen, and anti-tubular basement membrane nephritis: an 11-year follow-up. Am J Kidney Dis. 1998;32(6):1068–74. https://doi.org/10.1016/s0272-6386(98)70085-x. PMID: 9856526.

Kantarci S, Al-Gazali A, Hill RS, Donnai D, Black GCM, Bieth E, Chassaing N, Lacombe D, Devriendt K, Teebi A, Loscertales M, Robson C, Liu T, MacLaughlin DT, Noonan KM, Russell MK, Walsh CA, Donahoe PK, Pober BR. Mutations in LRP2, which encodes the multiligand receptor megalin, cause Donnai-Barrow and facio-oculo-acoustico-renal syndromes. Nat Genet. 2007;39:957–9. https://doi.org/10.1038/ng2063. Epub 2007 Jul 15. PMID: 17632512; PMCID: PMC2891728.

Katz A, Fish AJ, Santamaria P, Nevins TE, Kim Y, Butkowski RJ. Role of antibodies to tubulointerstitial nephritis antigen in human anti-tubular basement membrane nephritis associated with membranous nephropathy. Am J Med. 1992;93(6):691–8. https://doi.org/10.1016/0002-9343(92)90205-p. PMID: 1466368.

Kerjaschi D, Farquhar MG. Immunocytochemical localization of the Heymann nephritis antigen (GP330) in glomerular epithelial cells of normal Lewis rats. J Exp Med. 1983;157:667–86. https://doi.org/10.1084/jem.157.2.667. PMID: 6337231; PMCID: PMC2186920.

Kerjaschi D, Farquhar MG. The pathogenic antigen of Heymann nephritis is a membrane glycoprotein of the renal proximal tubule brush border. Proc Natl Acad Sci U S A. 1982;79:5557–61. https://doi.org/10.1073/pnas.79.18.5557. PMID: 6752952; PMCID: PMC346943.

Larsen CP, Trivin-Avillach C, Coles P, Collins AB, Merchant M, Ma H, Wilkey DW, Ambruzs JM, Messias NC, Cossey LN, Rosales IA, Wooldridge T, Walker PD, Colvin RB, Klein J, Salant DJ, Beck LH Jr. LDL receptor-related protein 2 (megalin) as a target antigen in human kidney anti-brush border antibody disease. J Am Soc Nephrol. 2018;29(2):644–53. https://doi.org/10.1681/ASN.2017060664. Epub 2017 Oct 26. PMID: 29074737; PMCID: PMC5791069.

Leheste JR, Rolinski B, Vorum H, Hilpert J, Nykjaer A, Jacobsen C, Aucouturier P, Moskaug J, Otto A, Christensen EI, Willnow TE. Megalin knockout mice as an animal model of low molecular weight proteinuria. Am J Pathol. 1999;155:1361–70. https://doi.org/10.1016/S0002-9440(10)65238-8. PMID: 10514418; PMCID: PMC1867027.

Morrison EB, Kozlowski EJ, McPhaul JJ Jr. Primary tubulointerstitial nephritis caused by antibodies to proximal tubular antigens. Am J Clin Pathol. 1981;75(4):602–9. https://doi.org/10.1093/ajcp/75.4.602. PMID: 7013472.

Rosales IA, Collins AB, do Carmo PA, Tolkoff-Rubin N, Smith RN, Colvin RB. Immune complex tubulointerstitial nephritis due to autoantibodies to the proximal tubule brush border. J Am Soc Nephrol. 2016;27(2):380–4. https://doi.org/10.1681/ASN.2015030334. Epub 2015 Sep 2. PMID: 26334028; PMCID: PMC4731130.

Storm T, Emma F, Verroust PJ, Hertz JM, Nielsen R. A patient with cubulin deficiency. N Engl J Med. 2011;364:89–91. https://doi.org/10.1056/NEJMc1009804. PMID: 21208123.

Zhu X, Tu L, Liu S, You H, Xue J, Hao C. Complete remission of nephrotic syndrome in a young woman with anti-LRP2 nephropathy after immunosuppressive therapy. BMC Nephrol. 2020;21(1):364. https://doi.org/10.1186/s12882-020-02027-w. PMID: 32831033; PMCID: PMC7446201.

Transplant Rejection and Infection Associated Tubulointerstitial Nephritis

Sam Kant, Serena Bagnasco, and Daniel C. Brennan

1 Introduction

Tubulointerstitial nephritis (TIN) in kidney allografts is the third most common biopsy proven pathology after rejection and calcineurin inhibitor toxicity. It can be caused by a myriad of etiologies including systemic diseases like lupus, sarcoidosis, other autoimmune diseases and hereditary tubulointerstitial kidney disease, but is most commonly from infections, drugs, and rejection. While the histological presence of an interstitial mononuclear infiltrate and tubulitis points towards the unifying pathological diagnosis of TIN- it can, however, be challenging to discern the presence of rejection from other causes. While there will be features with respect to patient history, characteristics, co-morbidities, and pathology that will aid in differentiating causes that lead to TIN, investigating with a broad differential diagnosis is essential. This chapter will review the etiologies associated with TIN in kidney transplants, with a focus on rejection and infection.

S. Kant (✉) · D. C. Brennan
Division of Nephrology, Department of Medicine, Johns Hopkins University School of Medicine, Baltimore, MD, USA

Comprehensive Transplant Center, Johns Hopkins University School of Medicine, Baltimore, MD, USA
e-mail: skant1@jhmi.edu; dbrenna4@jhmi.edu

S. Bagnasco
Department of Pathology, Johns Hopkins University School of Medicine, Baltimore, MD, USA
e-mail: sbagnas1@jhmi.edu

M. G. Atta, M. A. Perazella (eds.), *Tubulointerstitial Nephritis*,
https://doi.org/10.1007/978-3-030-93438-5_10

2 Transplant Rejection Associated Tubulointerstitial Nephritis

Organ rejection as a concept was introduced in 1902 by the French surgeon Alexis Carrel with use of the term *biologic incompatibility*. Histological descriptions of renal allograft rejections were first reported in 1967, however, a standardized classification for defining and grading of transplant rejection only came into effect in 1991 with the Banff working group. The pathology of renal allograft rejections can extend into an isolated or combined involvement of the four components of the kidney- glomeruli, tubules, interstitium and vessels. The damage to these structures as a consequence of rejection can be cellular or antibody mediated, with the terms "acute" or "chronic" used in context of the period post transplantation and rejection activity. Acute cellular and antibody mediated rejection can occur independently or simultaneously.

Rejection associated TIN is usually a consequence of T cell-mediated (cellular) rejection (TCMR). There is a concerted reaction of the T cells with natural killer (NK) cells and macrophages against histocompatibility antigens present not only in the tubules and interstitium, but also, the endothelium of vessels. Human leukocyte antigen (HLA) mismatch involving A/B/DR is the main predictor of acute TCMR, with no predictive effect extended by panel reactive antibody and repeat transplantation. In the post-transplant period, type and exposure of immunosuppressive therapy determines risk of ACR, with the use of rabbit thymocyte globulin, tacrolimus, and mycophenolate mofetil associated with lower risk of TCMR.

2.1 *Presentation*

Episodes of acute rejection-associated TIN mostly occur within 12 months of engraftment, while most episodes after 1 year of transplantation occur as a consequence of noncompliance or iatrogenic reduction in immunosuppression. Patients with acute rejection-associated TIN will mostly be asymptomatic and will be detected because of an explained worsening of renal function manifested by increase in serum creatinine with or without abnormalities on urinalysis (proteinuria, microscopic hematuria and or leukocyturia). Occasionally, patients may present with generalized malaise, fever, oliguria and/or graft pain.

Plasma levels of donor-derived cell free DNA (dd-cfDNA) may be elevated in patients with acute TCMR-associated TIN, with a cut off >1% predictive of ACR-positive and negative predictive value for active rejection of 61% and 84%, respectively. The dd-cfDNA may, therefore, serve as a non-invasive biomarker of ACR associated TIN.

Radiologic findings would be considered non-specific for discerning TCMR-associated TIN from other forms of rejection or acute kidney injury. Renal ultrasound may demonstrate increased graft size, with loss of corticomedullary junction, prominent hypoechoic pyramids, and decreased echogenicity of the renal sinus, with doppler studies showing elevated resistive indices. Kidney biopsy continues to be the gold standard for diagnosis of rejection-associated TIN.

2.2 *Pathology*

Interstitial inflammation and tubulitis are primary lesions associated with acute TCMR. This includes interstitial infiltration with mononuclear cells, and, occasionally eosinophils, and disruption of the tubular basement membranes by the infiltrating cells (ie, tubulitis).

Tubulitis can be a feature of acute and chronic active TCMR, characterized by presence of inflammatory cells between tubular epithelial cells. Tubulitis present in non-severely atrophic tubules would be indicative of acute TCMR (Fig. 1), whereas tubulitis involving both atrophic and non-atrophic tubules demonstrate evidence of chronic active TCMR. The dominant inflammatory cells present in tubulitis are monocytes and lymphocytes, and less commonly plasma cells.

Similar to tubulitis, interstitial inflammation can be present in both acute and chronic active TCMR. In acute TCMR, inflammatory cell infiltration is present in the edematous stroma, associated with tubulitis of non-severely atrophic tubules (Fig. 2). Inflammatory cells in both the edematous and fibrotic stroma accompanied by tubulitis of atrophic and non-atrophic tubules, indicates chronic active TCMR. The infiltrating cells are most often lymphocytes and monocytes, but plasma cells, neutrophils, or eosinophils can also be present. T cells tend to infiltrate diffusely or in scattered patterns, whereas B cells are often aggregated.

The presence of scattered mononuclear cell infiltrates without tubulitis can be an inconsequential finding in normal functioning renal allografts and in isolation is

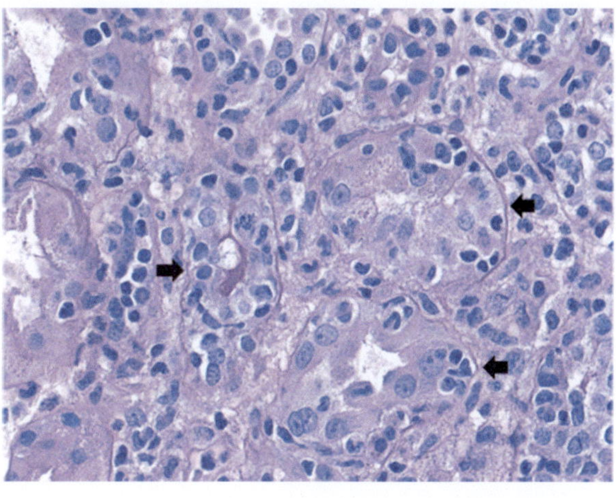

Fig. 1 T cell mediated rejection, severe tubulitis, with lymphocytes invading the epithelial tubular walls (arrow), associated with interstitial inflammation with lymphocytes (H&E, 160X). (Image courtesy of Dr. Serena Bagnasco)

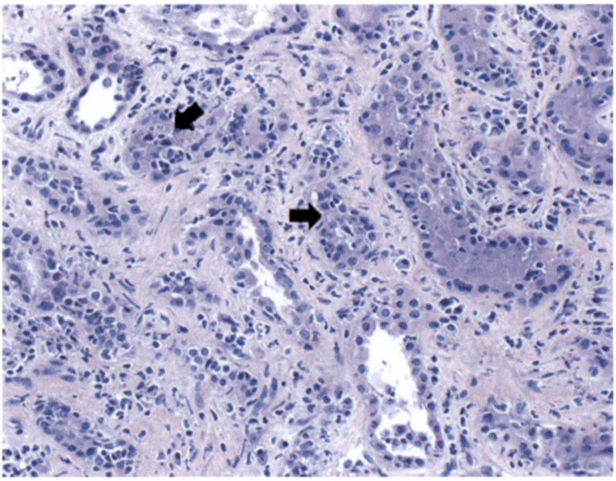

Fig. 2 T cell mediated rejection, interstitial inflammation and severe tubulitis (arrows) is present in non-severely atrophic cortical tubules. The interstitium shows active inflammation with lymphocytes and plasma cells and interstitial fibrosis (H&E 64X). (Image courtesy of Dr. Serena Bagnasco)

Table 1 Histologic criteria for diagnosing acute and chronic active T cell mediated rejection according to 2018 Banff guidelines

Active TCMR		
Type	Description	Banff scores
Borderline	Mild interstitial inflammation plus any tubulitis or significant interstitial inflammation	i0/i1 + t1/2/3 or i2/3 + t1
IA	Moderate tubulitis and at least moderate interstitial inflammation	t2i2 or t2i3
IB	Severe tubulitis and at least moderate interstitial inflammation	t3i2 or t3i3
IIA	Mild to moderate intimal arteritis	v1
IIB	Severe intimal arteritis (> 25% of the luminal area)	v2
III	Transmural arteritis and/or fibrinoid necrosis	v3
Chronic active TCMR		
IA	Moderate tubulitis and at least moderate total cortical inflammation and at least moderate scarred cortical inflammation and other known causes ruled out	t2, ti ≥ 2, and i-IFTA ≥ 2
IB	Severe tubulitis and at least moderate total cortical inflammation and at least moderate scarred cortical inflammation and other known causes ruled out	t3, ti ≥ 2, and i-IFTA ≥ 2
II	Arterial intimal fibrosis with mononuclear cell inflammation, formation of neointima	cv1, cv2, or cv3

Abbreviations: cv, arterial fibrous intimal thickening; i, interstitial inflammation; i-IFTA, tubulointerstitial inflammation (inflammation in areas of interstitial fibrosis and tubular atrophy); t, tubulitis; TCMR, T cell-mediated rejection; ti, tubulointerstitial inflammation (inflammation in total parenchyma, including scarred and non-scarred cortex); v, intimal arteritis

insufficient for a diagnosis of acute TCMR. The presence of neutrophils is uncommon and suggests the diagnosis of infection or ABMR.

Histologic criteria for diagnosing acute and chronic active TCMR according to Banff 2018 guidelines is presented in Table 1. A synopsis of threshold for Banff lesion scores in TCMR are highlighted in Table 2.

Table 2 Synopsis of threshold for Banff lesion scores in acute and chronic active T cell mediated rejection according to 2018 Banff guidelines

Banff lesion score	Abbreviation	0	1	2	3
Interstitial inflammation	*i*	<10%	10–25%	26–50%	>50%
Tubulitis	*t*	None	1–4 mononuclear cells/tubular cross section or 10 tubular epithelial cells	5–10	>10 or foci of tubular basement membrane destruction with i ≥ 2 and t2 elsewhere
Intimal arteritis	*v*	None	<25% luminal area lost	≥25% luminal area lost	Transmural and/or fibrinoid change and medial smooth muscle necrosis
Interstitial fibrosis	*ci*	≤5%	6–25%	26–50%	>50%
Tubular atrophy	*ct*	None	≤25%	26–50%	>50%
Vascular fibrous intimal thickening	*cv*	None	≤25%	26–50%	>50%
Total inflammation	*ti*	<10%	10–25%	26–50%	>50%
Inflammation in the area of interstitial fibrosis and tubular atrophy	*i-IFTA*	<10%	10–25%	26–50%	>50%

2.3 *Treatment*

Worse graft outcomes have been associated with higher histologic scores (i: interstitial inflammation, t: tubulitis, v: intimal arteritis) and a later onset of rejection (>3 months posttransplant). In addition, higher histologic severity of acute TCMR (ie, Banff grade greater than IA) is associated with lower response rates to therapy.

The diagnosis of acute TCMR requires a histologic score of at least t2 and i2. Any scores below this (e.g., i1+t2 or i2+t1) are considered to be borderline rejection. Following are treatment recommendations for Banff grades that have evidence of TIN:

1. Borderline [Mild interstitial inflammation (<25% of nonsclerotic cortical parenchyma; i0 or i1) plus any tubulitis (t1, t2, or t3) or significant interstitial inflammation (>25% of nonsclerotic cortical parenchyma; i2 or i3) plus foci of mild tubulitis (t1)]: the optimal strategy of treatment would be target higher calcineurin inhibitor levels with or without increment in mycophenolate mofetil and steroids. Some centers advocate treating borderline rejection as acute TCMR.
2. Type IA: administer pulse intravenous glucocorticoids with subsequent oral taper, along with augmenting maintenance immunosuppression
3. Type IB/II/III: in addition to treatment outlined for Banff IA, administer rabbit antithymocyte globulin for patients with no or few chronic histologic lesions (interstitial fibrosis/tubular atrophy [IF/TA], vascular intimal sclerosis, arteriolar hyaline thickening) presenting less than 1 year pots engraftment.

A successful reversal of rejection has been defined as decrease in serum creatinine to within 10% of baseline level. Allografts with evidence of chronic injury and fibrosis are expected to have lower likelihood of reversal of allograft dysfunction with treatment.

3 Transplant Infection Associated Tubulointerstitial Nephritis

Tubulointerstitial nephritis can be a consequence of graft infection, with both viral and bacterial etiologies. Cytomegalovirus (CMV), BK and adenovirus represent the primary viral causes, whereas gram negative bacteria causing acute pyelonephritis can lead to TIN. Patient characteristics, time elapsed post transplantation, immunosuppression regimen/exposure and histologic features can aid in distinguishing these etiologies, in addition to specific microbiologic data. In this section, our focus will be on viral causes of TIN in renal allografts.

3.1 Cytomegalovirus Associated TIN

The predominant risk factor for CMV infection is the CMV serologic status of the donor(D)/recipient(R) pair. There is substantial risk of CMV reactivation in both CMV D+/R- and CMV D+/R+ patients, but CMV D+/R- patients are at higher risk of developing CMV infection than CMV R+ patients- reflecting that the source of majority of CMV infections is a seropositive donor. In patients with CMV reactivation, peak CMV loads are highest among CMV D+/R- patients. The incidence of these infections has significantly reduced with widespread adoption of CMV prophylaxis during the early post-transplant phase.

3.2 Presentation

CMV associated TIN is usually a manifestation of tissue invasive CMV disease (clinical signs and symptoms of end organ disease) as opposed to CMV syndrome (presence of detectable viral replication in blood without invasive tissue disease).

Patients with TIN can present with fever, generalized malaise, arthralgia, leukopenia, and thrombocytopenia, with evidence of elevation of creatinine with or without abnormalities on urinalysis. Symptoms of other organ involvement could be evident and present as following:

1. Meningitis/encephalitis: headache, altered mental status; with demonstration of CMV in the cerebrospinal fluid.

2. Pneumonitis: cough, dyspnea; evidence interstitial infiltrates on radiologic imaging and demonstration of CMV in bronchial-alveolar lavage.
3. Gastrointestinal: nausea, vomiting and abdominal pain (colitis/enteritis, pancreatitis, hepatitis); elevation of lipase/amylase, alanine aminotransferase (ALT) and aspartate aminotransferase (AST).

The serum/blood fluid and tissue demonstration of the virus is important for diagnosis of CMV associated TIN, especially given high degree overlap of histologic features with rejection, drugs and other infectious processes. Tests of such as nucleic acid testing (NAT) using polymerase chain reaction (PCR) for CMV DNA is recommended over serologic testing or cell cultures.

CMV infection is associated with morbidity, allograft failure, and death in kidney transplant recipients.

3.3 Pathology

A scattered pleomorphic infiltrate with lymphocytes, plasma cells, and macrophages is present. Tubulitis occurs with characteristic intranuclear glassy-appearing basophilic inclusions with surrounding halo (owl's eye-type inclusion) and marked increase in the size of the cell (cytomegaly), particularly in tubular epithelial cells and in endothelial cells. A specific diagnosis is confirmed by immunohistochemical staining for CMV.

Acute TCMR-associated TIN can be distinguished from CMV by absence of viral cytopathic changes or positive CMV staining. Other viruses are diagnosed by specific immunohistochemistry or in situ hybridization.

3.4 Treatment

The treatment of CMV associated TIN is centered on reduction of immunosuppression and anti-viral treatment. Typically, cessation of anti-metabolites (mycophenolate mofetil or azathioprine) until completion of anti-viral therapy and eradication of the virus with re-initiation of lower doses only in those with very risk of rejection or recurrent glomerulonephritis with subsequent post-treatment monitoring of CMV is used. Commonly secondary prophylaxis with oral valganciclovir is used for 1–3 months.

3.5 BK Virus-Associated TIN

A member of the polyomavirus family, BK virus is present in renal tubular epithelial and uroepithelial cells devoid of any associated clinical consequences in the majority of individuals, with a worldwide seroprevalence of 80–90%. In immunocompromised hosts, its reactivation predominantly causes renal manifestations involving kidney, ureter, and bladder. Renal injury is mainly manifested histologically by TIN, with viral replication most commonly occurring in the first-year post engraftment. Based on multiple studies, it is estimated that 1–10% of kidney transplant recipients will develop BK virus associated nephropathy (BKVAN), with highest incidence being 2–6 months post transplantation.

3.5.1 Presentation

The earliest manifestation of BK virus infection is asymptomatic viruria (35%)-detected only on screening. The majority of cases do not progress to viremia, with viruria being a sensitive marker progression to BKVAN albeit non-specific. Viruria is followed by an asymptomatic viremia (15%), which if sustained (longer than 5 weeks), portends to a greater predictive value for development of BKVAN. The sensitivity, specificity, positive predictive value, and negative predictive values of a urine level of >9.5 log10 copies/mL were 70%, 70%, 53% and 83% for any viremia, and 91%, 66%, 33% and 98% for sustained viremia. TIN associated with BKVAN most commonly presents as asymptomatic elevation of creatinine with or without abnormal urinalysis. Urine microscopy may reveal renal tubular or uroepithelial cells containing intranuclear viral inclusions termed as decoy cells. Hemorrhagic cystitis and ureteral stenosis are rare manifestation of BK viral infection.

Unrelenting infection is associated with progressive allograft dysfunction and graft loss over period of months. Registry data showed that 3-year graft survival was significantly lower in recipients with BK nephropathy.

3.5.2 Pathology

The histology of BKVAN is represented by a patchy pleomorphic interstitial infiltrate with lymphocytes, plasma cells, and occasional neutrophils with accompanied interstitial edema, tubulitis, and tubular injury. The infected tubular epithelial cells have enlarged nuclei with amorphous inclusions, with a ground-glass appearance with irregular central clearing, or a coarse vesicular appearance. BKVAN associated TIN has a predilection for distal tubules are involved more often than proximal tubules.

Medullary involvement in may be present in early stages, with subsequent affliction of parietal epithelial cells. Infected epithelial cell nuclei stain with antibody to the large T antigen of the SV40 virus, which serves as a surrogate marker of human polyomavirus infection (Fig. 3). Positive staining may be seen in the absence of nuclear enlargement or inclusions.

On immunofluorescence microscopy, the tubular basement membrane (TBM) demonstrates granular staining for IgG, C3, and C4d may be present in up to 10–25% of cases. Polyomavirus particles (30–45 nm) are present in nuclei of infected cells, in a reticulate arrangement may be present on electron microscopy, with immune complex–type deposits are present along TBM (Latif et al. 199–207).

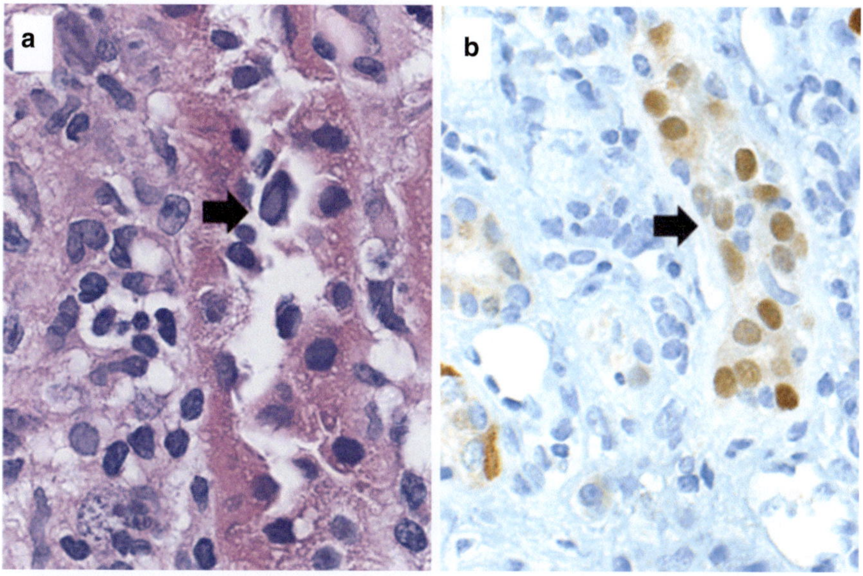

Fig. 3 BK polyoma virus nephropathy. (**a**) basophilic nuclear inclusion in a tubular cell (arrow). (**b**) Immunostain for SV40 is positive in the nucleus of tubular cells infected by BK virus. (Image courtesy of Dr. Serena Bagnasco)

3.5.3 Treatment

Reduction of immunosuppression in a stepwise fashion, as dictated by viral loads, is the initial recommended treatment in patients without concomitant rejection. This approach consists of immediate and indefinite discontinuation of the anti-metabolite, with subsequent reduction of the calcineurin inhibitor for sustained viremia which has been shown to be safe and effective up to 10 years after transplantation. Other adjunctive treatments include intravenous immunoglobulin given immunomodulatory properties. The use of cidofovir, leflunomide and quinolone antibiotics have been shown not to have clinical efficacy.

3.6 Adenovirus Associated TIN

The human adenovirus infection in patients with kidney transplants is usually a consequence of latent disease activation, with environmental or donor organ transmission being reported. Urinary tract involvement occurs in 5% of kidney transplant recipients. Of those with disease, onset was within the first 3 months in 75% of the patients, and 97% were reported within 1 year. Allograft involvement, manifested by severe granulomatous TIN, occurs in <1%.

3.6.1 Presentation

Initial presentation of an adenovirus-associated TIN is characterized by symptoms of a urinary tract infection. There is concomitant elevation of serum creatinine with sterile pyuria. Hemorrhagic cystitis is usually accompanied by allograft dysfunction. Confirmatory diagnostic testing involves adenovirus PCR quantification in urine and tissue biopsy.

Disseminated disease portends to high mortality. It can be present with extra-renal manifestations such as lymphopenia, pneumonitis, gastroenteritis and orchitis.

3.6.2 Pathology

Adenovirus associated TIN is evidenced by pleomorphic infiltrate composed of lymphocytes, histiocytes, plasma cells, and variable numbers of neutrophils, with interstitial edema and hemorrhage (Fig. 4). In addition, viral cytopathic changes comprise of smudgy basophilic intranuclear inclusions with enlarged nuclei of infected cells. Similar to BK, the virus has a propensity to effect distal tubules (medulla) in comparison to proximal tubules. Concomitant acute tubular injury is present with frank tubular necrosis and may be associated with necrotizing interstitial granulomas. Severe granulomatous TIN is characteristic of adenovirus infection and is unlikely to be present with CMV and BK infections. Focal wedge-shaped necrosis may occur in renal parenchyma. Immunostaining for adenovirus shows strong nuclear and cytoplasmic staining in infected cells. With respect to electron microscopy, viral particles are seen in infected epithelial nuclei and cytoplasm and are nonenveloped with hexagonal outline and a diameter of 70–110 nm, aggregated in a crystalline array.

3.6.3 Treatment

The treatment is similar to the stepwise approach of reduction in immunosuppression employed in BKVAN. Severe disseminated disease may require treatment with cidofovir, which requires close monitoring of renal and hematological indices. Cidofovir has activity against all adenovirus serotypes and has also been used in combination with intravenous immunoglobulin.

4 Conclusion

It is the imperative for transplant physicians to be able to distinguish between various causes of TIN. The spectrum of rejection to infection encompasses most of the pathologies that are encountered in transplant medicine in general. Being cognizant of distinguishing features of various presentations of TIN aids in expedient diagnosis and treatment, which in turn, leads to reduction in probability of short- and long-term graft dysfunction.

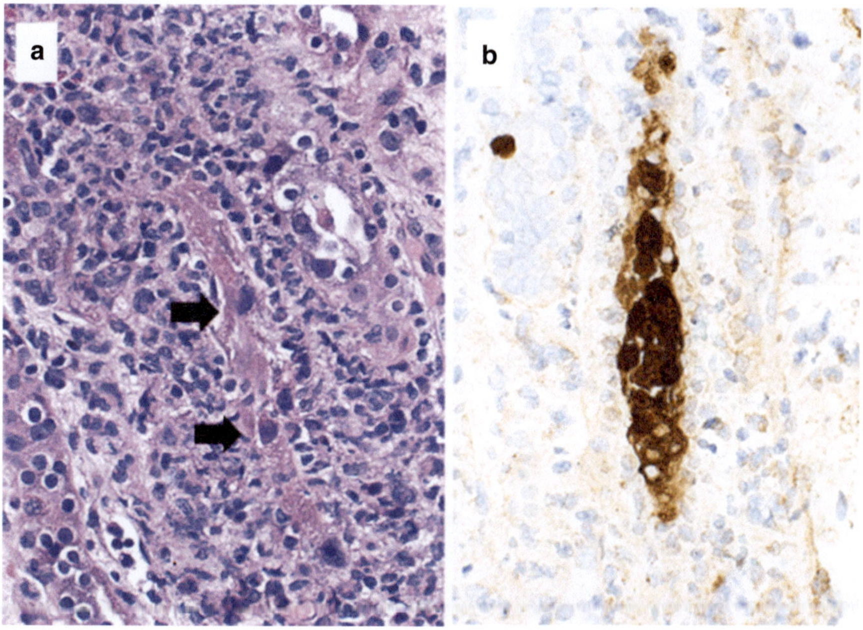

Fig. 4 Adenovirus infection. (**a**) An infected tubule shows tubular cells with a washed-out appearance, large nuclei without inclusion (arrows) and is surrounded by inflammatory cells including neutrophils (H&E, 160X). (**b**) Immunostain for Adenovirus show strong staining in nucleus and cytoplasm of infected tubular cells (160X). (Image courtesy of Dr. Serena Bagnasco)

Suggested Reading

Bloom RD, et al. Cell-free DNA and active rejection in kidney allografts. J Am Soc Nephrol. 2017;28(7):2221–32.

Brennan DC, et al. Incidence of BK with tacrolimus versus cyclosporine and impact of preemptive immunosuppression reduction. Am J Transplant. 2005;5(3):582–94.

Dharnidharka VR, Cherikh WS, Abbott KC. An OPTN analysis of national registry data on treatment of BK virus allograft nephropathy in the United States. Transplantation. 2009;87(7):1019–26.

Doyle AM, Lechler RI, Turka LA. Organ transplantation: halfway through the first century. J Am Soc Nephrol. 2004;15(12):2965–71.

Fogo AB, et al. AJKD atlas of renal pathology: cytomegalovirus infection. Am J Kidney Dis. 2016;68(6):e35–6.

Hardinger KL, et al. BK-virus and the impact of pre-emptive immunosuppression reduction: 5-year results. Am J Transplant. 2010;10(2):407–15.

Hart A, et al. OPTN/SRTR 2017 annual data report: kidney. Am J Transplant. 2019;19(S2):19–123.

Hartmann A, Sagedal S, Hjelmesoeth J. The natural course of cytomegalovirus infection and disease in renal transplant recipients. Hagerstown: Lippincott; 2006. p. S15–7.

Hatlen T, et al. Disseminated adenovirus nephritis after kidney transplantation. Kidney Int Rep. 2018;3(1):19–23.

Hirsch HH, et al. Prospective study of polyomavirus type BK replication and nephropathy in renal-transplant recipients. N Engl J Med. 2002;347(7):488–96.

Hofland CA, Eron LJ, Washecka RM. Hemorrhagic adenovirus cystitis after renal transplantation. Transplant Proc. 2004;36(10):3025–7.

Kean JM, et al. Seroepidemiology of human polyomaviruses. PLoS Pathog. 2009;5(3):e1000363.
Khoury JA, et al. Prophylactic versus preemptive oral valganciclovir for the management of cytomegalovirus infection in adult renal transplant recipients. Am J Transplant. 2006;6(9):2134–43.
Kincaid-Smith P. Histological diagnosis of rejection of renal homografts in man. The Lancet (British edition). 1967;2(7521):849–52.
Knowles WA, et al. Population-based study of antibody to the human polyomaviruses BKV and JCV and the simian polyomavirus SV40. J Med Virol. 2003;71(1):115–23.
Kozlowski T, Nickeleit V, Andreoni K. Donor-transmitted adenovirus infection causing kidney allograft nephritis and graft loss. Transpl Infect Dis. 2011;13(2):168–73.
Lamarche C, et al. Efficacy of acute cellular rejection treatment according to banff score in kidney transplant recipients: a systematic review. Transplant Direct. 2016;2(12):e115.
Latif S, et al. BK polyomavirus in renal transplants: role of electron microscopy and immunostaining in detecting early infection. Ultrastruct Pathol. 2007;31(3):199–207.
Lion T. Adenovirus infections in immunocompetent and immunocompromised patients. Clin Microbiol Rev. 2014;27(3):441–62.
Lusco MA, et al. AJKD atlas of renal pathology: polyomavirus nephropathy. Am J Kidney Dis. 2016;68(6):e37–8.
Lusco MA, et al. AJKD atlas of renal pathology: adenovirus infection. Am J Kidney Dis. 2018;71(1):e1–2.
Madden K, et al. Prediction of BK viremia by urine viral load in renal transplant patients: an analysis of BK viral load results in paired urine and plasma samples. Transpl Infect Dis. 2018;20(5):e12952.
Naesens M, et al. The histology of kidney transplant failure: a long-term follow-up study. Transplantation. 2014;98(4):427–35.
Nankivell BJ, et al. BK virus nephropathy: histological evolution by sequential pathology. Am J Transplant. 2017;17(8):2065–77.
Nickeleit V, et al. BK-virus nephropathy in renal transplants-tubular necrosis, MHC-class II expression and rejection in a puzzling game. Nephrol Dial Transplant. 2000;15(3):324–32.
Pham PTT, Nast, et al. Diagnosis and therapy of graft dysfunction. In: Periera BJG, Sayegh MH, Blake P, editors. Chronic kidney disease, dialysis and transplantation, vol. 2. Philadelphia: Elsevier Saunders; 2005. p. 641.
Sagedal S, et al. Impact of early cytomegalovirus infection and disease on long-term recipient and kidney graft survival. Kidney Int. 2004;66(1):329–37.
Schold JD, et al. Treatment for BK virus: incidence, risk factors and outcomes for kidney transplant recipients in the United States. Transpl Int. 2009;22(6):626–34.
Seifert ME, et al. Polyomavirus reactivation and immune responses to kidney-specific self-antigens in transplantation. J Am Soc Nephrol. 2017;28(4):1314–25.
Solez K, et al. International standardization of criteria for the histologic diagnosis of renal allograft rejection: the Banff working classification of kidney transplant pathology. Kidney Int. 1993;44(2):411–22.
Watcharananan SP, et al. Adenovirus disease after kidney transplantation: course of infection and outcome in relation to blood viral load and immune recovery. Am J Transplant. 2011;11(6):1308–14.
Wehmeier C, et al. Donor specificity but not broadness of sensitization is associated with antibody-mediated rejection and graft loss in renal allograft recipients. Am J Transplant. 2017;17(8):2092–102.
Woodle ES, et al. Tacrolimus therapy for refractory acute renal allograft rejection: definition of the histologic response by protocol biopsies. Transplantation. 1996;62(7):906–10.
Wu K, et al. The relationship of the severity and category of acute rejection with intimal arteritis defined in Banff classification to clinical outcomes. Transplantation. 2015;99(8):e105–14.

Part IV
Causes of non-Immune Mediated Tubulointerstitial Nephritis

Genetic Diseases Associated with Tubulointerstitial Nephritis

Matthias T. F. Wolf, Whitney Besse, Anthony J. Bleyer, and Neera K. Dahl

Genetic forms of tubulointerstitial kidney disease are an important cause of tubulointerstitial disease and may be more prevalent than currently recognized. Early diagnosis can help prevent inappropriate use of immunosuppressive therapy, help focus on extrarenal manifestations, and facilitate earlier planning for kidney transplantation.

1 Autosomal Dominant Tubulointerstitial Kidney Disease (ADTKD)

ADTKD is a clinical syndrome attributable to heterozygous mutations in at least 5 genes (Table 1). Clinical characteristics of ADTKD are shown in Table 2.

M. T. F. Wolf
Pediatric Nephrology, University of Texas Southwestern Medical Center, Dallas, TX, USA
e-mail: Matthias.Wolf@UTSouthwestern.edu

W. Besse · N. K. Dahl (✉)
Section of Nephrology, Yale School of Medicine, New Haven, CT, USA
e-mail: whitney.besse@yale.edu; neera.dahl@yale.edu

A. J. Bleyer
Section in Nephrology, Wake Forest School of Medicine, Winston-Salem, NC, USA
e-mail: ableyer@wakehealth.edu

M. G. Atta, M. A. Perazella (eds.), *Tubulointerstitial Nephritis*,
https://doi.org/10.1007/978-3-030-93438-5_11

Table 1 Clinical, laboratory, and pathological findings for the genetically-defined forms of ADTKD

Subclassification	ADTKD-*UMOD*	ADTKD-*MUC1*	ADTKD-*REN*	ADTKD-*HNF1B*	ADTKD-*SEC61A1*
Chromosome	16q12	1q22	1q32	17q12	3q21.3
OMIM ID	603860/191845	174000/158340	613092/179820	614227/189907	617056/609213
Clinical (additional findings beyond kidney disease are variable)	Early onset of gout Slow progressive CKD	No specific findings May have gout Slow progressive CKD	Mild hypotension, Risk for AKI↑ Slow progressive CKD Anemia	May have CAKUT Polyuria-polydipsia CKD in childhood in severe forms Diabetes Hyperparathyroidism Hypomagnesiumia Gout Genital abnormalities If 17q12 rearrangement, developmental, learning and psychiatric problems	Growth retardation, neutropenia, recurrent skin infections, congenital anemia, small, dysplastic, possibly cystic kidneys
Tissue expression	Kidney, TAL and DCT	Secretory epithelia (lungs, stomach, intestine, kidney)	Kidney (juxtaglomerular apparatus)	Kidney, pancreas, liver, lung, intestine, urogenital tract	Ubiquitous
Protein function	Uromodulin regulates ion channel transport, BP, urinary concentration, May protect against kidney stones & UTIs Regulation of innate immunity. Null mouse model without significant histologic consequence.	Mucin-1 plays a role in protection of epithelial barrier, immunomodulation, and signal transduction. Null mouse model without significant consequence if unperturbed. Pathogenic protein is a Mucin-1 with specific frameshift peptide (Muc1-fs)	Protease, cleaves angiotensinogen Role in renal development BP regulation	Transcription factor Involved in organ development (kidney, genital tract, pancreas, liver, lung, gut)	The major component of the SEC61 channel-forming complex which mediates, transport of protein precursors across the ER membrane.

Laboratory findings	Uric acid ↑ FEUrat <5%		Uric acid ↑ Hgb ↓ K^+↑	Uric acid ↑ Mg^{2+}↓ K^+ ↓ Abnormal LFTs Hyperparathyroidism	Anemia Neutropenia
Imaging	Occasional renal cysts	Occasional renal cysts	Small to normal-sized kidneys	Pre- and postnatal increased renal echogenicity Renal cysts Pancreatic hypoplasia Extra-renal cysts (liver, pancreas))	Small, dysplastic kidneys
Onset in childhood	Rare	Rare	Common	Common	Common
Histology	Intracellular accumulation of UMOD in TAL	Intracellular accumulation of MUC1-fs in distal nephron	Intracellular accumulation and/or impaired renin function in/from cells of the juxtaglomerular apparatus	Small-normal kidneys Dysplastic kidneys Glomerulocystic kidney disease	Multiple small foci of tubulointerstitial lesions and a glomerulocystic pattern

(continued)

Table 1 (continued)

Subclassification	ADTKD-*UMOD*	ADTKD-*MUC1*	ADTKD-*REN*	ADTKD-*HNF1B*	ADTKD-*SEC61A1*
Previously used terminology	Medullary cystic kidney disease type 2 Uromodulin-associated kidney disease (UAKD) Familial juvenile hyperuricemic nephropathy (FJHN) Uromodulin kidney disease Hereditary interstitial kidney disease Glomerulocystic kidney disease	Medullary cystic kidney disease type 1 Mucin-1 kidney disease Hereditary interstitial kidney disease	Familial juvenile hyperuricemic nephropathy Hereditary interstitial kidney disease	MODY5 (maturity onset diabetes mellitus of the young type 5) RCAD (renal cyst and diabetes syndrome) Familial juvenile hyperuricemic nephropathy Hereditary interstitial kidney disease	N/A
Genetic mutations	Heterozygous specific non-truncating mutations that impair maturation. Not caused by truncating/loss of function mutations.	Heterozygous specific frameshift mutations in VNTR region that replaces C-terminus of Mucin-1 with a frameshift peptide. Not caused by truncating/loss of function mutations.	Heterozygous. Mutations early in gene may have different effect that those late in gene	Heterozygous loss of function or deleterious mutations.	Heterozygous missense mutations reported. Too few reported cases to define spectrum.

AKI acute kidney injury, *BP* blood pressure, *DCT* distal convoluted tubule, *ER* endoplasmic reticulum, *FEUrat* fractional excretion of uric acid, *HNF1B* hepatocyte nuclear factor 1B, K^+ potassium, *LFT* liver function test, Mg^{2+} magnesium, *MUC1* Mucin-1, *REN* Renin; *SEC61A1* α1 subunit of transport protein SEC61, *TAL* thick ascending limb, *UMOD* Uromodulin; *VNTR* variable number of tandem repeats

Table 2 Characteristics of ADTKD

Autosomal dominant inheritance
Bland urine sediment
No proteinuria or only mild proteinuria
Progressive worsening of chronic kidney disease
Early-onset hyperuricemia or gout
Lack of significant hypertension in early stages
Urinary concentration defect, with polydipsia-polyuria in severe forms
Enuresis or nocturia in children
Early chronic kidney disease in severe forms in children
Normal or small-sized kidneys
Lack of exposure to medications causing tubulointerstitial nephritis

1.1 Clinical Description

ADTKD is characterized by elevated serum creatinine, family history of kidney disease, bland urine sediment, and normal to small kidneys, with—or more often without bilateral cysts on imaging. It should also be considered in the absence of family history when other causes of non-glomerular progressive kidney disease are excluded or when extrarenal features consistent with ADTKD genetic subtypes such as gout or anemia are noted. End-stage kidney disease (ESKD) has been reported in young children in ADTKD-*UMOD* but more commonly impaired kidney function is diagnosed in adolescence or early adulthood and ESKD occurs after age 30. Median age of ESKD is in the fifth decade for ADTKD-*UMOD* and ADTKD-*MUC1* and may be similar for other forms. A urinary concentration defect which can lead to enuresis is frequently present in cases of ADTKD-*UMOD*. This may contribute to mild, sub-clinical, chronic volume depletion that results in enhanced proximal tubule fluid and uric acid reabsorption, low fractional excretion of uric acid (FE_{Urate}) <5%, hyperuricemia and gout. Gout is a common finding in ADTKD, particularly in ADTKD-*UMOD*, ADTKD-*REN*, and ADTKD-*HNF1B,* and can present in childhood prior to the diagnosis of kidney disease. Gout occurs earlier in ADTKD-*UMOD* than in ADTKD-*MUC1* patients (30 vs. 67 years). There are no other extrarenal manifestations of ADTKD-*UMOD* or ADTKD-*MUC1*.

ADTKD is one of multiple potential phenotypes that can result from heterozygous *HNF1B* mutations (Table 3). ADTKD-*HNF1B*, a progressive tubulointerstitial kidney disease, typically manifests with bilateral kidney cysts, gout, hypomagnesemia and may have additional extra-renal manifestations. Extreme forms of ADTKD-*HNF1B* can present in utero with oligohydramnios, Potter's sequence, and severely enlarged polycystic kidneys that may resemble autosomal dominant or recessive polycystic kidney disease. This may be explained through the transcriptional role of HNF1β as a master regulator of *PKHD1* and *PKD2* genes. Milder forms may be diagnosed in adulthood and progress slowly. *HNF1B*-related extra-renal

Table 3 Kidney and extra-renal manifestations of *HNF1β* patients[a]

Organ	Comments
Kidney Bilateral hyperechogenic kidneys Bilateral cysts Glomerulocystic disease Multicystic dysplastic kidney Single kidney Horseshoe kidney Oligomeganephronia Hydronephrosis and megaureter Chronic kidney disease Hypomagnesemia Hypokalemia Chromophobe renal carcinoma (exceptional)	Most frequent cause of kidney dysplasia of monogenic origin Normal or small sized kidneys Amniotic fluid preserved in prenatal ultrasound Renal failure in adults, rare in children Electrolyte disorders mainly in adults
Development-psycho Epilepsy Autism spectrum disorder Developmental delay	Present when *HNF1β* loss is associated with 17q12 rearrangement
Genital Bicornate uterus Uterus didelphys Double vagina Vaginal hypoplasia & absent uterus Cryptorchidism Hypospadias Epididymal cysts Agenesis of the vas deferens	Mayer-Rokitansky-Küster-Hauser syndrome cases in *HNF1β* deletions
Endocrine Early-onset diabetes (MODY-5) New-onset diabetes after transplantation Pancreatic cysts Hypoplastic pancreatic body and tail Hyperparathyroidism	<5% of MODY-type diabetes Anticalcineuric drugs down-regulate HNF1β
Digestive Pancreatic exocrine dysfunction Elevated liver enzymes (common) Neonatal cholestasis (rare)	Casual finding, most patients asymptomatic
Others Early-onset gout (hyperuricemia)	Gout precedes chronic kidney disease

[a]Modified from Attanasio M et al. (2007)

manifestations include pancreatic hypoplasia, maturity onset diabetes of young type 5 (MODY5), abnormal liver function tests, hyperparathyroidism, and gynecologic structural abnormalities. *HNF1B* mutations were found to explain the previously named renal cysts and diabetes syndrome (RCAD). Affected family members may have a varied presentation. For example, one family member may be asymptomatic, another family member may have hypomagnesemia and diabetes, and another family member may have gout and chronic kidney disease.

HNF1B mutations may alternatively result in congenital anomalies of the kidney and urinary tract (CAKUT). This may include renal hypoplasia, agenesis, multicystic dysplastic kidneys, glomerulocystic kidney disease, horseshoe kidneys, and Müllerian duct abnormalities. When *HNF1B* loss is part of an approximately 1.5 MB microdeletion syndrome of chromosome 17q12, additional features including autism, attention-deficit/hyperactivity disorder (ADHD), and facial dysmorphism can also be seen.

ADTKD-*REN* is characterized by a slowly progressive chronic kidney disease, with most individuals proceeding to end-stage kidney disease after age 45 years, despite presenting in early childhood with CKD. Decreased production of normal renin results in mild hypotension, hyperkalemia, acidemia, hyperuricemia, and anemia. Many of the clinical manifestations of this disorder can be treated with fludrocortisone.

ADTKD-*SEC61A1* is a rare cause of ADTKD, with only two families described in the literature. Extrarenal features of one ADTKD-*SEC61A1* family included congenital anemia, intrauterine growth retardation, and variable findings of cleft palate, velo-pharyngeal insufficiency, pre-axial polydactyly, and mild cognitive impairment. The second family had diagnosis of CKD at a later age and neutropenia with recurrent cutaneous abscesses. Like ADTKD-*REN*, some cases had gout, and some showed evidence of hyperkalemia with inappropriately low renin and aldosterone when assayed.

1.2 Kidney Biopsy

Kidney biopsies show interstitial fibrosis, tubular atrophy, and thickened tubular basement membrane. Immunohistochemistry may show intracellular accumulation of the mutant protein, or in the case of ADTKD-*REN* reduced renin in the juxtaglomerular apparatus.

1.3 Epidemiology

The true prevalence of ADTKD remains unclear. ADTKD-*UMOD* accounted for 35.1% of ADTKD cases in one large cohort study, with ADTKD-*MUC1* accounting for 38.4% of UMOD-negative cases. *HNF1B*, *REN*, and particularly *SEC61A1* are more rare causes of ADTKD; together they explain an undefined fraction of the remaining 30–40% of cases. In a cohort of 3315 patient with chronic kidney disease (CKD), 65% of whom had ESKD, 9.3% of all patients were found to have a monogenetic etiology, and *UMOD* was the sixth most common gene affected, explaining 0.3% of the cohort. A study from England estimated that ADTKD-*UMOD* contributes to 1% of all CKD stage 3–5 patients, 2% of all ESKD, 9% of inherited kidney disease, and 56% of ADTKD, with an estimated population prevalence of 16 per million for ADTKD and 9 per million for ADTKD-*UMOD*. These data make ADTKD the most common monogenetic kidney disease after ADPKD and collagen IV-related diseases. Overcoming challenges with molecular diagnosis, clinician recognition, and discovering additional disease genes will help to clarify the prevalence of this disease.

1.4 Pathophysiology

ADTKD-*UMOD*, ADTKD-*MUC1*, ADTKD-*REN*, and possibly other forms of ADTKD have intracellular accumulation of abnormal forms of highly expressed proteins and thus may be considered protein storage diseases. Uromodulin, also known as Tamm Horsfall protein, encoded by *UMOD,* is the most abundant protein in human urine. *UMOD* is highly expressed in the thick ascending loop of Henle (TAL) and early distal convoluted tubule (DCT). Approximately 60% of all pathogenic *UMOD* mutations affect cysteine residues and therefore potentially affect disulfide bonds. Mucin-1, encoded by the *MUC1* gene, is a heavily glycosylated protein strongly expressed along the distal nephron that can form polymers in the urine. Normally uromodulin and mucin-1 undergo membrane anchoring, folding, glycosylation, and quality control assessment in the endoplasmic reticulum (ER) and Golgi apparatus before trafficking to the apical membrane where a final extracellular fragment is cleaved into the urine. Mutant uromodulin, or mucin-1 with a modified C-terminus (MUC1-fs) accumulate in cells. Further, mutant uromodulin has a dominant negative effect on wild-type uromodulin from the unaffected allele. *In vitro*, as well as mouse models of ADTKD, pathogenic mutations in *Umod* or *Muc1* show activation of the unfolded protein response (UPR) pathway, ER stress, and at least in the case of *Umod* models, mitochondrial dysfunction. This is accompanied by transcriptional evidence of upregulation of inflammatory and fibrotic pathways.

ADTKD-*REN* results in intracellular accumulation of abnormal renin, leading to ER stress, and subsequent apoptosis. Subtypes have been defined based on whether the pathogenic mutation affects the signal peptide, pro-segment, or mature protein. Mutations in the mature protein have later onset of ESKD (mean age 63) without the anemia commonly seen in other forms. Extrarenal manifestations are attributable to impaired renin response to physiologic stimuli. Renin is an activator of the RAAS and is important during kidney development, blood pressure regulation, thirst regulation, and modification of erythropoiesis. Renin-producing cells enhance erythropoietin secretion.

SEC61A1 encodes the core protein of the mammalian heteromeric ER translocation pore (translocon) through which newly generated secretory proteins enter the ER lumen and ER membrane. ADTKD-*SEC61A1* cases with missense variants had mislocalization of SEC61A1 protein in the ER-Golgi intermediate compartment (ERGIC) and in the Golgi apparatus. A dysfunctional translocon may contribute to abnormal conformation, post-translational modifications, and trafficking of secretory proteins including uromodulin, mucin-1, and renin. Truncating variants in *SEC61A1* are reported to cause monogenic plasma cell deficiency or severe congenital neutropenia.

HNF1B, also known as *TCF2*, encodes the Hepatocyte nuclear factor 1β (HNF1β). ADTKD-*HNF1B* pathology is notably not due to protein accumulation, but from heterozygous loss of function, deleterious, or deletion mutations resulting in haploinsufficiency. HNF1β is a DNA-binding transcription factor which regulates tissue-specific gene expression particularly during development of the kidney, the pancreas, genital organs, and to a lesser extent liver, during embryogenesis. HNF1β is required for branching morphogenesis, nephrogenesis, nephron patterning, and tubulogenesis;. Kidney-specific loss of *Hnf1b* in mice results in polycystic kidney disease. Moreover, HNF1β is involved in epithelial-mesenchyme transition (EMT) pathways, Wnt signaling, and kidney fibrosis via the *TWIST2* transcriptional network, and abnormal TGF-β as has been shown in other forms of ADTKD.

1.5 Molecular Genetic Diagnosis

UMOD, MUC1, REN, HNF1B, and *SEC61A1* are responsible for approximately two thirds of clinically suspected ADTKD cases, with other genetic causes yet to be identified. Typical next-generation sequencing-based methods, such as targeted gene panels or whole exome sequencing, reliably identify pathogenic variants in each of these genes except for pathogenic *MUC1* variants. The most common pathogenic *MUC1* variant is a cytosine duplication in the variable number of tandem repeats (VNTR) region of the gene that results in a specific frameshift peptide (MUC1-fs). Because this is not detected by usual methods, *MUC1* clinical genetic testing is typically performed only after a negative ADTKD gene panel. MUC1 genetic testing is available without cost from the Broad Institute. Contact ableyer@wakehealth.edu for information.

For ADTKD-*UMOD*, biopsy detection of intracellular uromodulin or reduction of urinary uromodulin has also been proposed; the former may not be reliable, however the latter is recommended in an algorithm for UMOD-score. Penetrance for the most well studied forms of ADTKD, ADTKD-*UMOD* and ADTKD-*MUC1*, is typically close to 100%. *De novo* variants in ADTKD genes may explain cases with apparent negative family history and are seen in up to 40% of all *HNF1B* -related cases. In cases where the pattern of inheritance is unknown, genetic causes of adolescent forms of nephronophthisis should also be considered.

Decision making regarding genetic testing of children with this disorder is complex, and input from a genetics counselor is important. In general, children should not undergo genetic testing for disorders in which there are no specific treatments available. Thus, for ADTKD-*MUC1* and families with a later clinical presentation of ADTKD-*UMOD*, genetic testing should wait until the individual can fully participate in decision making. For ADTKD-*UMOD*, genetic testing may be performed in childhood to prevent gout. For ADTKD-*REN*, genetic testing is advisable in childhood due to many potential therapies. Genetic testing should also be considered for ADTKD-*HNF1B*, since early detection of extrarenal manifestations can be beneficial. As *HNF1B* can occur as part of the 17q12 deletion syndrome, a chromosomal microarray, multiplex ligation-dependent probe amplification (MLPA), or careful copy number variation analysis of high read depth next-generation sequencing is required.

1.6 Therapies

Currently no specific therapies for ADTKD are available. Allopurinol for hyperuricemia and gout in ADTKD may slow disease progression but low purine diets are not recommended. *In vitro* studies showed colchicine, probenecid, topiroxostat, and the chaperone and ER-stress reducer Na^+-4-phenylbutyrate (4-PBA) partially rescued accumulation of mutant uromodulin. The effect of 4-PBA could not be confirmed *in vivo*. Blocking the TNF-α signaling improved kidney function compared to untreated mutant mice. Topiroxostat, a xanthine oxidase inhibitor reduced apoptosis. Inhibitors of the mTOR pathway enhance autophagy and secretion of mutant UMOD. For ADTKD-*MUC1*, a small molecule named BRD4780 was shown to enhance secretion of MUC1-fs secretion by targeting a cargo receptor called TMED9.

ADTKD-*HNF1B* patients may need treatment of hyperuricemia, hypomagnesemia, pancreatic dysfunction, and genital tract malformations. ADTKD-*HNF1B* patients may have a higher risk of new-onset diabetes after a kidney transplant (NODAT) as hypomagnesemia is an independent risk factor for NODAT. These patients may benefit from other immunosuppression strategies such as belatacept, steroid-sparing regimens, or mTOR inhibitors.

ADTKD-*REN* and ADTKD-*SEC61A1* patients benefit from erythropoietin therapy to addresses anemia, and in some cases fludrocortisone to address volume depletion, acidosis, and hyperkalemia due to insufficient renin. During puberty anemia often improves due to increased synthesis of sexual steroids. There is no risk of recurrence of the underlying kidney disease following kidney transplant in ADTKD.

2 Nephronophthisis

Nephonophthisis (NPHP) is an autosomal recessive kidney disease and one of the most common genetic reasons for ESKD in the pediatric cohort. Over 20 disease genes, encoding proteins known as nephrocystins contribute to this disease complex. Nearly all nephrocystins localize to the membrane-bound sensory organelle known as the primary cilium, or its associated centrosome or basal body. As such, NPHP is classified as a ciliopathy.

2.1 Epidemiology and Clinical Description

The reported incidence of NPHP varies from 1 in 50,000 to one in a million. Patients typically present with profound anemia, a urinary concentration defect with polyuria and polydipsia, sometimes secondary enuresis, and short stature. Onset of CKD is subtle and NPHP is often only diagnosed when patients present with symptoms of ESKD. The majority of NPHP patients have only kidney involvement. However, 15–20% of all NPHP patients present with a multi-organ disease involving, the eyes, liver, heart, CNS, or bones (Table 4) reflecting the role of the unique nephrocystin in the cilia during development and maintenance of ciliary function. Extrarenal symptoms can include retinal degeneration (with Senior-Løken syndrome, which is the most common extrarenal manifestation with 10–15%), cerebellar vermis aplasia (Joubert syndrome), bone-related phenotypes (Mainzer-Saldino,

Table 4 Extrarenal manifestations associated with NPHP and resulting syndromes associated with *NPHP* mutations

Ophthalmologic disorder	**Syndrome**
Retinitis pigmentosa	Senior-Løken syndrome (SLSN) Arima syndrome (cerebro-oculo-hepato-renal syndrome) Alstrom (RP, obesity, DM type 2, hearing impairment) RHYNS (RP, hypopituitarism, skeletal dysplasia)
Oculomotor apraxia Nystagmus Coloboma	Cogan syndrome Joubert syndrome/Joubert syndrome related disorders Joubert syndrome/Joubert syndrome related disorders
Skeletal disorder Short ribs Cone-shaped epiphysis Postaxial polydactyly	Jeune syndrome/asphyxiating thoracic dystrophy Mainzer-Saldino syndrome Joubert syndrome/Joubert syndrome related disorders Bardet-Biedl syndrome (NPHP, RP, obesity, deafness) Ellis van Creveld
Skeletal dysplasia	Sensenbrenner syndrome / cranioectodermal dysplasia Ellis van Creveld
Hepatic disorder Liver fibrosis	Boichis syndrome Meckel-Gruber syndrome (occipital encephaolocele, NPHP) Arima syndrome (cerebro-oculo-hepato-renal syndrome) Joubert syndrome/Joubert syndrome related disorders Meckel-Gruber syndrome (occipital encephalocele, NPHP) Joubert syndrome/Joubert syndrome related disorders RHYNS (RP, hypopituitarism, skeletal dysplasia)
Neurological disorder Encephalocele Vermis aplasia Hypopituitarism	
Others *Situs inversus* Cardiac malformation Bronchiectasis Ulcerative colitis	

RP retinitis pigmentosa/retinal degeneration, *DM* diabetes mellitus, *NPHP* nephronophthisis

Sensenbrenner, and Jeune syndromes), oculomotor apraxia (Cogan syndrome), *situs inversus*, and liver fibrosis. An extreme form of NPHP is Meckel-Gruber syndrome, which is usually a lethal condition with developmental defects, occipital encephalocele, liver fibrosis, microophthalmia, and polydactyly. NPHP is characterized as infantile, juvenile, or adolescent/adult depending on the age of ESKD. Juvenile NPHP is the most common and the mean age of ESKD is 13 years. NPHP diagnosed in young adults or later in life was thought to be extremely rare, although a recent study suggested that a whole-gene deletion of *NPHP1* may be a more common cause of undiagnosed ESKD in adulthood than previously recognized.

2.2 Laboratory Studies and Kidney Biopsy

Urinary osmolality may be low. Hemoglobin and reticulocytes are reduced disproportionally to the degree of CKD. Kidneys may be initially normal sized but usually decrease due to fibrosis over time and show increased echogenicity. Histologic findings in NPHP are nonspecific, including tubular atrophy, thickened tubular basement membrane, and interstitial fibrosis along the cortico-medullary border. Cysts are present in 70% of patients but are not required for the diagnosis. In the infantile form of NPHP kidneys are enlarged and have widespread cysts. An eye exam, LFTs, and a liver ultrasound may help to identify eye and liver involvement.

2.3 Physiology and Pathophysiology

Primary cilia are present in most mammalian cells and are considered a sensory organelle. In contrast to motile cilia which have 9 + 2 microtubular doublets, primary cilia contain 9 + 0 microtubular doublets. Over 20 genes are known to cause about 63% of all NPHP cases (Table 5). Through their role in primary cilia maintenance and function, nephrocystin loss may affect important signaling pathways such as planar cell polarity, Wnt, signaling, Sonic hedgehog signaling, the DNA damage response pathway, Hippo signaling, cAMP, and mTOR. Perturbations in these pathways may underly pathogenesis, but mechanisms are not entirely known.

2.4 Diagnosis

Specific diagnosis is made by genetic testing. This can be efficiently accomplished using commercially available next-generation sequencing gene panels for ciliopathy and tubulointerstitial kidney disease, or whole exome sequencing, although some genes such as *RPGRIP1L* may have low coverage and therefore a risk for false negative results. Copy number variation (CNV) analysis is necessary to detect whole gene deletions such as the most common *NPHP1* variant and typically is accomplished by commercial testing but sensitivity may be variable between labs.

Table 5 Summary of *NPHP1-NPHP18 and NHPH1L and NPHP2L* genes, gene products, chromosomal localization, phenotypes, extrarenal symptoms, and interaction partners

Gene (protein)	Chromosome	Extrarenal symptoms	Phenotype (mean age at ESRD)	Interaction partners
NPHP1 (Nephrocystin-1)	2q13	RP (10%), OMA (2%), JBTS and LF (rarely)	NPHP (13 years)	Inversin, nephrocystins-3-5, nephrocystin-8/ RPGRIPL, RPGR, polycystin-1, filamin A and B, tensin, PALS1/PATJ, Par6, β-tubulin, PTK2B, p130(Cas), Pyk2
NPHP2/INVS (inversin)	9q31	RP (10%), LF, *situs inversus*, CHD	Infantile NPHP (<4 years)	Nephrocystin-1, 3, 5, 9, and 16, calmodulin, catenins, β-tubulin, APC2, RPGR
NPHP3 (Nephrocystin-3)	3q22	LF, RP (10%), situs inversus, MKS, CHD	Infantile and adolescent NPHP	Nephrocystin-1, 9, 16, Inversin
NPHP4 (Nephrocystin-4)	1p36	RP (10%), OMA, LF	NPHP (21 years)	Nephrocystin-1, 6, 8, 9, BCAR1, PALS1/ PATJ, Par6, p130(Cas), Pyk2, PTK2B, Jade-1, Lats1, TAZ, α-tubulin, RPGR, RPGRIP1, TMEM107, 237
NPHP5/IQCB1 (Nephrocystin-5)	3q21	Early-onset RP, SLNS	NPHP (13 years)	Calmodulin, RPGR, nephrocystin-6
NPHP6/CEP290 (Nephrocystin-6/ CEP290)	12q21	JBTS, MKS, LF, LCA	NPHP	ATF4, nephrocystin-5, Rab8a, Rkip, MKKS, FAM161A, RPGR, CC2D2A, Tectin1
NPHP7/GLIS2 (Nephrocystin-7/ GLIS2)	16p	–	NPHP	TRIM32, p120 catenin, β catenin CtBP1, HDAC3
NPHP8/RPGRIP1L (Nephrocystin-8/ RPGRIP1L)	16q	JBTS, MKS, LCA	NPHP	Nephrocystin-1, 4, 6, RPGR, CSPP, Nek4, Pmsd2
NPHP9/NEK8 (Nephrocystin-9/ NEK8)	17q11	LF, CHD	Infantile NPHP	Nephrocystin-1, 3, 4, 16, Inversin, TAZ, Anks3

(continued)

Table 5 (continued)

Gene (protein)	Chromosome	Extrarenal symptoms	Phenotype (mean age at ESRD)	Interaction partners
NPHP10/SDCCAG8 (Nephrocystin-10/ SDCCAG8)	1q43	RP (SLS), BBS-like	Juvenile NPHP	OFD1, FAM161A, AZI1, RABEP2
NPHP11/TMEM67/ MKS3 (Nephrocystin-11/ Meckelin)	8q22.1	JBTS, MKS, LF	NPHP	MKS1, nephrocystin-1, 4, 6, nesprin-2, TMEM216, filamin A
NPHP12/TTC21B// JBTS11 (Nephrocystin-12/ IFT139)	2q24.3	JATD, MKS, JBTS, BBS-like	Early onset NPHP, juvenile NPHP	IFT121, NPHP13/ IFT144, ciliopathy modifier
NPHP13/WDR19 (Nephrocystin-13/ IFT144)	4p14	JATD, SBS, CED, RP, Caroli, BBS-like	NPHP	Presumed IFT139 and IFT140 interaction
NPHP14/ZNF423 (Nephrocystin-14/ ZNF423)	16q12.1	JBTS, *situs inversus*	Infantile NPHP, PKD	PARP1, nephrocystin-6, ZNF521
NPHP15/CEP164 (Nephrocystin-15 centrosomal protein 164 kDa)	11q23.3	RP, JBTS, LF, obesity	NPHP (8 years)	Nephrocystin-3, 4, 18, ATRIP, CCDC92, TTBK2, Dvl3, INPP5, Chibby
NPHP16/ANKS6 (Nephrocystin-16/ ANKS6)	9q22.33	LF, *situs inversus*, CHD cardiovascular abnorm.	Infantile and juvenile NPHP	INVS, nephrocystin-3, 9, HIF1AN, BICC1, ANKS3
NPHP17/IFT172 (Nephrocystin-17/ IFT172)	2p23.3	JATD, MZSDS, JBTS	NPHP	IFT140, IFT38, IFT57, IFT80, MKS1
NPHP18/CEP83 (Nephrocystin-18/ centrosomal protein 83 kDa)	12q22	Learning disability, hydrocephalus, LF	Early-onset NPHP (3 years)	Nephrocystin-15, IFT20
NPHP19/DCDC2 (Nephrocystin-19/ doublecortin domain-containing 2)	6p22	LF	NPHP	Dishevelled-3
NPHP20/MAPKBP1 (Nephrocystin-20/ mitogen activated protein kinase binding protein 1)	15q1		NPHP	JNK2, WDR62

Table 5 (continued)

Gene (protein)	Chromosome	Extrarenal symptoms	Phenotype (mean age at ESRD)	Interaction partners
NPHP21/ADAMTS9 (Nephrocystin-21/a disintegrin and metalloproteinase with thrombospondin type 1 motif)	3p14.1	JBTS, CHD, deafness, coloboma, short stature, hepatosplenomegaly	NPHP	
NPHP1L/XPNPEP3 (Nephrocystin-1 L/ XPNPEP3)	22q13	Cardiomyopathy, seizures	NPHP	Cleaves LRRC50, ALMS1, nephrocystin-6
NPHP2L/SLC41A1 (Nephrocystin-2 L/ SLC41A1)	1q32.1	Bronchiectasis	NPHP	

ATF4 activating transcription factor 4, *APC2* anaphase-promoting complex 2, *BCAR1* breast cancer anti-estrogen resistance 1, *CAD* cranioectodermal dysplasia, *CC2D2A* coiled-coil and C2 domain containing 2A, *CHD* congenital heart disease, *JATD* jeune asphyxiating thoracic dysplasia, *JBTS* joubert syndrome, *LCA* leber congenital amaurosis, *LF* liver fibrosis, *MKS* Meckel-Gruber syndrome, *OMA* oculomotor apraxia, *PTK2B* protein tyrosine kinase 2B, *RP* retinitis pigmentosa, *RPGR* retinitis pigmentosa GTPase regulator, *SBS* Sensenbrenner syndrome

2.5 Therapies

There are no specific therapies for NPHP. Therapeutic avenues in development include targeting cAMP with Vasopressin 2 receptor antagonists such as tolvaptan; and targeting the cyclin-dependent kinase pathway of the DNA damage response with Roscovitone or S-CR-8. Other approaches include targeting the hedgehog signaling pathway. Rapamycin ameliorated kidney cyst formation in mouse and zebrafish models.

3 Differential Diagnosis

Whereas NPHP usually presents early in life, ADTKD more commonly presents later in adulthood. There is overlap in age of onset and phenotype between some forms of each and thus both must be considered if inheritance pattern is unclear. Rarely, NPHP presents in adults or is inherited in a pseudo-dominant fashion. Specific extrarenal manifestations may also help to distinguish ADTKD from NPHP. In utero diagnosis of cystic kidneys can require genetic diagnosis to distinguish NPHP from autosomal recessive polycystic kidney disease (ARPKD), or severe ADTKD-*HNF1B*. Biopsy findings in ADTKD can also resemble drug-induced tubulointerstitial kidney disease (calcineurin inhibitors, lithium, NSAIDs), autoimmune processes, or tubulointerstitial nephritis with uveitis syndrome (TINU).

4 Other Genetic Diseases of Interest

Heterozygous *DNAJB11* mutations can present with slow progressive CKD with kidney failure late in life, normal sized kidneys, kidney fibrosis, and variable manifestations of multiple kidney cysts that may be clinically diagnosed as autosomal dominant polycystic kidney disease (ADPKD) or ADKTD. Homozygous *DNAJB11* mutations cause Ivermark II syndrome, a form of renal-hepatic-pancreatic dysplasia, which presents with severe oligohydramnios, interstitial fibrosis, and kidney cysts. *PAX2* mutations and mutations in mitochondrial DNA also can contribute to tubulointerstitial kidney disease. The ocular findings in patients with *PAX2* mutations (aka renal coloboma syndrome) should help to differentiate these patients from ADTKD. In a mitochondrial disease, only maternal transmission would be anticipated.

5 Conclusion

Genetic forms of tubulointerstitial kidney disease may be more prevalent than presently recognized. Recognition of these tubulointerstitial diseases is critical to preventing unnecessary exposure to immunosuppressive therapy and facilitating kidney transplantation. Clinicians should be familiar with the clinical features, epidemiology, pathogenesis, diagnosis, therapies, and need for ongoing research in ADTKD and NPHP.

Acknowledgements MTW is supported by Children's Clinical Research Advisory Committee (CCRAC), Department of Defense (W81XWH1910205), and the NIH (P30 DK079328-11, R01DK119631). WB is supported by a Robert E. Leet and Clara Guthrie Patterson Trust mentored research award and the NIH (K08DK119642).

Suggested Reading

Adalat S, Woolf AS, Johnstone KA, Wirsing A, Harries LW, Long DA, et al. HNF1B mutations associate with hypomagnesemia and renal magnesium wasting. J Am Soc Nephrol. 2009;20(5):1123–31.

Attanasio M, Uhlenhaut NH, Sousa VH, O'Toole JF, Otto E, Anlag K, et al. Loss of GLIS2 causes nephronophthisis in humans and mice by increased apoptosis and fibrosis. Nat Genet. 2007;39(8):1018–24.

Augusto JF, Subra JF, Duveau A, Rakotonjanahary J, Dussaussoy C, Picquet J, et al. Relation between pretransplant magnesemia and the risk of new onset diabetes after transplantation within the first year of kidney transplantation. Transplantation. 2014;97(11):1155–60.

Bellanné-Chantelot C, Chauveau D, Gautier JF, Dubois-Laforgue D, Clauin S, Beaufils S, et al. Clinical spectrum associated with hepatocyte nuclear factor-1beta mutations. Ann Intern Med. 2004;140(7):510–7.

Bergmann C. Genetics of autosomal recessive polycystic kidney disease and its differential diagnoses. Front Pediatr. 2017;5:221.

Bernascone I, Janas S, Ikehata M, Trudu M, Corbelli A, Schaeffer C, et al. A transgenic mouse model for uromodulin-associated kidney diseases shows specific tubulo-interstitial damage, urinary concentrating defect and renal failure. Hum Mol Genet. 2010;19(15):2998–3010.

Bernascone I, Vavassori S, Di Pentima A, Santambrogio S, Lamorte G, Amoroso A, et al. Defective intracellular trafficking of uromodulin mutant isoforms. Traffic. 2006;7(11):1567–79.

Bingham C, Ellard S, Van't Hoff WG, Simmonds HA, Marinaki AM, Badman MK, et al. Atypical familial juvenile hyperuricemic nephropathy associated with a hepatocyte nuclear factor-1beta gene mutation. Kidney Int. 2003;63(5):1645–51.

Bleyer AJ, Hart TC, Shihabi Z, Robins V, Hoyer JR. Mutations in the uromodulin gene decrease urinary excretion of Tamm-Horsfall protein. Kidney Int. 2004;66(3):974–7.

Bleyer AJ, Woodard AS, Shihabi Z, Sandhu J, Zhu H, Satko SG, et al. Clinical characterization of a family with a mutation in the uromodulin (Tamm-Horsfall glycoprotein) gene. Kidney Int. 2003;64(1):36–42.

Bleyer AJ, Zivná M, Hulková H, Hodanová K, Vyletal P, Sikora J, et al. Clinical and molecular characterization of a family with a dominant renin gene mutation and response to treatment with fludrocortisone. Clin Nephrol. 2010;74(6):411–22.

Blowey DL, Querfeld U, Geary D, Warady BA, Alon U. Ultrasound findings in juvenile nephronophthisis. Pediatr Nephrol. 1996;10(1):22–4.

Bolar NA, Golzio C, Zivna M, Hayot G, Van Hemelrijk C, Schepers D, et al. Heterozygous loss-of-function SEC61A1 mutations cause autosomal-dominant tubulo-interstitial and glomerulocystic kidney disease with anemia. Am J Hum Genet. 2016;99(1):174–87.

Bollee G, Dahan K, Flamant M, Moriniere V, Pawtowski A, Heidet L, et al. Phenotype and outcome in hereditary tubulointerstitial nephritis secondary to UMOD mutations. Clin J Am Soc Nephrol. 2011;6(10):2429–38.

Bower MA, Schimmenti LA, Eccles MR. PAX2-related disorder. In: Adam MP, Ardinger HH, Pagon RA, Wallace SE, LJH B, Stephens K, et al., editors. GeneReviews(®). Seattle: University of Washington, Seattle; 1993.

Braun DA, Hildebrandt F. Ciliopathies. Cold Spring Harb Perspect Biol. 2017;9(3):a028191.

Chaki M, Airik R, Ghosh AK, Giles RH, Chen R, Slaats GG, et al. Exome capture reveals ZNF423 and CEP164 mutations, linking renal ciliopathies to DNA damage response signaling. Cell. 2012;150(3):533–48.

Chan SC, Zhang Y, Shao A, Avdulov S, Herrera J, Aboudehen K, et al. Mechanism of fibrosis in HNF1B-related autosomal dominant tubulointerstitial kidney disease. J Am Soc Nephrol. 2018;29(10):2493–509.

Choi HJ, Lin JR, Vannier JB, Slaats GG, Kile AC, Paulsen RD, et al. NEK8 links the ATR-regulated replication stress response and S phase CDK activity to renal ciliopathies. Mol Cell. 2013;51(4):423–39.

Choi SW, Ryu OH, Choi SJ, Song IS, Bleyer AJ, Hart TC. Mutant tamm-horsfall glycoprotein accumulation in endoplasmic reticulum induces apoptosis reversed by colchicine and sodium 4-phenylbutyrate. J Am Soc Nephrol. 2005;16(10):3006–14.

Chung EM, Conran RM, Schroeder JW, Rohena-Quinquilla IR, Rooks VJ. From the radiologic pathology archives: pediatric polycystic kidney disease and other ciliopathies: radiologic-pathologic correlation. Radiographics. 2014;34(1):155–78.

Clissold RL, Hamilton AJ, Hattersley AT, Ellard S, Bingham C. HNF1B-associated renal and extra-renal disease-an expanding clinical spectrum. Nat Rev Nephrol. 2015;11(2):102–12.

Connor TM, Hoer S, Mallett A, Gale DP, Gomez-Duran A, Posse V, et al. Mutations in mitochondrial DNA causing tubulointerstitial kidney disease. PLoS Genet. 2017;13(3):e1006620.

Cornec-Le Gall E, Olson RJ, Besse W, Heyer CM, Gainullin VG, Smith JM, et al. Monoallelic mutations to DNAJB11 cause atypical autosomal-dominant polycystic kidney disease. Am J Hum Genet. 2018;102(5):832–44.

Dahan K, Devuyst O, Smaers M, Vertommen D, Loute G, Poux JM, et al. A cluster of mutations in the UMOD gene causes familial juvenile hyperuricemic nephropathy with abnormal expression of uromodulin. J Am Soc Nephrol. 2003;14(11):2883–93.

Dahan K, Fuchshuber A, Adamis S, Smaers M, Kroiss S, Loute G, et al. Familial juvenile hyperuricemic nephropathy and autosomal dominant medullary cystic kidney disease type 2: two facets of the same disease? J Am Soc Nephrol. 2001;12(11):2348–57.

Decramer S, Parant O, Beaufils S, Clauin S, Guillou C, Kessler S, et al. Anomalies of the TCF2 gene are the main cause of fetal bilateral hyperechogenic kidneys. J Am Soc Nephrol. 2007;18(3):923–33.

Devuyst O, Olinger E, Rampoldi L. Uromodulin: from physiology to rare and complex kidney disorders. Nat Rev Nephrol. 2017;13(9):525–44.

Devuyst O, Olinger E, Weber S, Eckardt KU, Kmoch S, Rampoldi L, et al. Autosomal dominant tubulointerstitial kidney disease. Nat Rev Dis Primers. 2019;5(1):60.

Dvela-Levitt M, Kost-Alimova M, Emani M, Kohnert E, Thompson R, Sidhom EH, et al. Small molecule targets TMED9 and promotes lysosomal degradation to reverse Proteinopathy. Cell. 2019;178(3):521–35.e23.

Eckardt KU, Alper SL, Antignac C, Bleyer AJ, Chauveau D, Dahan K, et al. Autosomal dominant tubulointerstitial kidney disease: diagnosis, classification, and management-a KDIGO consensus report. Kidney Int. 2015;88(4):676–83.

Ekici AB, Hackenbeck T, Moriniere V, Pannes A, Buettner M, Uebe S, et al. Renal fibrosis is the common feature of autosomal dominant tubulointerstitial kidney diseases caused by mutations in mucin 1 or uromodulin. Kidney Int. 2014;86(3):589–99.

Faguer S, Decramer S, Chassaing N, Bellanné-Chantelot C, Calvas P, Beaufils S, et al. Diagnosis, management, and prognosis of HNF1B nephropathy in adulthood. Kidney Int. 2011;80(7):768–76.

Fanni D, Iacovidou N, Locci A, Gerosa C, Nemolato S, Van Eyken P, et al. MUC1 marks collecting tubules, renal vesicles, comma- and S-shaped bodies in human developing kidney tubules, renal vesicles, comma- and s-shaped bodies in human kidney. Eur J Histochem. 2012;56(4):e40.

Ferre S, Bongers EM, Sonneveld R, Cornelissen EA, van der Vlag J, van Boekel GA, et al. Early development of hyperparathyroidism due to loss of PTH transcriptional repression in patients with HNF1beta mutations? J Clin Endocrinol Metab. 2013;98(10):4089–96.

Fischer E, Legue E, Doyen A, Nato F, Nicolas JF, Torres V, et al. Defective planar cell polarity in polycystic kidney disease. Nat Genet. 2006;38(1):21–3.

Frank V, Habbig S, Bartram MP, Eisenberger T, Veenstra-Knol HE, Decker C, et al. Mutations in NEK8 link multiple organ dysplasia with altered hippo signalling and increased c-MYC expression. Hum Mol Genet. 2013;22(11):2177–85.

Gagnadoux MF, Bacri JL, Broyer M, Habib R. Infantile chronic tubulo-interstitial nephritis with cortical microcysts: variant of nephronophthisis or new disease entity? Pediatr Nephrol. 1989;3(1):50–5.

Garg N, Weinberg J, Ghai S, Bradauskaite G, Nuhn M, Gautam A, et al. Lower magnesium level associated with new-onset diabetes and pre-diabetes after kidney transplantation. J Nephrol. 2014;27(3):339–44.

Gast C, Marinaki A, Arenas-Hernandez M, Campbell S, Seaby EG, Pengelly RJ, et al. Autosomal dominant tubulointerstitial kidney disease-UMOD is the most frequent non polycystic genetic kidney disease. BMC Nephrol. 2018;19(1):301.

Gattone VH 2nd, Sinders RM, Hornberger TA, Robling AG. Late progression of renal pathology and cyst enlargement is reduced by rapamycin in a mouse model of nephronophthisis. Kidney Int. 2009;76(2):178–82.

Gattone VH 2nd, Wang X, Harris PC, Torres VE. Inhibition of renal cystic disease development and progression by a vasopressin V2 receptor antagonist. Nat Med. 2003;9(10):1323–6.
Gresh L, Fischer E, Reimann A, Tanguy M, Garbay S, Shao X, et al. A transcriptional network in polycystic kidney disease. EMBO J. 2004;23(7):1657–68.
Groopman EE, Marasa M, Cameron-Christie S, Petrovski S, Aggarwal VS, Milo-Rasouly H, et al. Diagnostic utility of exome sequencing for kidney disease. N Engl J Med. 2019;380(2):142–51.
Haghighi A, Savaj S, Haghighi-Kakhki H, Benoit V, Grisart B, Dahan K. Identification of an NPHP1 deletion causing adult form of nephronophthisis. Ir J Med Sci. 2016;185(3):589–95.
Halbritter J, Diaz K, Chaki M, Porath JD, Tarrier B, Fu C, et al. High-throughput mutation analysis in patients with a nephronophthisis-associated ciliopathy applying multiplexed barcoded array-based PCR amplification and next-generation sequencing. J Med Genet. 2012;49(12):756–67.
Hanisch FG, Muller S. MUC1: the polymorphic appearance of a human mucin. Glycobiology. 2000;10(5):439–49.
Hart TC, Gorry MC, Hart PS, Woodard AS, Shihabi Z, Sandhu J, et al. Mutations of the UMOD gene are responsible for medullary cystic kidney disease 2 and familial juvenile hyperuricaemic nephropathy. J Med Genet. 2002;39(12):882–92.
Hecking M, Werzowa J, Haidinger M, Hörl WH, Pascual J, Budde K, et al. Novel views on new-onset diabetes after transplantation: development, prevention and treatment. Nephrol Dial Transplant. 2013;28(3):550–66.
Heidet L, Decramer S, Pawtowski A, Morinière V, Bandin F, Knebelmann B, et al. Spectrum of HNF1B mutations in a large cohort of patients who harbor renal diseases. Clin J Am Soc Nephrol. 2010;5(6):1079–90.
Hiesberger T, Bai Y, Shao X, McNally BT, Sinclair AM, Tian X, et al. Mutation of hepatocyte nuclear factor-1beta inhibits Pkhd1 gene expression and produces renal cysts in mice. J Clin Invest. 2004;113(6):814–25.
Hildebrandt F, Attanasio M, Otto E. Nephronophthisis: disease mechanisms of a ciliopathy. J Am Soc Nephrol. 2009;20(1):23–35.
Hildebrandt F, Benzing T, Katsanis N. Ciliopathies. N Engl J Med. 2011;364(16):1533–43.
Hildebrandt F, Otto E. Cilia and centrosomes: a unifying pathogenic concept for cystic kidney disease? Nat Rev Genet. 2005;6(12):928–40.
Hoefele J, Nayir A, Chaki M, Imm A, Allen SJ, Otto EA, et al. Pseudodominant inheritance of nephronophthisis caused by a homozygous NPHP1 deletion. Pediatr Nephrol. 2011;26(6):967–71.
Huang JW, Famure O, Li Y, Kim SJ. Hypomagnesemia and the risk of new-onset diabetes mellitus after kidney transplantation. J Am Soc Nephrol. 2016;27(6):1793–800.
Hudson R, Patel C, Hawley CM, O'Shea S, Snelling P, Ho G, et al. Adult-diagnosed nonsyndromic nephronophthisis in Australian families caused by biallelic NPHP4 variants. Am J Kidney Dis. 2020;76(2):282–7.
Husson H, Moreno S, Smith LA, Smith MM, Russo RJ, Pitstick R, et al. Reduction of ciliary length through pharmacologic or genetic inhibition of CDK5 attenuates polycystic kidney disease in a model of nephronophthisis. Hum Mol Genet. 2016;25(11):2245–55.
Hynes AM, Giles RH, Srivastava S, Eley L, Whitehead J, Danilenko M, et al. Murine Joubert syndrome reveals hedgehog signaling defects as a potential therapeutic target for nephronophthisis. Proc Natl Acad Sci U S A. 2014;111(27):9893–8.
Johnson BG, Dang LT, Marsh G, Roach AM, Levine ZG, Monti A, et al. Uromodulin p.Cys147Trp mutation drives kidney disease by activating ER stress and apoptosis. J Clin Invest. 2017;127(11):3954–69.
Jordan P, Arrondel C, Bessières B, Tessier A, Attié-Bitach T, Guterman S, et al. Ivemark II syndrome, a renal-hepatic-pancreatic dysplasia. Kidney Int. 2020;99(2):405–9.
Kanda S, Morisada N, Kaneko N, Yabuuchi T, Nawashiro Y, Tada N, et al. New-onset diabetes after renal transplantation in a patient with a novel HNF1B mutation. Pediatr Transplant. 2016;20(3):467–71.

Kemter E, Frohlich T, Arnold GJ, Wolf E, Wanke R. Mitochondrial dysregulation secondary to endoplasmic reticulum stress in autosomal dominant tubulointerstitial kidney disease - UMOD (ADTKD-UMOD). Sci Rep. 2017;7:42970.

Kemter E, Prueckl P, Sklenak S, Rathkolb B, Habermann FA, Hans W, et al. Type of uromodulin mutation and allelic status influence onset and severity of uromodulin-associated kidney disease in mice. Hum Mol Genet. 2013;22(20):4148–63.

Kemter E, Rathkolb B, Rozman J, Hans W, Schrewe A, Landbrecht C, et al. Novel missense mutation of uromodulin in mice causes renal dysfunction with alterations in urea handling, energy, and bone metabolism. Am J Physiol Renal Physiol. 2009;297(5):F1391–8.

Kemter E, Sklenak S, Rathkolb B, Hrabe de Angelis M, Wolf E, Aigner B, et al. No amelioration of uromodulin maturation and trafficking defect by sodium 4-phenylbutyrate in vivo: studies in mouse models of uromodulin-associated kidney disease. J Biol Chem. 2014;289(15):10715–26.

Kidd K, Vylet'al P, Schaeffer C, Olinger E, Živná M, Hodaňová K, et al. Genetic and clinical predictors of age of ESKD in individuals with autosomal dominant tubulointerstitial kidney disease due to UMOD mutations. Kidney Int Rep. 2020;5(9):1472–85.

Kirby A, Gnirke A, Jaffe DB, Baresova V, Pochet N, Blumenstiel B, et al. Mutations causing medullary cystic kidney disease type 1 lie in a large VNTR in MUC1 missed by massively parallel sequencing. Nat Genet. 2013;45(3):299–303.

Konig J, Kranz B, Konig S, Schlingmann KP, Titieni A, Tonshoff B, et al. Phenotypic spectrum of children with nephronophthisis and related ciliopathies. Clin J Am Soc Nephrol. 2017;12(12):1974–83.

Kurt B, Paliege A, Willam C, Schwarzensteiner I, Schucht K, Neymeyer H, et al. Deletion of von Hippel-Lindau protein converts renin-producing cells into erythropoietin-producing cells. J Am Soc Nephrol. 2013;24(3):433–44.

Leroy X, Copin MC, Devisme L, Buisine MP, Aubert JP, Gosselin B, et al. Expression of human mucin genes in normal kidney and renal cell carcinoma. Histopathology. 2002;40(5):450–7.

Luyten A, Su X, Gondela S, Chen Y, Rompani S, Takakura A, et al. Aberrant regulation of planar cell polarity in polycystic kidney disease. J Am Soc Nephrol. 2010;21(9):1521–32.

Ma L, Liu Y, El-Achkar TM, Wu XR. Molecular and cellular effects of Tamm-Horsfall protein mutations and their rescue by chemical chaperones. J Biol Chem. 2012;287(2):1290–305.

Ma L, Liu Y, Landry NK, El-Achkar TM, Lieske JC, Wu XR. Point mutation in D8C domain of Tamm-Horsfall protein/uromodulin in transgenic mice causes progressive renal damage and hyperuricemia. PLoS One. 2017;12(11):e0186769.

Madariaga L, García-Castaño A, Ariceta G, Martínez-Salazar R, Aguayo A, Castaño L. Variable phenotype in HNF1B mutations: extrarenal manifestations distinguish affected individuals from the population with congenital anomalies of the kidney and urinary tract. Clin Kidney J. 2019;12(3):373–9.

Madariaga L, Morinière V, Jeanpierre C, Bouvier R, Loget P, Martinovic J, et al. Severe prenatal renal anomalies associated with mutations in HNF1B or PAX2 genes. Clin J Am Soc Nephrol. 2013;8(7):1179–87.

McBride MB, Simmonds HA, Ogg CS, Cameron JS, Rigden S, Rees L, et al. Efficacy of allopurinol in ameliorating the progressive renal disease in familial juvenile hyperuricaemic nephropathy (FJHN). A six-year update. Adv Exp Med Biol. 1998;431:7–11.

McKenzie JK, McQueen EG. Immunofluorescent localization of Tamm-Horsfall mucoprotein in human kidney. J Clin Pathol. 1969;22(3):334–9.

Mefford HC, Clauin S, Sharp AJ, Moller RS, Ullmann R, Kapur R, et al. Recurrent reciprocal genomic rearrangements of 17q12 are associated with renal disease, diabetes, and epilepsy. Am J Hum Genet. 2007;81(5):1057–69.

Mitchel MW, Moreno-De-Luca D, Myers SM, Levy RV, Turner S, Ledbetter DH, et al. 17q12 recurrent deletion syndrome. In: Adam MP, Ardinger HH, Pagon RA, Wallace SE, Bean LJH, Stephens K, et al., editors. GeneReviews(®). Seattle: University of Washington, Seattle; 2020.

Moreno-De-Luca D, Mulle JG, Kaminsky EB, Sanders SJ, Myers SM, Adam MP, et al. Deletion 17q12 is a recurrent copy number variant that confers high risk of autism and schizophrenia. Am J Hum Genet. 2010;87(5):618–30.

Moskowitz JL, Piret SE, Lhotta K, Kitzler TM, Tashman AP, Velez E, et al. Association between genotype and phenotype in uromodulin-associated kidney disease. Clin J Am Soc Nephrol. 2013;8(8):1349–57.

Nasr SH, Lucia JP, Galgano SJ, Markowitz GS, D'Agati VD. Uromodulin storage disease. Kidney Int. 2008;73(8):971–6.

Nie M, Bal MS, Yang Z, Liu J, Rivera C, Wenzel A, et al. Mucin-1 increases renal TRPV5 activity in vitro, and urinary level associates with calcium nephrolithiasis in patients. J Am Soc Nephrol. 2016;27(11):3447–58.

Olinger E, Hofmann P, Kidd K, Dufour I, Belge H, Schaeffer C, et al. Clinical and genetic spectra of autosomal dominant tubulointerstitial kidney disease due to mutations in UMOD and MUC1. Kidney Int. 2020;98(3):717–31.

Otto EA, Hurd TW, Airik R, Chaki M, Zhou W, Stoetzel C, et al. Candidate exome capture identifies mutation of SDCCAG8 as the cause of a retinal-renal ciliopathy. Nat Genet. 2010;42(10):840–50.

Pennica D, Kohr WJ, Kuang WJ, Glaister D, Aggarwal BB, Chen EY, et al. Identification of human uromodulin as the Tamm-Horsfall urinary glycoprotein. Science. 1987;236(4797):83–8.

Piret SE, Olinger E, Reed AAC, Nesbit MA, Hough TA, Bentley L, et al. A mouse model for inherited renal fibrosis associated with endoplasmic reticulum stress. Dis Model Mech. 2017;10(6):773–86.

Rampoldi L, Caridi G, Santon D, Boaretto F, Bernascone I, Lamorte G, et al. Allelism of MCKD, FJHN and GCKD caused by impairment of uromodulin export dynamics. Hum Mol Genet. 2003;12(24):3369–84.

Schaeffer C, Merella S, Pasqualetto E, Lazarevic D, Rampoldi L. Mutant uromodulin expression leads to altered homeostasis of the endoplasmic reticulum and activates the unfolded protein response. PLoS One. 2017;12(4):e0175970.

Schäffer P, Gombos E, Meichelbeck K, Kiss A, Hart PS, Bleyer AJ. Childhood course of renal insufficiency in a family with a uromodulin gene mutation. Pediatr Nephrol. 2010;25(7):1355–60.

Schubert D, Klein MC, Hassdenteufel S, Caballero-Oteyza A, Yang L, Proietti M, et al. Plasma cell deficiency in human subjects with heterozygous mutations in Sec61 translocon alpha 1 subunit (SEC61A1). J Allergy Clin Immunol. 2018;141(4):1427–38.

Schueler M, Halbritter J, Phelps IG, Braun DA, Otto EA, Porath JD, et al. Large-scale targeted sequencing comparison highlights extreme genetic heterogeneity in nephronophthisis-related ciliopathies. J Med Genet. 2016;53(3):208–14.

Scolari F, Caridi G, Rampoldi L, Tardanico R, Izzi C, Pirulli D, et al. Uromodulin storage diseases: clinical aspects and mechanisms. Am J Kidney Dis. 2004;44(6):987–99.

Shahani S, Braga-Basaria M, Maggio M, Basaria S. Androgens and erythropoiesis: past and present. J Endocrinol Investig. 2009;32(8):704–16.

Shao A, Chan SC, Igarashi P. Role of transcription factor hepatocyte nuclear factor-1β in polycystic kidney disease. Cell Signal. 2020;71:109568.

Sikri KL, Foster CL, MacHugh N, Marshall RD. Localization of Tamm-Horsfall glycoprotein in the human kidney using immuno-fluorescence and immuno-electron microscopical techniques. J Anat. 1981;132(Pt 4):597–605.

Simons M, Gloy J, Ganner A, Bullerkotte A, Bashkurov M, Kronig C, et al. Inversin, the gene product mutated in nephronophthisis type II, functions as a molecular switch between Wnt signaling pathways. Nat Genet. 2005;37(5):537–43.

Snoek R, van Setten J, Keating BJ, Israni AK, Jacobson PA, Oetting WS, et al. NPHP1 (Nephrocystin-1) gene deletions cause adult-onset ESRD. J Am Soc Nephrol. 2018;29(6):1772–9.

Srivastava S, Ramsbottom SA, Molinari E, Alkanderi S, Filby A, White K, et al. A human patient-derived cellular model of Joubert syndrome reveals ciliary defects which can be rescued with targeted therapies. Hum Mol Genet. 2017;26(23):4657–67.

Thornley C, Dawnay A, Cattell WR. Human Tamm-Horsfall glycoprotein: urinary and plasma levels in normal subjects and patients with renal disease determined by a fully validated radioimmunoassay. Clin Sci (Lond). 1985;68(5):529–35.

Tobin JL, Beales PL. Restoration of renal function in zebrafish models of ciliopathies. Pediatr Nephrol. 2008;23(11):2095–9.

Tokonami N, Takata T, Beyeler J, Ehrbar I, Yoshifuji A, Christensen EI, et al. Uromodulin is expressed in the distal convoluted tubule, where it is critical for regulation of the sodium chloride cotransporter NCC. Kidney Int. 2018;94(4):701–15.

Tramma D, Samourkasidou D. Hyperuricemia and early-onset chronic kidney disease in a 7-year-old child. Indian Pediatr. 2020;57(8):765.

Tran PV, Talbott GC, Turbe-Doan A, Jacobs DT, Schonfeld MP, Silva LM, et al. Downregulating hedgehog signaling reduces renal cystogenic potential of mouse models. J Am Soc Nephrol. 2014;25(10):2201–12.

Trudu M, Schaeffer C, Riba M, Ikehata M, Brambilla P, Messa P, et al. Early involvement of cellular stress and inflammatory signals in the pathogenesis of tubulointerstitial kidney disease due to UMOD mutations. Sci Rep. 2017;7(1):7383.

Tudorache E, Sellier-Leclerc AL, Lenoir M, Tubiana-Rufi N, Bensman A, Bellanne-Chantelot C, et al. Childhood onset diabetes posttransplant in a girl with TCF2 mutation. Pediatr Diabetes. 2012;13(6):e35–9.

Ulinski T, Lescure S, Beaufils S, Guigonis V, Decramer S, Morin D, et al. Renal phenotypes related to hepatocyte nuclear factor-1beta (TCF2) mutations in a pediatric cohort. J Am Soc Nephrol. 2006;17(2):497–503.

Utami SB, Mahati E, Li P, Maharani N, Ikeda N, Bahrudin U, et al. Apoptosis induced by an uromodulin mutant C112Y and its suppression by topiroxostat. Clin Exp Nephrol. 2015;19(4):576–84.

Van Nieuwenhove E, Barber JS, Neumann J, Smeets E, Willemsen M, Pasciuto E, et al. Defective Sec61α1 underlies a novel cause of autosomal dominant severe congenital neutropenia. J Allergy Clin Immunol. 2020;146(5):1180–93.

Verhave JC, Bech AP, Wetzels JF, Nijenhuis T. Hepatocyte nuclear factor 1beta-associated kidney disease: more than renal cysts and diabetes. J Am Soc Nephrol. 2016;27(2):345–53.

Vylet'al P, Kublova M, Kalbacova M, Hodanova K, Baresova V, Stiburkova B, et al. Alterations of uromodulin biology: a common denominator of the genetically heterogeneous FJHN/MCKD syndrome. Kidney Int. 2006;70(6):1155–69.

Waldherr R, Lennert T, Weber HP, Fodisch HJ, Scharer K. The nephronophthisis complex. A clinicopathologic study in children. Virchows Arch A Pathol Anat Histol. 1982;394(3):235–54.

Williams SE, Reed AA, Galvanovskis J, Antignac C, Goodship T, Karet FE, et al. Uromodulin mutations causing familial juvenile hyperuricaemic nephropathy lead to protein maturation defects and retention in the endoplasmic reticulum. Hum Mol Genet. 2009;18(16):2963–74.

Wolf MT, Beck BB, Zaucke F, Kunze A, Misselwitz J, Ruley J, et al. The Uromodulin C744G mutation causes MCKD2 and FJHN in children and adults and may be due to a possible founder effect. Kidney Int. 2007;71(6):574–81.

Wolf MT, Hildebrandt F. Nephronophthisis. Pediatr Nephrol. 2011;26(2):181–94.

Zivna M, Hulkova H, Matignon M, Hodanova K, Vylet'al P, Kalbacova M, et al. Dominant renin gene mutations associated with early-onset hyperuricemia, anemia, and chronic kidney failure. Am J Hum Genet. 2009;85(2):204–13.

Živná M, Kidd K, Zaidan M, Vyleťal P, Barešová V, Hodaňová K, et al. An international cohort study of autosomal dominant tubulointerstitial kidney disease due to REN mutations identifies distinct clinical subtypes. Kidney Int. 2020;98(6):1589–604.

Cystinosis

Francesco Emma and Elena Levtchenko

1 Introduction

Cystinosis is a rare monogenic autosomal recessive disease caused by mutations in the *CTNS* gene that encodes for cystinosin, a lysosomal H^+/cystine symporter. Heterozygous carriers are asymptomatic, and display half the maximum cystine transport across their lysosomal membranes. In cystinosis, cysteine produced in lysosomes by the hydrolysis of proteins or taken up from the cytosol is oxidized to cystine and accumulates in virtually all organs; in several tissues cystine crystals form with time. Studies performed in the past two decades have revealed cell abnormalities that are related to defects in the cystinosin protein *per se*, independently from its transport activity. In addition to lysosomal cystine accumulation, the current view of cell dysfunction in cystinosis includes impaired intracellular trafficking and endolysosomal dynamics, abnormal autophagy, altered mTORC1 signaling, cell oxidation, mitochondrial damage, and increased susceptibility to apoptosis. It remains unclear, which of the above abnormalities are primary events, and which are consequences.

F. Emma (✉)
Department of Pediatric Subspecialties, Division of Nephrology, Bambino Gesù Children's Hospital – IRCCS, Rome, Italy
e-mail: francesco.emma@opbg.net

E. Levtchenko
Department of Pediatric Nephrology and Development and Regeneration, University Hospitals Leuven, Leuven, Belgium
e-mail: elena.levtchenko@uzleuven.be

M. G. Atta, M. A. Perazella (eds.), *Tubulointerstitial Nephritis*,
https://doi.org/10.1007/978-3-030-93438-5_12

2 Genetics

The incidence of cystinosis is estimated at 1 in 100,000–200,000 live births, with few hot spots in some regions such as Britany or Quebec, where the incidence is 4–6 time higher (a carrier frequency of 1:370 has recently been estimated in Germany). The *CTNS* gene is located on chromosome 17p13 and has been identified in 1998. It is composed of 12 exons and encodes for a 367-amino acid seven transmembrane domain cystine transporter. More than 160 different *CTNS* mutations, including deletions, insertions, nonsense, missense, and splice site mutations, have been reported. The most common mutation in Northern Europe is a 57 KB deletion that arouse in Germany around 500 AD and involves the first 10 exons of the *CTNS* and the neighboring the CARKL and the TRPV1 genes.

Three different phenotypes of cystinosis have been described. The most frequent form, termed infantile nephropathic cystinosis (INC) (OMIM 219800), accounts for more than 95% of cases. No phenotype-genotype correlation has been reported to date among individuals with this form of the disease. Rarely, patients present with a milder form, termed intermediate cystinosis (alternative designations: juvenile or adolescent cystinosis) (OMIM 219900), which is usually diagnosed in late childhood or adolescence in patients with asymptomatic proteinuria. The classic tubulopathy of the infantile form is mild or absent, but most patients eventually progress to end-stage kidney disease (ESKD). Exceptionally, patients are diagnosed with ocular cystinosis (alternative designations: adult or benign cystinosis) (OMIM 219750). These patients only present corneal and bone marrow cystine crystals and complain of photophobia. From the genetic standpoint, individuals with intermediate cystinosis carry one severe and one mild *CTNS* mutation; individuals with ocular cystinosis always have one or two mild *CTNS* mutations. The remaining of the text focus only on the most frequent INC.

3 Kidney Pathology

Excessive cystine accumulation results in formation of cystine crystals, which can be seen by phase contrast microscopy in virtually all organs of cystinosis patients. On electron microscopy, these crystals have hexagonal or rectangular shape and are localized in the lysosomes.

The kidneys are the first affected organs and demonstrate pathological changes during the first year of life. Renal tubules show remarkable irregularities of the tubular epithelium that is characterized by the presence within the same section of simplified flat cells and of enlarged cells with a prominent hyperchromatic cytoplasm. At the tubular-glomerular junction, cells typically undergo atrophy, causing the formation of the so-called swan-neck deformity that leads to the formation of “atubular glomeruli”. At early stages of the disease, the glomeruli appear normal, although giant multinucleated podocytes are frequently observed (Fig. 1). During

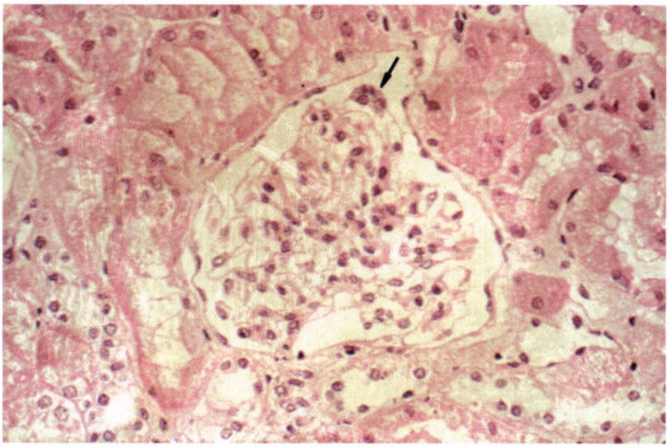

Fig. 1 Kidney tissue of 7-year-old male with cystinosis and renal Fanconi syndrome. Large multi-nucleated podocytes (arrow) and irregular tubular epithelial cells are characteristic for early disease stages

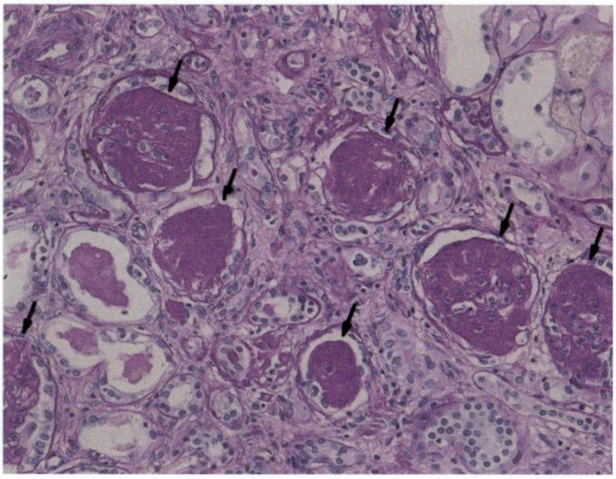

Fig. 2 End stage kidney tissue of 12-year-old female which was nephrectomized after kidney transplantation shows the total collapse of glomeruli (arrow), pronounced tubular atrophy and interstitial fibrosis

disease progression, patients develop focal and segmental glomerulosclerosis and extensive tubulo-interstitial lesions with tubular atrophy and interstitial fibrosis leading to kidney failure (Fig. 2).

4 Clinical Manifestations

4.1 Kidney Disease

INC is the most common cause of renal Fanconi syndrome in very young children. Patients usually develop growth retardation and other renal symptoms related to the proximal tubulopathy in the first year of life, mostly around 6 months of age. Clinical symptoms vary in severity and include rickets if treatment is not started rapidly. From the metabolic standpoint, the Fanconi syndrome is almost always complete, including polyuria, metabolic acidosis, electrolytes disturbances, hyperphosphaturia, hypermagnesuria, aminoaciduria, glucosuria, and low molecular weight proteinuria. Hypocalcemia is frequent and may cause secondary hyperparathyroidism. Patients may suffer from dehydration, in particular during acute illnesses. Overtime, kidney damage develops. Chronic interstitial inflammation secondary to cystine crystal depositions is always present. Progressive glomerular injury also contributes to proteinuria and to the decline in kidney function. Without cysteamine therapy, patients progress to ESKD around 10 years of age. If well treated, kidney function survival improves on average by 7–10 years.

4.2 Ocular Involvement

Corneal crystals start accumulating in the anterior third of the cornea during the first year of life and are always present at 16 months of age on slit lamp examination. They are diagnostic for INC, in particular if children have Fanconi syndrome. Without topical cysteamine therapy, children develop photophobia around 5–10 years of age. Non-compliant patients may present blepharospasm, and in some cases corneal ulcerations in adulthood. Retinal accumulation of crystals may also occur. These complications are now rarely observed in compliant patients.

4.3 Growth Impairment

Patients with INC are born with normal height and weight, but rapidly develop failure to thrive, which often leads to the diagnosis. Growth retardation in INC is multifactorial, including malnutrition, rickets, acidosis, electrolyte imbalances, and CKD. Children with INC are on average shorter compared to children with kidney failure secondary to other causes, suggesting an intrinsic bone defect. This is further supported by experimental data showing poor growth of cystinotic mice in the absence of glomerular and tubular damage and by persistently impaired bone metabolism in patients with INC after successful kidney transplantation.

4.4 Other Clinical Findings

Cystinosis children usually have poor appetite and complain of nausea and vomiting. Approximately one-third of young adults have mild hepatomegaly. Patients have decreased skin pigmentation; Caucasian individuals are frequently blond. Most patients manifest decreased production of sweat, tears and saliva. Idiopathic intracranial hypertension and *pseudotumor cerebri* secondary to non-absorptive hydrocephalus has been reported in several patients. Approximately half of patients not treated with cysteamine develop hypothyroidism during childhood and nearly all in adulthood. After kidney transplantation, many develop insulin-dependent diabetes mellitus. Exocrine pancreatic insufficiency is rare.

Puberty is delayed by 1–3 years in most patients; untreated adult males have hypogonadotropic hypogonadism. Well-treated men can achieve normal sexual development, but most have azoospermia. To date, only one male patient with INC has fathered twins after testicular sperm aspiration combined with intracytoplasmic sperm injection. Female patients with preserved kidney function have normal ovulatory function and sex hormone levels, with several of them having given birth to normal children.

One of the most severe complications of INC that occurs primarily in untreated patients, is progressive development of a life-threatening vacuolar myopathy that begins distally in the hands and progresses centrally. Patients progressively develop hypophonic speech, swallowing difficulties, and restrictive lung disease due to weakness of the thoracic musculature. Untreated adults often develop other neurological symptoms, including seizures, memory losses, cognitive defects, stroke episodes, inability to walk, and loss of speech .

5 Diagnosis and Treatment

5.1 Symptomatic Therapy

All patients with renal Fanconi syndrome should be investigated for cystinosis. Corneal crystals on slit lamp examination are diagnostic but may only appear in the second year of life. The diagnosis is based on the demonstration of elevated leukocyte cystine concentrations and mutations in the *CTNS* gene. Cystine levels should be measured preferentially using a purified granulocyte fractions and is only available in specialized laboratories. To date, newborn screening programs have not been developed, although early treatment is crucial to improve the prognosis of kidney disease.

Symptomatic treatment includes the replacement of kidney losses secondary to the Fanconi syndrome. Patients often require nasogastric tubes or gastrostomies in their first years of life to receive large amounts of supplements and medications. Nutritional support is critical to guarantee appropriate and well-balanced caloric intake. Some patients, especially in Europe, are treated in the first years of life with indomethacin to reduce urinary volume losses. L-thyroxine supplementation should be prescribed to patients with hypothyroidism and insulin is generally required for patients developing diabetes mellitus. Rickets requires treatment with vitamin D and phosphate supplementation. Same patients also need calcium supplements. Growth retarded patients do not have growth hormone deficiency, but they can benefit from growth hormone therapy, in particular if they have CKD, after correcting rickets, metabolic acidosis, and after providing adequate nutrition. Caution should be used in children with hyperparathyroidism. Physical exercise should be encouraged in all patients.

Patients reaching ESKD can undergo kidney transplantation. The overall kidney graft survival is excellent and is, on average, superior to that for other conditions. Nonetheless, INC patients should receive standard antirejection therapy. The disease does not recur in the transplanted graft, but occasionally, cystine crystals originating from infiltrating monocytes can be observed in the transplant kidney biopsy.

5.2 Specific Treatment

From the 1980's, the prognosis of INC has dramatically improved after introducing cysteamine for the treatment of this disease. Oral cysteamine penetrates the lysosomal membranes and interacts with cystine to produce cysteine and a cysteine-cysteamine mixed disulfide that can exit the organelle using other lysosomal carriers. Cysteamine bitartrate (Cystagon®) was approved in the US for treatment of cystinosis in 1994 and in Europe in 1997. The recommended dose is 60–90 mg/kg/day or 1.3–1.95 g/m^2/day, divided in 4 doses to be administered every 6 h. In 2013, an enteric-coated delayed-release formulation of cysteamine bitartrate (Procysby®) that can be administered every 12 h has been approved for clinical use in the US and in Europe. The doses of cysteamine should be titrated to maintain leukocyte cystine levels less than 1.0–1.5 nmol half-cystine/mg protein. The main side effects include gastric discomfort that can be attenuated with acid reducing therapy, and foul odor that significantly decreases compliance, particularly in adolescents. Exceptionally, patients have develop reactive angioendotheliomatosis skin lesions, *striae rubrae*, bone pain, and/or myalgia. Other infrequent side effects include drug-induced lupus, neutropenia, seizures, lethargy, somnolence and drug rash. Cysteamine is contraindicated in pregnant women.

Despite its very beneficial effects on kidney function, early initiation of cysteamine therapy delays but does not prevent progression to ESKD. In addition, cysteamine has little effect on the renal Fanconi syndrome. Treatment significantly improves growth and delays or even prevent all other complications of the disease. Patients treated with cysteamine since diagnosis are only entering in their forties now, and most are still in their twenties and thirties. More data are needed to assess the very long-term benefits of this therapy.

Systemic therapy does not reach the cornea. Therefore, patients need to use a cysteamine collyrium that is not well tolerated and needs to be employed very frequently. Two commercial preparations have recently been introduced in the US and in Europe. CYSTARAN® is a 0.44% cysteamine eye drop solution with increased stability and tolerability, and CYSTADROPS® is a 0.55% viscous solution that can be applied four times per day and has shown long-term benefits on corneal crystal deposition.

Promising preclinical data have been obtained after bone marrow transplantation in cystinosis mice. The benefits of this therapy are related to infiltrating hematopoietic stem cell-derived macrophages that can clear cystine crystals and rescue neighboring cells by direct cell-cell contact mediated by tunneling nanotubes. An allogenic hematopoietic stem cell transplantation has been performed in a 16-year-old boy; the patient unfortunately expired after complications related to the transplantation, but evidence of engraftment and improvement could be demonstrated. A phase I/II clinical trial (NCT03897361) using gene-corrected autologous hematopoietic stem cells is currently underway.

Suggested Reading

Adelmann CH, Traunbauer AK, Chen B, Condon KJ, Chan SH, Kunchok T, et al. MFSD12 mediates the import of cysteine into melanosomes and lysosomes. Nature. 2020;588(7839):699–704.

Ariceta G, Lara E, Camacho JA, Oppenheimer F, Vara J, Santos F, et al. Cysteamine (Cystagon(R)) adherence in patients with cystinosis in Spain: successful in children and a challenge in adolescents and adults. Nephrol Dial Transplant. 2015;30(3):475–80.

Attard M, Jean G, Forestier L, Cherqui S, van't Hoff W, Broyer M, et al. Severity of phenotype in cystinosis varies with mutations in the CTNS gene: predicted effect on the model of cystinosin. Hum Mol Genet. 1999;8(13):2507–14.

Besouw MT, Bowker R, Dutertre JP, Emma F, Gahl WA, Greco M, et al. Cysteamine toxicity in patients with cystinosis. J Pediatr. 2011;159(6):1004–11.

Besouw MT, Kremer JA, Janssen MC, Levtchenko EN. Fertility status in male cystinosis patients treated with cysteamine. Fertil Steril. 2010;93(6):1880–3.

Blakey H, Proudfoot-Jones J, Knox E, Lipkin G. Pregnancy in women with cystinosis. Clin Kidney J. 2019;12(6):855–8.

Brodin-Sartorius A, Tete MJ, Niaudet P, Antignac C, Guest G, Ottolenghi C, et al. Cysteamine therapy delays the progression of nephropathic cystinosis in late adolescents and adults. Kidney Int. 2012;81(2):179–89.

Chandra M, Stokes MB, Kaskel F. Multinucleated podocytes: a diagnostic clue to cystinosis. Kidney Int. 2010;78(10):1052.

Cherqui S, Courtoy PJ. The renal Fanconi syndrome in cystinosis: pathogenic insights and therapeutic perspectives. Nat Rev Nephrol. 2017;13(2):115–31.

Cherqui S, Sevin C, Hamard G, Kalatzis V, Sich M, Pequignot MO, et al. Intralysosomal cystine accumulation in mice lacking cystinosin, the protein defective in cystinosis. Mol Cell Biol. 2002;22(21):7622–32.

Chik CL, Friedman A, Merriam GR, Gahl WA. Pituitary-testicular function in nephropathic cystinosis. Ann Intern Med. 1993;119(7 Pt 1):568–75.

Cohen C, Charbit M, Chadefaux-Vekemans B, Giral M, Garrigue V, Kessler M, et al. Excellent long-term outcome of renal transplantation in cystinosis patients. Orphanet J Rare Dis. 2015;10:90.

Corden BJ, Schulman JD, Schneider JA, Thoene JG. Adverse reactions to oral cysteamine use in nephropathic cystinosis. Dev Pharmacol Ther. 1981;3(1):25–30.

David D, Princiero Berlingerio S, Elmonem MA, Oliveira Arcolino F, Soliman N, van den Heuvel B, et al. Molecular basis of cystinosis: geographic distribution, functional consequences of mutations in the CTNS gene, and potential for repair. Nephron. 2019;141(2):133–46.

Dogulu CF, Tsilou E, Rubin B, Fitzgibbon EJ, Kaiser-Kupper MI, Rennert OM, et al. Idiopathic intracranial hypertension in cystinosis. J Pediatr. 2004;145(5):673–8.

Elmonem MA, Veys K, Oliveira Arcolino F, Van Dyck M, Benedetti MC, Diomedi-Camassei F, et al. Allogeneic HSCT transfers wild-type cystinosin to nonhematological epithelial cells in cystinosis: first human report. Am J Transplant. 2018;18(11):2823–8.

Elmonem MA, Veys KR, Soliman NA, van Dyck M, van den Heuvel LP, Levtchenko E. Cystinosis: a review. Orphanet J Rare Dis. 2016;11:47.

Emma F, Nesterova G, Langman C, Labbe A, Cherqui S, Goodyer P, et al. Nephropathic cystinosis: an international consensus document. Nephrol Dial Transplant. 2014;29(Suppl 4):iv87–94.
Eroglu FK, Besbas N, Ozaltin F, Topaloglu R, Ozen S. Lupus in a patient with cystinosis: is it drug induced? Lupus. 2015;24(13):1452–4.
Ewert A, Leifheit-Nestler M, Hohenfellner K, Buscher A, Kemper MJ, Oh J, et al. Bone and mineral metabolism in children with nephropathic cystinosis compared with other CKD entities. J Clin Endocrinol Metab. 2020;105(8):e2738–e2752.
Fivush B, Flick JA, Gahl WA. Pancreatic exocrine insufficiency in a patient with nephropathic cystinosis. J Pediatr. 1988;112(1):49–51.
Fivush B, Green OC, Porter CC, Balfe JW, O'Regan S, Gahl WA. Pancreatic endocrine insufficiency in posttransplant cystinosis. Am J Dis Child. 1987;141(10):1087–9.
Gahl WA, Balog JZ, Kleta R. Nephropathic cystinosis in adults: natural history and effects of oral cysteamine therapy. Ann Intern Med. 2007;147(4):242–50.
Gahl WA, Bashan N, Tietze F, Schulman JD. Lysosomal cystine counter-transport in heterozygotes for cystinosis. Am J Hum Genet. 1984a;36(2):277–82.
Gahl WA, Dalakas MC, Charnas L, Chen KT, Pezeshkpour GH, Kuwabara T, et al. Myopathy and cystine storage in muscles in a patient with nephropathic cystinosis. N Engl J Med. 1988;319(22):1461–4.
Gahl WA, Hubbard VS, Orloff S. Decreased sweat production in cystinosis. J Pediatr. 1984b;104(6):904–5.
Gahl WA, Kuehl EM, Iwata F, Lindblad A, Kaiser-Kupfer MI. Corneal crystals in nephropathic cystinosis: natural history and treatment with cysteamine eyedrops. Mol Genet Metab. 2000;71(1–2):100–20.
Gahl WA, Reed GF, Thoene JG, Schulman JD, Rizzo WB, Jonas AJ, et al. Cysteamine therapy for children with nephropathic cystinosis. N Engl J Med. 1987;316(16):971–7.
Gahl WA, Thoene JG, Schneider JA. Cystinosis. N Engl J Med. 2002;347(2):111–21.
Gahl WA. Early oral cysteamine therapy for nephropathic cystinosis. Eur J Pediatr. 2003;162(Suppl 1):S38–41.
Galarreta CI, Forbes MS, Thornhill BA, Antignac C, Gubler MC, Nevo N, et al. The swan-neck lesion: proximal tubular adaptation to oxidative stress in nephropathic cystinosis. Am J Physiol Renal Physiol. 2015;308(10):F1155–66.
Geelen JM, Monnens LA, Levtchenko EN. Follow-up and treatment of adults with cystinosis in the Netherlands. Nephrol Dial Transplant. 2002;17(10):1766–70.
Gubler MC, Lacoste M, Sich M, Broyer M. The pathology of the kidney in cystinosis. In: Broyer M, editor. Cystinosis. Amsterdam: Elsevier; 1999. p. 42–8.
Hohenfellner K, Bergmann C, Fleige T, Janzen N, Burggraf S, Olgemoller B, et al. Molecular based newborn screening in Germany: follow-up for cystinosis. Mol Genet Metab Rep. 2019;21:100514.
Huynh N, Gahl WA, Bishop RJ. Cysteamine ophthalmic solution 0.44% for the treatment of corneal cystine crystals in cystinosis. Expert Rev Ophthalmol. 2013;8(4):341–5.
Ivanova EA, Arcolino FO, Elmonem MA, Rastaldi MP, Giardino L, Cornelissen EM, et al. Cystinosin deficiency causes podocyte damage and loss associated with increased cell motility. Kidney Int. 2016;89(5):1037–48.
Jonas AJ, Conley SB, Marshall R, Johnson RA, Marks M, Rosenberg H. Nephropathic cystinosis with central nervous system involvement. Am J Med. 1987;83(5):966–70.
Kalatzis V, Cherqui S, Antignac C, Gasnier B. Cystinosin, the protein defective in cystinosis, is a H(+)-driven lysosomal cystine transporter. EMBO J. 2001;20(21):5940–9.
Kizilbash SJ, Snyder J, Vock DM, Chavers BM. Trends in kidney transplant outcomes in children and young adults with cystinosis. Pediatr Transplant. 2019;23(8):e13572.
Krischock L, Horsfield C, D'Cruz D, Rigden SP. Drug-induced lupus and antiphospholipid syndrome associated with cysteamine therapy. Nephrol Dial Transplant. 2009;24(6):1997–9.

Langman CB, Barshop BA, Deschenes G, Emma F, Goodyer P, Lipkin G, et al. Controversies and research agenda in nephropathic cystinosis: conclusions from a "Kidney Disease: Improving Global Outcomes" (KDIGO) Controversies Conference. Kidney Int. 2016;89(6):1192–203.
Liang H, Labbe A, Baudouin C, Plisson C, Giordano V. Long-term follow-up of cystinosis patients treated with 0.55% cysteamine hydrochloride. Br J Ophthalmol. 2020;608–13.
Liang H, Labbe A, Le Mouhaer J, Plisson C, Baudouin C. A new viscous cysteamine eye drops treatment for ophthalmic cystinosis: an open-label randomized comparative phase III pivotal study. Invest Ophthalmol Vis Sci. 2017;58(4):2275–83.
Mahoney CP, Striker GE. Early development of the renal lesions in infantile cystinosis. Pediatr Nephrol. 2000;15(1–2):50–6.
Markello TC, Bernardini IM, Gahl WA. Improved renal function in children with cystinosis treated with cysteamine. N Engl J Med. 1993;328(16):1157–62.
Martin-Begue N, Alarcon S, Wolley-Dod C, Lara LE, Madrid A, Cano P, et al. Intracranial hypertension in cystinosis is a challenge: experience in a children's hospital. JIMD Rep. 2017;35:17–22.
Naphade S, Sharma J, Gaide Chevronnay HP, Shook MA, Yeagy BA, Rocca CJ, et al. Brief reports: lysosomal cross-correction by hematopoietic stem cell-derived macrophages via tunneling nanotubes. Stem Cells. 2015;33(1):301–9.
Patrick AD, Lake BD. Cystinosis: electron microscopic evidence of lysosomal storage of cystine in lymph node. J Clin Pathol. 1968;21(5):571–5.
Prencipe G, Caiello I, Cherqui S, Whisenant T, Petrini S, Emma F, et al. Inflammasome activation by cystine crystals: implications for the pathogenesis of cystinosis. J Am Soc Nephrol. 2014;25(6):1163–9.
Sadjadi R, Sullivan S, Grant N, Thomas SE, Doyle M, Hammond C, et al. Clinical myopathy in patients with nephropathic cystinosis. Muscle Nerve. 2020;61(1):74–80.
Schulman JD, Bradley KH, Seegmiller JE. Cystine: compartmentalization within lysosomes in cystinotic leukocytes. Science. 1969;166(3909):1152–4.
Servais A, Saitovitch A, Hummel A, Boisgontier J, Scemla A, Sberro-Soussan R, et al. Central nervous system complications in adult cystinosis patients. J Inherit Metab Dis. 2020;43(2):348–56.
Shotelersuk V, Larson D, Anikster Y, McDowell G, Lemons R, Bernardini I, et al. CTNS mutations in an American-based population of cystinosis patients. Am J Hum Genet. 1998;63(5):1352–62.
Syres K, Harrison F, Tadlock M, Jester JV, Simpson J, Roy S, et al. Successful treatment of the murine model of cystinosis using bone marrow cell transplantation. Blood. 2009;114(12):2542–52.
Theodoropoulos DS, Krasnewich D, Kaiser-Kupfer MI, Gahl WA. Classic nephropathic cystinosis as an adult disease. JAMA. 1993;270(18):2200–4.
Town M, Jean G, Cherqui S, Attard M, Forestier L, Whitmore SA, et al. A novel gene encoding an integral membrane protein is mutated in nephropathic cystinosis. Nat Genet. 1998;18(4):319–24.
Van Stralen KJ, Emma F, Jager KJ, Verrina E, Schaefer F, Laube GF, et al. Improvement in the renal prognosis in nephropathic cystinosis. Clin J Am Soc Nephrol. 2011;6(10):2485–91.
Veys KR, D'Hauwers KW, van Dongen A, Janssen MC, Besouw MTP, Goossens E, et al. First successful conception induced by a male cystinosis patient. JIMD Rep. 2018;38:1–6.
Veys KR, Elmonem MA, Arcolino FO, van den Heuvel L, Levtchenko E. Nephropathic cystinosis: an update. Curr Opin Pediatr. 2017;29(2):168–78.

Chronic Tubulointerstitial Nephritis: Hypokalemia, Hyperoxaluria, and Hyperuricemia

Carmen Elena Cervantes and Mohamed G. Atta

1 Introduction

Non-immune metabolic diseases are an important cause of chronic interstitial nephritis. These include metabolic disorders such as hypokalemia, hyperoxaluria and hyperuricemia/hyperuricosuria. Tubulointerstitial injury develops from various mechanisms and results in chronic kidney disease from interstitial fibrosis. For example, medullary ammonia accumulation activates the alternative complement pathway in hypokalemic interstitial nephritis. In contrast, excessive concentrations of urinary oxalate and uric acid lead to crystal formation and intra-renal deposition. In addition to tubular obstruction and direct tubular toxicity, these crystals activate the NALP-3 inflammasome in the interstitial cells, resulting in maturation of proinflammatory IL-1β and IL-18. Also, uric acid directly stimulates the nuclear factor-κB (NF-κB) signaling pathway. In this chapter, these metabolic causes are discussed. Table 1 summarizes these causes of tubulointerstitial nephritis.

2 Hypokalemic Chronic Interstitial Nephritis

2.1 Epidemiology

Hypokalemic chronic interstitial nephritis was first described in the mid 1950's, particularly in patients with anorexia nervosa. It is more common in women than men and it is usually identified by the age of 25 years with an estimated prevalence of 15–20% among patients with eating disorders. In a 21 year follow up study of

C. E. Cervantes (✉) · M. G. Atta
Division of Nephrology, Johns Hopkins University, Baltimore, MD, USA
e-mail: ccervan2@jhmi.edu; matta1@jhmi.edu

M. G. Atta, M. A. Perazella (eds.), *Tubulointerstitial Nephritis*,
https://doi.org/10.1007/978-3-030-93438-5_13

Table 1 Summary of metabolic causes of chronic interstitial nephritis

Metabolic cause of chronic interstitial nephritis	Etiologies	Mechanism	Clinical presentation	Treatment
Hypokalemia	Eating disorders (e.g., anorexia nervosa) Primary or secondary hyperaldosteronism Bartter and Gittelman syndromes Herbs (glycyrrhiza species)	Ammoniagenesis in the proximal tubules ➔ NH_3 accumulation in the medullary interstitium causes alternative complement pathway activation via C3	Low plasma potassium, high aldosterone, and variable renin levels Low molecular weight proteinuria Medullary renal cysts Kidney biopsy: focal lymphocytic cellular infiltrate, vacuoles in the proximal and distal tubular cells, hypertrophy, and hyperplasia of the juxtaglomerular apparatus	Potassium repletion Potassium sparing diuretics Focused on the underlying etiology

Table 1 (continued)

Metabolic cause of chronic interstitial nephritis	Etiologies	Mechanism	Clinical presentation	Treatment
Calcium oxalate	Primary oxaluria ➔ defective enzyme activity resulting in endogenous production of oxalate Secondary forms ➔ enteric hyperoxaluria, with fat malabsorption being the most common one, followed by high dietary oxalate intake Medications such as ascorbic acid and orlistat Juicing drinks Ethylene glycol	Crystal dependent mechanism ➔ NALP3 inflammasome pathway activation	Proteinuria Hematuria Urinary oxalate crystals Kidney biopsy: mononuclear interstitial infiltration, calcium oxalate crystals in the tubules and interstitium, periglomerular and interstitial fibrosis	Diet: Increased fluid and calcium, and decreased fat and oxalate intakes Unproven benefit: cholestyramine In primary oxaluria type 1: Lumasiran, pyridoxine Novel therapies under study: substrate reduction therapies (siRNA, inhibitors, or gene silencing) and replacement therapies (enzyme replacement, cell, or gene therapy Liver-kidney transplantation for primary hyperoxaluria type 1 Restoration of bowel continuity in secondary forms related to bariatric surgery

(continued)

Table 1 (continued)

Metabolic cause of chronic interstitial nephritis	Etiologies	Mechanism	Clinical presentation	Treatment
Uric acid	High dietary intake of purines or food high in carbohydrates and salt High cell turnover states (e.g., tumor lysis syndrome) Chronic kidney disease, diuretics, Mesoamerican nephropathy UMOD mutation	Crystal independent mechanism ➔ NF-κB signaling pathway activation in the tubular cells and oxidative stress Crystal dependent mechanism ➔ NALP3 inflammasome pathway activation	Bland urine sediment, mild proteinuria, and hyperuricemia Medullary cysts – in patients with UMOD mutation Kidney biopsy: glomerulosclerosis, tubulointerstitial fibrosis, and uric acid crystal deposition in the tubules and medulla	Allopurinol, febuxostat and urine alkalinization (unproven benefit)

patients with anorexia nervosa, 5.2% developed end-stage kidney disease (ESKD) after diagnosis.

Other causes of severe hypokalemia linked to interstitial nephritis include chronic vomiting, laxative or diuretic abuse, Bartter and Gitelman syndromes, primary hyperaldosteronism or conditions that mimic an aldosterone excess, such as those associated with the consumption of herbs containing glycyrrhiza species.

2.2 Pathophysiology

Low potassium nephropathy is characterized by a state of mineralocorticoid excess in its primary forms or secondary to hypovolemia, which results in maintenance of hypokalemia. Chronic exposure of the kidney to the downstream effects of hypokalemia can ultimately result in tubulointerstitial injury and fibrosis—the essence of hypokalemic nephropathy.

In the proximal tubule, hypokalemia increases the production of ammonia (NH_3) from the cellular metabolism of glutamine. This process generates ammonium (NH_4^+), which is secreted to the lumen by the Na^+/H^+ exchanger and subsequently reabsorbed via the apical Na^+-$K^+(NH_4^+)$-$2Cl^-$ cotransporter and basolateral Na^+-$H^+(NH_4^+)$ exchanger 4 in the thick ascending limb of the Loop of Henle. The net effect is an increased concentration of NH_4^+ in the medullary interstitium, which in turn dissociates into H^+ and NH_3 (Fig. 1). The latter induces alternative complement pathway activation. Under normal conditions, complement activation is dampened by complement factor regulators, but the excessive amount of ammonia saturates the system, culminating in uncontrolled complement terminal pathway activation, tissue injury, inflammation, and subsequent fibrosis.

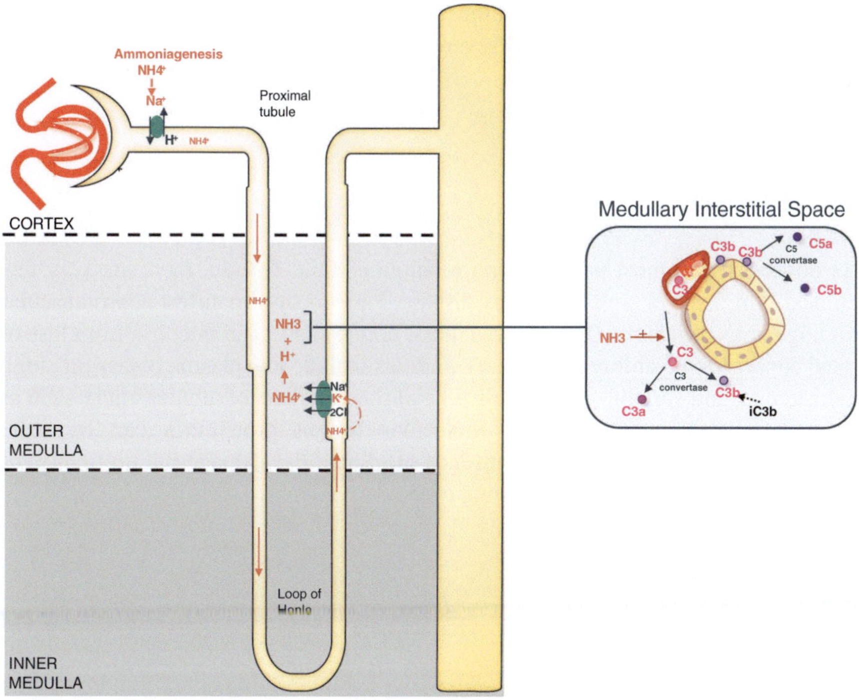

Fig. 1 Mechanism of interstitial nephritis in hypokalemia. Severe hypokalemia induces ammoniagenesis in the proximal tubule. Ammonium (NH_4^+) is secreted to the lumen by the Na^+/H^+ exchanger and it is reabsorbed via the apical Na^+-$K^+(NH_4^+)$-$2Cl^-$ cotransporter and basolateral $Na^+(NH_4^+)$-H^+ exchanger 4 in the thick ascending limb of the Loop of Henle. The net effect is an increased concentration of NH_4^+ in the medullary interstitium, which will dissociate into H^+ and NH_3. Ammonia induces alternative complement pathway activation via C3. Under normal conditions, C3b inhibitor (iC3b) maintains a balance, but the excessive amount of ammonia saturates the system, culminating in complement activation. Abbreviations: Ammonium (NH_4^+), ammonia (NH_3), C3b inhibitor(iC3b)

Another mechanism that may be playing a role in hypokalemic chronic interstitial nephritis is collecting tubular cell hyperplasia. In animal models, a decrease in extracellular potassium concentration with the subsequent intracellular acidosis promotes protein synthesis via an increase in growth factors. The resulting hyperplasia of the collecting-tubule cells in the outer medulla obstructs the tubular lumen, creating tubular dilatation, and medullary cysts.

2.3 *Histopathology*

Almost 75% of the cases of hypokalemic chronic interstitial nephritis show a focal lymphocytic cellular infiltrate in the interstitial space. Other characteristic pathologic findings include vacuolar formation in the proximal and distal tubular cells, and hypertrophy and hyperplasia of the juxtaglomerular apparatus. The latter occurs at least 1 month after the onset of severe hypokalemia and may be reversible with potassium repletion.

2.4 Clinical Picture

As observed with most patients with tubulointerstitial disease, there are very few clinical symptoms or signs of kidney disease. Patients may manifest neuromuscular findings of hypokalemia (muscle weakness, cramps, etc.) and nocturia from loss of renal concentrating ability. Laboratory findings include low plasma potassium, high aldosterone, and variable renin levels. In addition, markers of tubular injury such as urine β_2-microglobulin and low molecular weight proteinuria can be seen. Albuminuria is infrequent due to absence of glomerular damage but up to 44% of these patients develop medullary renal cysts.

2.5 Treatment

The therapy should be focused on addressing the underlying condition. Potassium repletion, potassium-sparing diuretics like epithelial sodium channel blockers (e.g., amiloride, triamterene), or mineralocorticoid antagonists (e.g., spironolactone, eplerenone) can be used.

3 Oxalate Nephropathy

3.1 Epidemiology

Oxalate nephropathy is a well-recognized entity that can present with kidney stone formation and/or chronic kidney disease (CKD). Acute oxalate nephropathy may also be seen. The etiology of hyperoxaluria can be primary from inherited diseases or secondary to a variety of disorders (gastric bypass procedures, gastrointestinal diseases, pancreatic insufficiency, drugs, etc.).

Primary hyperoxaluria usually presents at a mean age of 9.5 years. Three genetic types have been described, but the most common and severe one is caused by an autosomal recessive defect in the vitamin B6 dependent hepatic peroxisomal enzyme alanine glyoxalate aminotransferase, which results in an increased endogenous production of oxalate. ESKD develops in approximately 43% of the patients with type 1 primary hyperoxaluria within 30 years following the diagnosis. The prevalence of primary oxaluria is highest in countries with high rate of consanguinity such as Middle Eastern countries.

In contrast, secondary forms present at a mean age of 56 years and up to 58% of these patients progress to ESKD. Secondary hyperoxaluria is commonly caused by fat malabsorption (75%), followed by high dietary oxalate intake, and less frequently decreased intestinal oxalate degradation, and increased colonic permeability to oxalate. Medications such as high-dose ascorbic acid, various high oxalate containing juicing drinks, intoxicants such as ethylene glycol, and the gastrointestinal-lipase inhibitor orlistat are associated with oxalate nephropathy.

3.2 Pathophysiology

Oxalate is derived from the hepatic metabolism of glyoxylate, amino acids, and carbohydrates or from exogenous dietary sources. It is primarily filtered by the glomeruli and secreted by the proximal tubules without expected renal reabsorption. In hyperoxaluria, the solute-linked carrier 26 A1 (SLC26A1) transporter is overexpressed on the basolateral side of the proximal tubules to enhance its secretion into the lumen via the Cl^-/oxalate exchanger (SLC26A6) expressed on the brush-border membrane of proximal tubular cells.

Urinary oxalate binds with calcium and in higher concentrations, it causes calcium oxalate supersaturation and crystal formation. This can take the form of stones (nephrolithiasis) and/or tissue calcifications (nephrocalcinosis). Calcium oxalate crystals have toxic effects on the interstitial, epithelial and tubular cells. As shown in Fig. 2, the nucleotide-binding domain leucine-rich repeat inflammasome (NALP3) proteins are stimulated in response to high oxalate levels and lead to maturation of proinflammatory IL-1β and IL-18. The inflammasomes are intracellular protein complexes, part of the innate immune system, that lead to activation of pro-inflammatory caspase 1, thereby mediating apoptosis, interstitial inflammation, and fibrosis.

3.3 Histopathology

In acute settings, acute tubular injury and mononuclear interstitial infiltration are seen. Other findings include calcium oxalate crystals in the tubules and interstitium (Fig. 3), and approximately 70% of patients already have evidence of chronicity, such as interstitial fibrosis, mesangial matrix expansion and periglomerular fibrosis.

3.4 Clinical Presentation

Patients generally present with symptoms and signs of nephrolithiasis with flank pain and hematuria. Acute or chronic kidney disease may also be seen. Common urinary findings include proteinuria (69%), followed by hematuria (32%), and

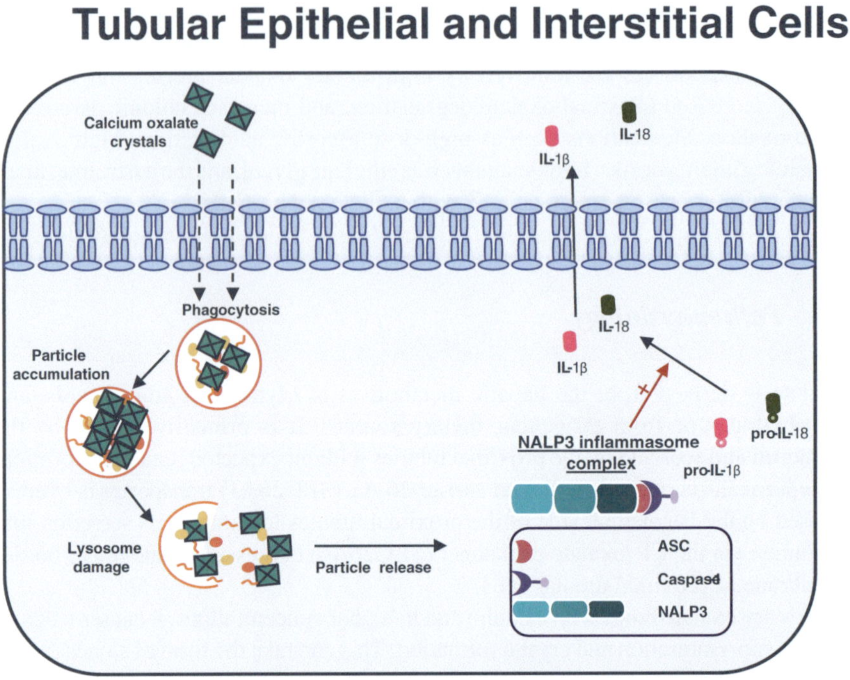

Fig. 2 Mechanism of interstitial nephritis in oxalate nephropathy. Calcium oxalate crystals have toxic effects on interstitial, epithelial, and tubular cells. Human kidney cells have the ability to phagocytose crystals, but given the urinary and tissue supersaturation of calcium oxalate, particle accumulation and lysosomal damage occur. This results in a release of cytotoxic substances such as lysosomal enzymes and crystals that culminate on the activation of NALP3. This molecule recruits the adaptor ASC and caspase 1, which cleaves pro-inflammatory cytokines and allow for maturation of IL-1β and IL-18. Subsequently, these interleukins will be released through membrane pores into the interstitial space, amplifying the inflammatory response. Abbreviations: Nucleotide-binding domain leucine-rich repeat (NALP3), inflammasome adaptor protein (ASC)

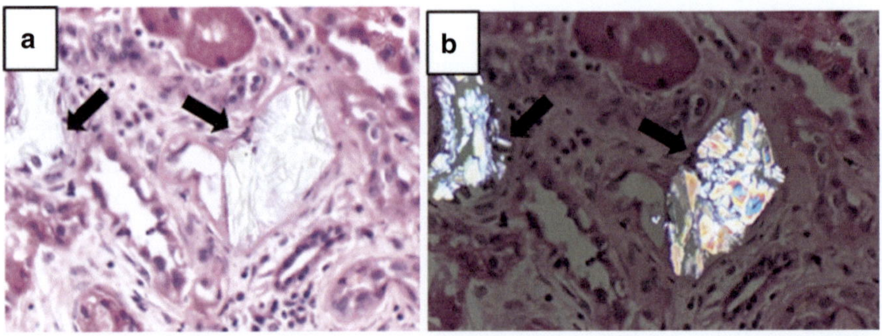

Fig. 3 (**a**) shows intratubular calcium oxalate crystals with gray-white and spiculated appearance (arrows). Under polarized light the crystals show positive birefringence (arrows) as seen in (**b**). (Images courtesy of Gabriel Giannini, MD)

urinary calcium oxalate crystals (26%). The finding of calcium oxalate crystal casts is diagnostic of oxalate nephropathy, although a kidney biopsy may be required in some cases. High oxalate levels in the serum (>9 mmol/l) and urine (>45 mg/24 h) are also described.

3.5 Treatment

General management includes supportive measures such as increased fluid, citrate, and calcium intake, along with decreased fat and oxalate consumption. Therapies with unproven benefit include cholestyramine and microbiome manipulation. Using RNA interference technology, the new agent Lumasiran has been demonstrated to reduce levels of glycolate oxidase (GO) enzyme by targeting the hydroxyacid oxidase 1 (HAO1) messenger ribonucleic acid (mRNA) in hepatocytes. Decreased GO enzyme levels reduce the amount of available glyoxylate, a substrate for oxalate production. Administered subcutaneously as a loading dose, based on body weight, followed by monthly or quarterly dosing scheme, it reduces urinary oxalate excretion by about 50% at 6 months compared to placebo.

Pyridoxine (B6) at 20 mg/kg/d has been shown to also decrease urinary oxalate excretion by approximately 30% on patients with primary hyperoxaluria type 1, specifically in those with the p.Gly170Arg mutation. Combined liver-kidney transplantation can be used for primary hyperoxaluria type 1 with systemic oxalosis and end organ damage as it prevents disease recurrence in the kidney allograft. Other agents are being tested to treat all types of primary hyperoxaluria including substrate reduction therapies (siRNA, inhibitors, or gene silencing) and replacement therapies (enzyme replacement, cell or gene therapy). Restoration of bowel continuity has been implemented in secondary forms related to bariatric surgery.

4 Uric Acid Nephropathy

4.1 Epidemiology

Approximately 20% of the US population has hyperuricemia, defined as uric acid levels greater than 7 mg/dL in men and 6.0 mg/dL in women. Although higher levels are both a cause and a consequence of kidney disease, most studies support the role of hyperuricemia as an independent risk factor for CKD, with a 2-to 10-fold increased risk, especially among women.

Exogenous sources of purines such as meats, alcohol, and fructose, and endogenous ones, like high cell turnover states (i.e., tumor lysis syndrome) can lead to hyperuricemia. Further, genetic mutation in the uromodulin (UMOD) gene can cause autosomal dominant tubulointerstitial nephritis, leading to ESKD by age 54.

In Mesoamerican nephropathy, although the cause of CKD remains uncertain, hyperuricemia and hypokalemia are common findings.

4.2 Pathophysiology

Uric acid can be generated from amino acid precursors in the liver by the action of xanthine oxidase, or through purine degradation (e.g., nucleic acids). Due to the absence of urate oxidase in humans, serum uric acid is mostly excreted by the renal and gastrointestinal systems.

In the kidneys, more than 90% of filtered urate is reabsorbed in the proximal tubules via the apical URAT1 (SLC22A12) and the basolateral transporter GLUT9 (SCLC2A9). Interestingly, later in the proximal tubule, it undergoes extensive secretion.

Uric acid induces inflammation through crystal dependent and independent mechanisms. Similar to oxalate nephropathy, the NALP3 inflammasome is activated by monosodium urate crystals and promotes tubular-interstitial inflammation through IL-1β and IL-18. Further, urate directly activates the nuclear factor- κB (NF-κB) signaling pathway in the tubular cells, resulting in T cell and macrophage accumulation in tubular epithelial cells and more predominantly in tubular interstitial spaces (Fig. 4). Consequently, the release of pro-inflammatory cytokines such as TNF-α, MCP-1 and RANTES amplifies the initial inflammatory response, oxidative stress, and apoptosis. Eventually, pro-fibrotic cytokines activate matrix-producing cells and transforms renal tubular cells to a mesenchymal phenotype capable of producing prorenin and activating the renin angiotensin aldosterone system. This leads to glomerular hypertrophy and tubulointerstitial inflammation even in the absence of crystal deposition.

4.3 Histopathology

Kidney biopsy shows arteriolosclerosis, glomerulosclerosis, tubulointerstitial fibrosis, and uric acid crystal deposition in the tubules and medulla (Fig. 5). The intrarenal crystals can generate a granulomatous reaction and micro-tophi, especially within the medulla.

4.4 Clinical Presentation

Urate nephropathy has nonspecific features, including decreased kidney function, bland urine sediment, mild proteinuria, and hyperuricemia. However, uric acid crystals (Fig. 5) may be seen and may point to the diagnosis of uric acid nephropathy in

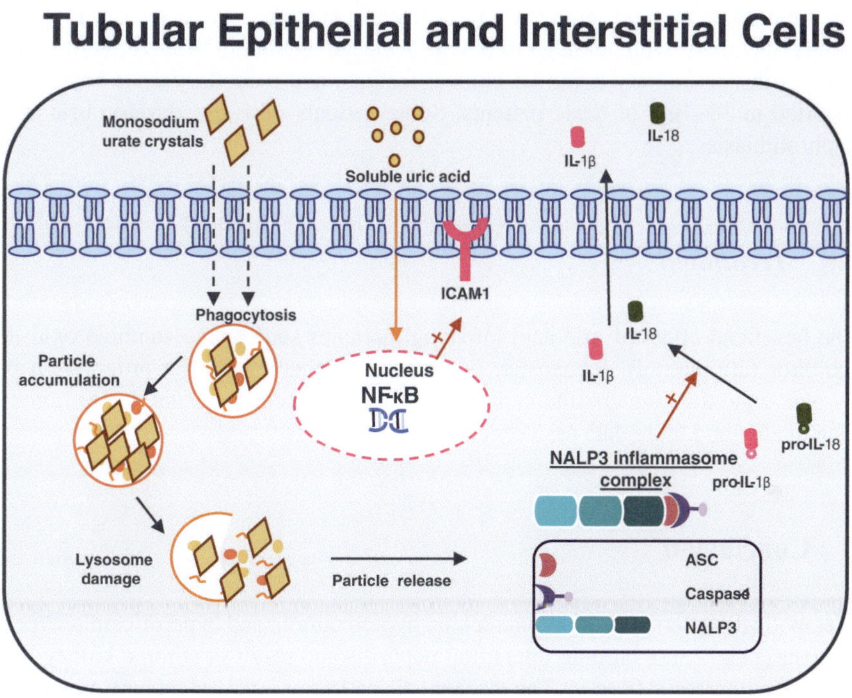

Fig. 4 Mechanism of interstitial nephritis in hyperuricemia. Uric acid induces inflammation through crystal dependent and independent mechanisms. Monosodium urate crystals activate the NALP3 inflammasome as described in Fig. 2, which induces the maturation of IL-1β and IL-18. Soluble uric acid directly activates the nuclear factor- κB (NF-κB) signaling pathway in the tubular cells to increase ICAM-1 expression. The net effect is T cell and macrophage accumulation in tubular epithelial cells and more predominantly in tubular interstitial spaces. Abbreviations: Nucleotide-binding domain leucine-rich repeat (NALP3), inflammasome adaptor protein (ASC), intercellular adhesion molecule-1 (ICAM-1)

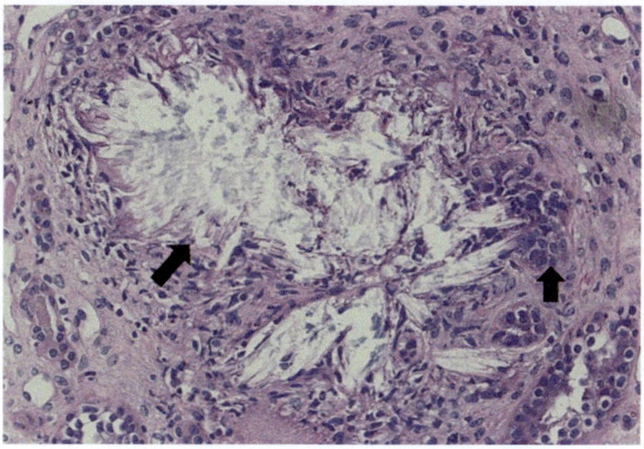

Fig. 5 H&E stain shows uric acid deposits in the renal medulla, with the typical needle-like crystals surrounded by some mononuclear inflammatory reaction (arrows). (Image courtesy of Serena Bagnasco, MD)

the appropriate clinical setting. CKD of unclear etiology can be seen in multiple family members with undiagnosed UMOD gene mutation. Hyperuricemia and gouty arthritis are very common clinical features and medullary cysts have been reported in 30–70% of these patients. Some patients may also develop uric acid nephrolithiasis.

4.5 Treatment

The beneficial effect of uric acid lowering therapies such as the xanthine oxidase inhibitor (allopurinol), febuxostat, or urine alkalinization on the progression of chronic urate tubulointerstitial nephropathy have been controversial due to limited data quality and more data are needed.

5 Conclusion

Metabolic disorders such as hypokalemia, hyperoxaluria, and hyperuricemia/hyperuricosuria can cause chronic interstitial nephritis and result in chronic kidney disease from interstitial fibrosis. The mechanistic pathways involved include medullary ammonia accumulation followed by alternative complement pathway activation in hypokalemic interstitial nephritis; and direct tubular toxicity and activation of the NALP-3 inflammasome by oxalate and uric acid crystals. The development of end-stage kidney disease has been described in all these conditions. Therefore, it is important to identify these metabolic disorders in a timely manner, especially since newer therapies are now available and can prevent kidney related morbidity.

Suggested Reading

Bhasin B, Ürekli HM, Atta MG. Primary and secondary hyperoxaluria: understanding the enigma. World J Nephrol. 2015;4(2):235–44.

Bobulescu IA, Moe OW. Renal transport of uric acid: evolving concepts and uncertainties. Adv Chronic Kidney Dis. 2012;19(6):358–71.

Bouquegneau A, Dubois BE, Krzesinski JM, Delanaye P. Anorexia nervosa and the kidney. Am J Kidney Dis. 2012;60(2):299–307.

Brar JE, Quigg RJ. Complement activation in the tubulointerstitium: AKI, CKD, and in between. Kidney Int. 2014;86(4):663–6.

Canos HJ, Hogg GA, Jeffery JR. Oxalate nephropathy due to gastrointestinal disorders. Can Med Assoc J. 1981;124(6):729–33.

Devresse A, Cochat P, Godefroid N, Kanaan N. Transplantation for primary Hyperoxaluria type 1: designing new strategies in the era of promising therapeutic perspectives. Kidney Int Rep. 2020;5(12):2136–45.

Ejaz AA, Nakagawa T, Kanbay M, Kuwabara M, Kumar A, Garcia Arroyo FE, et al. Hyperuricemia in kidney disease: a major risk factor for cardiovascular events, vascular calcification, and renal damage. Semin Nephrol. 2020;40(6):574–85.

Garrelfs SF, Frishberg Y, Hulton SA, Koren MJ, O'Riordan WD, Cochat P, et al. Lumasiran, an RNAi therapeutic for primary Hyperoxaluria type 1. N Engl J Med. 2021;384(13):1216–26.

Glew RH, Sun Y, Horowitz BL, Konstantinov KN, Barry M, Fair JR, et al. Nephropathy in dietary hyperoxaluria: a potentially preventable acute or chronic kidney disease. World J Nephrol. 2014;3(4):122–42.

Han KH. Mechanisms of the effects of acidosis and hypokalemia on renal ammonia metabolism. Electrolyte Blood Press. 2011;9(2):45–9.

Hudson JI, Hiripi E, Pope HG, Kessler RC. The prevalence and correlates of eating disorders in the National Comorbidity Survey Replication. Biol Psychiatry. 2007;61(3):348–58.

Iseki K, Ikemiya Y, Inoue T, Iseki C, Kinjo K, Takishita S. Significance of hyperuricemia as a risk factor for developing ESRD in a screened cohort. Am J Kidney Dis. 2004;44(4):642–50.

Isnard Bagnis C, Deray G, Baumelou A, Le Quintrec M, Vanherweghem JL. Herbs and the kidney. Am J Kidney Dis. 2004;44(1):1–11.

Johnson RJ, Wesseling C, Newman LS. Chronic kidney disease of unknown cause in agricultural communities. Reply. N Engl J Med. 2019;381(7):689.

Karniski LP, Lötscher M, Fucentese M, Hilfiker H, Biber J, Murer H. Immunolocalization of sat-1 sulfate/oxalate/bicarbonate anion exchanger in the rat kidney. Am J Phys. 1998;275(1):F79–87.

Knauf F, Asplin JR, Granja I, Schmidt IM, Moeckel GW, David RJ, et al. NALP3-mediated inflammation is a principal cause of progressive renal failure in oxalate nephropathy. Kidney Int. 2013;84(5):895–901.

Lumlertgul N, Siribamrungwong M, Jaber BL, Susantitaphong P. Secondary oxalate nephropathy: a systematic review. Kidney Int Rep. 2018;3(6):1363–72.

Maekawa K, Fujimoto T, Shiiki H, Kanauchi M, Fujii Y, Dohi K, et al. A case of Bartter's syndrome with chronic renal failure due to chronic interstitial nephritis. Nihon Jinzo Gakkai Shi. 1998;40(4):309–14.

Novak-Hofer I, Küng W, Eppenberger U. Role of extracellular electrolytes in the activation of ribosomal protein S6 kinase by epidermal growth factor, insulin-like growth factor 1, and insulin in ZR-75-1 cells. J Cell Biol. 1988;106(2):395–401.

Relman AS, Schwartz WB. The nephropathy of potassium depletion; a clinical and pathological entity. N Engl J Med. 1956;255(5):195–203.

Riemenschneider T, Bohle A. Morphologic aspects of low-potassium and low-sodium nephropathy. Clin Nephrol. 1983;19(6):271–9.

Torres VE, Young WF, Offord KP, Hattery RR. Association of hypokalemia, aldosteronism, and renal cysts. N Engl J Med. 1990;322(6):345–51.

Zhao F, Bergstralh EJ, Mehta RA, Vaughan LE, Olson JB, Seide BM, et al. Predictors of incident ESRD among patients with primary Hyperoxaluria presenting prior to kidney failure. Clin J Am Soc Nephrol. 2016;11(1):119–26.

Zhou Y, Fang L, Jiang L, Wen P, Cao H, He W, et al. Uric acid induces renal inflammation via activating tubular NF-κB signaling pathway. PLoS One. 2012;7(6):e39738.

Zipfel S, Löwe B, Reas DL, Deter HC, Herzog W. Long-term prognosis in anorexia nervosa: lessons from a 21-year follow-up study. Lancet. 2000;355(9205):721–2.

Non-immunological Causes of Tubulointerstitial Disease

Cody Cobb, Joshua King, and Bernard G. Jaar

1 Historical Perspectives

Environmental and occupational exposures of nephrotoxic substances have been studied extensively since the onset of the industrial age. As early as the nineteenth century, physicians understood that lead exposure was associated with kidney disease. Notable cases of large-scale industrial and environmental exposures have helped define the scope and degree of some kidney diseases, although the true contribution of individual toxic exposures to kidney disease remains a challenge to determine. Investigations in children in Queensland, Australia exposed to

C. Cobb
Division of Renal Diseases and Hypertension, McGovern Medical School at University of Texas – Houston, Houston, TX, USA
e-mail: cody.m.cobb@uth.tmc.edu

J. King
Department of Medicine, University of Maryland, Baltimore, MD, USA

Department of Pharmacy, University of Maryland, Baltimore, MD, USA

Maryland Poison Center, Baltimore, MD, USA
e-mail: jdking@som.umaryland.edu

B. G. Jaar (✉)
Division of Nephrology, Department of Medicine, Johns Hopkins University School of Medicine, Baltimore, MD, USA

Department of Epidemiology, Johns Hopkins Bloomberg School of Public Health, Baltimore, MD, USA

Welch Center for Prevention, Epidemiology and Clinical Research, Johns Hopkins University, Baltimore, MD, USA

Nephrology Center of Maryland, Baltimore, MD, USA
e-mail: bjaar@aol.com

M. G. Atta, M. A. Perazella (eds.), *Tubulointerstitial Nephritis*,
https://doi.org/10.1007/978-3-030-93438-5_14

lead-based paints between 1890 and 1930 helped determine the extent and properties of lead-induced nephropathy. In the early twentieth century, residents in Toyama, Japan suffered from mass-exposure to cadmium giving rise to *itai-itai* ("Ouch Ouch") disease. The etiology of Balkan Endemic Nephropathy remained a mystery for several decades until a series of case reports in the early 1990s documenting acute toxicity from medicinal herbs containing *Aristolochia* revived an old hypothesis of aristolochic acid as the causative agent, linking together the chronic condition of Balkan Endemic Nephropathy with the acute condition of Chinese Herb Nephropathy. The toxicological literature is limited by its nature, with a heavy reliance on case reports, case series and animal models; similarly, diagnosis of toxin-induced kidney disease relies at least as much on careful history-taking as it does upon biological markers of toxin-specific disease, with some exposures (e.g., lithium, ionizing radiation) producing chronic kidney disease (CKD) years or decades in the future.

2 Heavy Metal Toxicity

A number of metals are able to cause tubulointerstitial nephritis (TIN), generally due to tubular damage from reactive oxygen species or interruption of normal metabolic processes. Tubulointerstitial disease caused by heavy metal toxicity is a complication of prolonged exposure, largely in occupational settings; while blood and urine levels of metals may be helpful, exposure history is key to the diagnosis. Heavy metals primarily affect the kidney through the proximal tubules and may induce generalized proximal tubular dysfunction (e.g., Fanconi syndrome) in earlier stages of toxicity, with TIN generally as a later finding. Common sources and extrarenal toxicities of selected heavy metals are listed in Table 1.

Table 1 Heavy metals implicated in development of tubulointerstitial nephritis

Metal	Example sources	Extrarenal disease
Arsenic	Groundwater, manufacturing (plywood, others)	Hair loss, blood dyscrasias, cancer (skin; many others), peripheral vascular disease
Cadmium	Mining; environmental runoff	Bone disease and fractures
Chromium	Mining, electroplating	Lung, liver, skin disease
Lead	Mining, refining, paint; battery manufacture; moonshine	Hypertension, gout, anemia, peripheral neuropathy
Mercury	Manufacturing (batteries, light bulbs); cosmetics; traditional medicines	Neuropsychiatric disease
Uranium	Mining; contaminated groundwater; warfare	Radiological toxicity (cancer, multiorgan disease)

2.1 Lead

Tubulointerstitial nephritis due to lead toxicity, known as lead nephropathy, is a complication of years (5–30) of exposure to high levels of lead (blood lead levels exceeding 60 μg/dL). Lead nephropathy is rare in developed countries; with removal of lead from paints and automotive fuels, blood lead levels in the United States rarely exceed 5 μg/dL in the modern era, and occupational controls mandate removal from the workplace for workers with lead levels greater than 50 μg/dL. While lead is ubiquitous in the environment, most kidney disease associated with lead is related to occupations such as mining and ore refining, work involving batteries, smelting, and welding, among others. In such settings, multiple prospective studies have supported the causative role of lead in the development of CKD. Historically, acute childhood lead poisoning related to ingestion of lead-containing paint may lead to TIN, as seen in an early twentieth century epidemic in Australia; in the modern era, this is rarely seen due to reduced household lead exposures, childhood lead level screening, and treatment of lead toxicity with chelation.

Lead nephropathy should be considered in the setting of chronic kidney disease of unclear etiology typically associated with a normal urine sediment, hypertension and gout. Ultimately, the diagnosis relies on a history of current or prior lead exposure, along with a host of extrarenal effects including anemia, peripheral neuropathy, neurodevelopmental issues, and others. Whole blood lead measurement is needed but level may not be high if dose exposure has significantly declined or ceased. In certain circumstances, diagnostic chelation may be needed but best performed by a clinician with expertise in the field because of potential associated side effects. Of note, generalized proximal tubular dysfunction may result from acute lead poisoning, often resolving with avoidance and treatment if needed.

2.2 Cadmium

Common exposures to cadmium include food grown with contaminated water or soil, cigarette smoke, and occupational exposure including agricultural fertilizers, and industrial processes (e.g., batteries, pigments, and welding). A well-known incident of large-scale contamination of groundwater with cadmium-containing industrial waste in the Toyama city of Japan gave rise to the disease entity known as Itai-Itai ("Ouch-Ouch" disease) in the early-to-mid twentieth century, characterized by kidney disease, osteomalacia and osteoporosis, and bone fractures.

Cadmium toxicity affects a wide range of organs, including skeletal, respiratory, cardiovascular, hepatic, and renal systems. After initial exposure, cadmium is bound to albumin in plasma, where it is subsequently transported to the liver; the Cadmium-Albumin complex is degraded, releasing free cadmium which induces the production of hepatic metallothioneins, low molecular weight proteins which bind physiological and xenobiotic heavy metals to prevent tissue injury from generation of reactive oxygen species. After hepatic injury, Cadmium-metallothionein (Cd-MT) complexes enter systemic circulation where they are freely filtered in the glomerulus and readily reabsorbed in the proximal tubules. Cd-MT complexes are degraded by the renal proximal tubules cell lysosome system, releasing cadmium ions which then induce synthesis of renal metallothionein proteins. This process continues until the ability of proximal tubule cells to synthesize metallothionein proteins is exhausted, after which free cadmium ions generate locally destructive reactive oxygen species. Continued insult of the proximal tubules with cadmium presents clinically with Fanconi syndrome: glucosuria, aminoaciduria, low molecular weight proteinuria.

2.2.1 Diagnosis of Cadmium Toxicity

Low molecular weight proteins such as beta2-microglobulin, retinol binding protein, and N-acetyl-Beta-D-glucosaminidase are sensitive urinary markers for tubular dysfunction in patients exposed to cadmium. Importantly, these urine proteins are not detected on standard urine dipstick assays. Previously, total body cadmium was estimated with urine cadmium (U-Cd) levels based on published associations of U-Cd levels with kidney cortex cadmium (K-Cd) in industrial workers with heavy inhalation exposures. A systemic review in 2015 did not reveal evidence for progression to CKD in workers and the general population exposed to cadmium.

2.2.2 Treatment of Cadmium Toxicity

The mainstay of toxic exposure management is removal from source and avoidance of further exposure. Unlike the comparatively better-studied chelation therapy protocols for lead toxicity, the benefit of chelation therapy for cadmium toxicity is controversial. Not all experts agree with the use of chelation therapy for acute cadmium toxicity, as mobilization of total body cadmium stores may exacerbate acute kidney injury by exposing the kidney to even higher concentrations of cadmium. However, greater evidence exists for the benefit of chelation therapy in chronic exposure, which is best discussed with an occupational physician with expertise in heavy metal toxicity.

2.3 *Arsenic*

Arsenic poisoning is of great historical significance, with a number of occupational – and intentional (i.e., murders) – poisonings prior to the twentieth century. Inorganic arsenic is significantly toxic, with mechanisms of toxicity involving production of reactive oxygen species and interference with cellular energy pathways. In contrast, organic arsenic is frequently found in seafood and ingested regularly, with little to no observable toxicity. Acute and chronic arsenic toxicity can affect nearly every organ system.

Arsenic has been shown to cause kidney disease in animal models. However, arsenic has very weak association with tubulointerstitial nephritis, with only a single case report in humans; to further complicate the utility of this case, there was no clear source of arsenic, and inorganic arsenic was not clearly delineated from total urinary arsenic levels (i.e., it is possible that TIN in this case was misattributed to arsenic). Given the rarity and uncertainty of arsenic's role in causing TIN, the utility of chelation is not established.

2.4 Chromium

Hexavalent chromium is a cytotoxic substance which has been implicated in kidney disease, largely through animal studies and population studies of exposed occupational workers, but with a somewhat unclear causative role in the development of CKD. Significant chromium exposure primarily occurs through mining and electroplating industries; chromium has significant extrarenal toxicity including lung, skin, and liver disease in chronic exposure, as well as caustic injury and multiorgan failure in acute poisoning. Kidney damage due to Tubulointerstitial disease has largely been demonstrated in animal models. The nephrotoxicity of chromium seems to worsen with concomitant lead and cadmium exposure.

2.5 Mercury

Mercury naturally occurs in three forms: elemental, inorganic, and organic. Inorganic and elemental mercury poisoning largely occurs in industrial settings: manufacturing of technical instruments, electroplating, mining, and refining; these forms of mercury are most associated with kidney disease. The most prominent (and generally most concerning) manifestations of elemental mercury poisoning are neurological, with uncommon cases of kidney disease; inorganic mercury poisoning is more associated with gastrointestinal and kidney toxicity. Organic mercury compounds are largely found in contaminated seafood, and primarily cause neurological disease.

While tubulointerstitial nephritis has been reported, mercury is more commonly implicated in causing glomerular disease (largely membranous nephropathy) and proximal tubular dysfunction. Studies of workers exposed to mercury largely reveal elevated kidney injury markers without decrease in glomerular filtration rate (GFR). While removal from source is paramount, the role of chelation in TIN related to mercury exposure is not clearly defined.

2.6 Uranium

Chronic uranium exposure has been associated with TIN, although human exposure studies are less definitive than animal studies demonstrating proximal tubular disease. While studies in occupational settings did not suggest decrease in GFR from uranium exposure, elevated kidney injury markers have been noted in patients exposed to uranium through occupational, environmental, and military settings. Depending on the source, uranium may be radioactive, leading to a combination of chemical toxicity (largely affecting the kidneys) and radiological toxicity (increase in frequencies of bone and other cancers). Management of uranium poisoning is best handled by providers with expertise in both chemical and radiation toxicity; chelation is sometimes employed.

2.7 Treatment of Heavy Metal Toxicity

The mainstay of therapy for heavy metal toxicity is removal from the source of poisoning; this generally involves removal from the workplace and industrial controls to limit worker exposure to metals. Chelation may be indicated for certain heavy metals, with indications best established in management of lead toxicity; however, the clinical utility of chelating agents is often poorly established. The decision to chelate is best made in consultation with an expert in occupational medicine or medical toxicology. Referral to these specialists is recommended for initial management of toxicity, as well as subsequent management which generally involves follow-up monitoring of blood or urine metal levels. Various chelating agents, which may be used for specific metals are summarized in Table 2.

Table 2 Chelating agents used to treat heavy metals causing TIN

Metal	Usual chelator of choice	Alternate agent(s)
Arsenic	Dimercaprol	DMPS (non-US)
Cadmium	Chelation not recommended	
Chromium	Chelation not recommended	
Lead	Succimer	Sequential dimercaprol + EDTA (in lead encephalopathy); D-penicillamine
Mercury	Succimer	Dimercaprol
Uranium	DTPA	EDTA, bicarbonate

DTPA diethylenetriaminepentaacetic acid, *EDTA* ethylenediaminetetraacetic acid, *DMPS* dimercaptopropanesulfonic acid

3 Plants, Mushrooms, and Herbal Medications

A number of dietary and traditional medicinal compounds have been associated with kidney disease, often through development of TIN. In Europe and elsewhere, foraging and consumption of *Cortinarius orellanus* and *Omphalatus orarius* which contain orellanine and similar toxins can cause acute kidney injury (AKI) due to generation of reactive oxygen species; this may lead to development of CKD and end-stage kidney disease (ESKD) from TIN. Similarly, the toxin allenic norleucine from *Amanita smithiana* mushrooms in the northwestern United States may lead to tubular damage ultimately resulting in TIN. Herbal medications have been implicated in a relatively large proportion of kidney disease in sub-Saharan Africa; it is not clear whether this is due to TIN. Aristolochic acid-containing plants and medications are widely recognized to cause kidney disease.

Aristolochic Acid Nephropathy (AAN) is the collective term for Balkan Endemic Nephropathy (BEN) and Chinese Herb Nephropathy (CHN), conditions attributed to chronic (BEN) or acute (CHN) exposure to aristolochic acid (AA). Chronic AA exposure results in insidious onset of kidney disease, characterized by tubular dysfunction and later atrophy, tubular proteinuria, aseptic leukocyturia, a more precocious anemia than expected for given stage of kidney disease (likely due to early destruction of erythropoietin-secreting peritubular cells), and, often, the absence of hypertension in contrast to most kidney disease. Acute AA toxicity, however, is more pronounced, with rapid decline of kidney function noted. Kidney damage is almost invariably irreversible.

The mechanism of AA nephrotoxicity is still uncertain, although the formation of AA-DNA adducts and interference of endocytosis of tubular cells is thought to play a role. Roughly 30–50% of individuals with AAN also develop urothelial cancers, typically along the upper urinary tract transitional epithelium (renal pelvis and ureters). AA-DNA adducts have also been implicated in the creation of T → A and A → T missense mutations of p53 tumor suppressor genes linked with the urological malignancies seen in AAN patients.

Aristolochic acid is the causative agent for two similar tubulointerstitial disease processes: BEN, a chronic kidney disease associated with upper urinary tract cancers from chronic exposure to grain contaminated with *Aristolochia clematitis* (European birthwort), and CHN, an acute toxicity attributed to use of herbal supplements containing extracts of plants from the *Aristolochiaceae* family (birthworts), including cosmopolitan genera *Aristolochia* and *Asarum* (wild ginger).

Balkan Endemic Nephropathy was first recognized in the mid-twentieth century in communities living along the Danube River in Serbia, Bulgaria, Romania, Croatia, and Bosnia and Herzegovina. Several different agents, including mycotoxins and heavy metals, were suspected as the etiology of BEN for decades before AA was finally determined to be the causative agent in the 1990s and 2000s based on the presence of DNA-AA adducts in the kidneys of all affected individuals.

Interestingly, a significant clue to the etiology of BEN occurred in 1993 when several women in Belgium under the age of 50 years suffered acute toxicity and profound kidney disease after a dietary supplement which was supposed to contain *Stephania tetrandra* ("hang fang ji") erroneously contained *Aristolochia fangchi* ("guang fang ji") instead. Subsequent investigations revealed similarities between patients with acute AA toxicity and patients with BEN.

Management of AAN needs to consider both urothelial cancers and kidney disease. Because of the high risk of urothelial cancers, urinary cytology surveillance for abnormal cells is strongly recommended. However, whether bilateral nephroureterectomies need to be performed prior to kidney transplantation remain uncertain. There is no proven therapy to slow progression of kidney disease in this setting, but recurrence post transplantation seems unlikely.

4 Therapeutic Agents

A large proportion of chemotherapeutic agents used in the treatment of cancer are nephrotoxic, with potential to cause acute kidney injury and chronic kidney disease; a large French study noted that nephrotoxic chemotherapy was used in 80% of cancer patients. Many of these agents produce tubular damage and may result in TIN and CKD. Due to space limitations, we will focus this discussion on platinum-based agents, cisplatin in particular; but also, lithium salts and analgesic nephropathy.

Platinum-Based Agents Platinum-based agents used for chemotherapy include cisplatin, carboplatin, and oxaliplatin; of these drugs, cisplatin use is most often associated with development of kidney disease. Cisplatin primarily acts through damaging and inhibiting the synthesis of deoxyribonucleic acid via generation of highly reactive metabolites, leading to apoptosis. Organic ion transporters in the proximal tubule avidly take up cisplatin, resulting in tubular damage, proximal tubular dysfunction which may manifest as Fanconi syndrome, and subsequently development of TIN due to tubular cell apoptosis and necrosis. The risk of development of cisplatin-induced CKD and AKI is primarily associated with patient's age and cisplatin dose; hypertension and hypoalbuminemia are also associated with increased risk for cisplatin nephrotoxicity. While pre-existing CKD is surprisingly not strongly correlated with risk for cisplatin nephrotoxicity, use of platinum agents is often avoided in patients with baseline kidney dysfunction. Roughly one-third of patients treated with cisplatin develop AKI; however, the large majority of patients treated with cisplatin with a baseline GFR > 60 mL/min/1.73 m^2 do not develop substantial long-term CKD.

Lithium Salts Chronic use of lithium salts is strongly associated with the development of TIN. Lithium, the smallest known therapeutic substance, is avidly reabsorbed by the kidney through a variety of sodium channels. Despite more than a century of use, the therapeutic and toxic mechanisms of lithium are not well understood; however, mechanisms of nephrotoxicity are thought to include widespread changes in intracellular signaling pathways. Roughly 15–20% of patients chronically taking lithium may develop CKD over the duration of use. Lithium-induced TIN progresses slowly, with an average drop in GFR found to be 2.3 mL/min per year in one study; development of ESKD from lithium use is generally seen after decades of use. In addition to TIN, microcyst development (potentially related to tubular damage) is seen histologically and on kidney imaging studies in many cases of lithium-induced nephropathy. Management of lithium-induced TIN involves cessation of lithium; due to its efficacy in controlling psychiatric disease; however, this is not always possible.

Analgesic Nephropathy Analgesic nephropathy refers to the development of TIN, often with evidence of renal papillary necrosis and kidney calcifications, linked to long-term use of high-dose non-opioid analgesic agents. Historically, analgesic nephropathy is largely linked to the use of combination analgesic agents containing phenacetin; after the withdrawal of phenacetin from markets in developed countries, the rates of analgesic nephropathy as a cause for ESKD fell from as high as 10–20% in parts of the United States, Europe, and Australia to nearly insignificant numbers after the year 2000. Development of analgesic nephropathy is largely seen in adults in the fifth or greater decade of life and is classically associated with irregular kidney contours and calcifications of the renal papillae. The pathogenesis is thought to involve both reactive oxygen species generation by metabolites of phenacetin and possibly acetaminophen, coupled to reduced renal blood flow caused by non-steroidal anti-inflammatory drugs (NSAIDs) and aspirin. Cessation of analgesics usually leads to stabilization of kidney function, although less so for patients with other risk factors or advanced kidney disease. Notably, NSAIDs use is associated with TIN from immune-related acute interstitial nephritis described elsewhere in this textbook.

5 Radiation

Ionizing radiation induces acute and chronic kidney damage in patients receiving high degrees of acute radiation for treatment of cancer, in nuclear plant accidents, warfare, high background radiation, or occupational radiation exposure. Disease caused by radiation is determined by the type of ionizing radiation; gamma and X-ray radiation have greater tissue penetrance and are most likely to cause kidney disease. Radiation induces oxygen radicals which damage DNA, ultimately leading to cell death. Compared to other manifestations of acute radiation syndrome such as myelosuppression, hair loss, gastrointestinal disease, and neuritis, acute radiation nephritis is a comparably late phenomenon, largely manifesting with TIN and associated symptoms 3–12 months after radiation exposure. Hypertension and anemia are often disproportionately present relative to other forms of kidney disease, and hypertensive encephalopathy may occur; notably, renin-mediated hypertension may be a consequence of unilateral kidney radiation even in the absence of development of CKD. Chronic radiation nephropathy typically occurs more than 18 months after radiation exposure.

The threshold dose for radiation nephropathy is 18–23 gray (Gy), with a 5% risk of radiation injury to the kidneys at this dose; as the dose of radiation to the kidneys increases to 28 Gy, the rate of radiation-induced kidney disease rises to 50%. However, smaller doses of radiation may induce CKD decades later; some survivors of the atomic bombs in Nagasaki and Hiroshima developed CKD 60 years after exposure to an estimated dose of <0.2 Gy. While there is no specific treatment for radiation nephropathy, consideration of other late-presenting complications of ionizing radiation (e.g., cancer) may be warranted.

6 Chronic Kidney Disease of Unknown Etiology (CKDu)

The term CKD of uncertain etiology (CKDu) refers to a number of seemingly epidemic cases of CKD, which cannot be attributed to traditionally known risk factors for CKD such as diabetes mellitus or infectious agents. Most of these cases are clustered in countries in the global tropics in Central America (e.g., El Salvador, Nicaragua) and South Asia (e.g., India and Sri Lanka), and CKDu in Central America is largely interchangeable with the disease entity known as Mesoamerican nephropathy. Kidney biopsy findings generally reveal TIN with associated glomerulosclerosis. There is a much higher prevalence of CKDu in males working in agriculture, suggesting that CKDu is largely an occupational disease. Multiple toxicologic causes have been posited, such as chronic use of NSAIDs, high consumption of fructose, agrochemicals including a variety of pesticides, and environmental exposure heavy metals such as arsenic; while these have varying degrees of support from epidemiological data and are biologically plausible, no clear single toxin has been associated with the disorder. There is growing concern that environmental heat exposure also plays a large part in development of CKDu, perhaps in combination with toxicologic and/or infectious causes.

7 Conclusion

Tubulointerstitial disease induced by toxic and radiation exposures is heterogeneous in nature, and often poorly responsive to treatment relative to immune-mediated TIN. As with all disease related to toxic exposures, avoidance (through occupational controls or other mitigating factors) and removal from the source of toxin forms the cornerstone of management of toxin and radiation-induced TIN.

Suggested Reading

Alarcon WA, State Adult Blood Lead Epidemiology and Surveillance (ABLES) Program Investigators. Elevated blood lead levels among employed adults - United States, 1994-2013. MMWR Morb Mortal Wkly Rep. 2016;63(55):59.

Amrit P, Singh R, Kumar G, Tajpreet K. Mechanisms pertaining to arsenic toxicity. Toxicol Int. 2011;18(2):87–93.

Arzuaga X, Rieth SH, Bathija A, Cooper GS. Renal effects of exposure to natural and depleted uranium: a review of the epidemiologic and experimental data. J Toxicol Environ Health B Crit Rev. 2010;13(7–8):527–45.

Baloch S, Kazi TG, Baig JA, Afridi HI, Arain MB. Occupational exposure of lead and cadmium on adolescent and adult workers of battery recycling and welding workshops: adverse impact on health. Sci Total Environ. 2020;720:137549.

Bendz H, Aurell M, Balldin J, Mathé AA, Sjödin I. Kidney damage in long-term lithium patients: a cross-sectional study of patients with 15 years or more on lithium. Nephrol Dial Transplant. 1994;9(9):1250.

Bernard A. Confusion about cadmium risks: the unrecognized limitations of an extrapolated paradigm. Environ Health Perspect. 2016;124(1):1–5.

Bernhoft RA. Cadmium toxicity and treatment. Sci World J. 2013;2013:1–7.

Bocchetta A, Ardau R, Carta P, Ligas F, Sardu C, Pani A, Del Zompo M. Duration of lithium treatment is a risk factor for reduced glomerular function: a cross-sectional study. BMC Med. 2013;11:33.

Boton R, Gaviria M, Batlle DC. Prevalence, pathogenesis, and treatment of renal dysfunction associated with chronic lithium therapy. Am J Kidney Dis. 1987;10(5):329.

Boulikas T, Vougiouka M. Cisplatin and platinum drugs at the molecular level. (Review). Oncol Rep. 2003;10(6):1663.

But PP-H, Atherton David J, Rustin Malcolm H, Brostoff J. Need for correct identification of herbs in herbal poisoning. Lancet. 1993;341(8845):637–8.

Byber K, Lison D, Verougstraete V, Dressel H, Hotz P. Cadmium or cadmium compounds and chronic kidney disease in workers and the general population: a systematic review. Crit Rev Toxicol. 2015;46(3):191–240.

Centers for Disease Control. Fourth national report on human exposure to environmental chemicals. https://www.cdc.gov/exposurereport. Accessed 18 May 2021.

Cohen EP, Lawton CA, Moulder JE, Becker CG, Ash RC. Clinical course of late onset bone marrow transplant nephropathy. Nephron. 1993;64:626–35.

Cohen EP, Robbins MEC. Radiation nephropathy. Semin Nephrol. 2003;23(5):486–99.

Cosyns J-P, Jadoul M, Squifflet J-P, Plaen J-F d, Ferluga D, de Strihou CVY d. Chinese herbs nephropathy: a clue to Balkan endemic nephropathy? Kidney Int. 1994;45(6):1680–8.

Cosyns JP, Jadoul M, Squifflet JP, Wese FX, van Ypersele de Strihou C. Urothelial lesions in Chinese-herb nephropathy. Am J Kidney Dis. 1999;33(6):1011.

Crummy AB Jr, Hellman S, Stansel HC Jr, Hukill PB. Renal hypertension secondary to unilateral radiation damage relieved by nephrectomy. Radiology. 1965;84:108–11.

Dawson LA, Kavanagh BD, Paulino AC, Das SK, Miften M, Li XA, Pan C, Ten Haken RK, Schultheiss TE. Radiation-associated kidney injury. Int J Radiat Oncol Biol Phys. 2010;76:S108–15.

De Broe ME, Elseviers MM. Over-the-counter analgesic use. J Am Soc Nephrol. 2009;20(10):2098.

Dhaliwal RS, Adelman RD, Turner E, Russo JC, Ruebner B. Radiation nephritis with hypertension and hyperreninemia: cure by nephrectomy. J Pediatr. 1980;96:68–70.

Dharma-wardana MWC. Fertilizer usage and cadmium in soils, crops and food. Environ Geochem Health. 2018;40(6):2739–59.

Diamond GL, Zalups RK. Understanding renal toxicity of heavy metals. Toxicol Pathol. 1998;26(1):92–103.

Duggin GG. Combination analgesic-induced kidney disease: the Australian experience. Am J Kidney Dis. 1996;28(1 Suppl 1):S39.
Evans M, Discacciati A, Quershi AR, et al. End-stage renal disease after occupational lead exposure: 20 years of follow-up. Occup Environ Med. 2017;74:396.
Foulkes EC. Renal tubular transport of cadmium-metallothionein. Toxicol Appl Pharmacol. 1978;45(2):505–12.
Frumkin H, Letz R, Williams PL, Gerr F, Pierce M, Sanders A, Elon L, Manning CC, Woods JS, Hertzberg VS, Mueller P, Taylor BB. Health effects of long-term mercury exposure among chloralkali plant workers. Am J Ind Med. 2001;39(1):1.
Gault MH, Wilson DR. Analgesic nephropathy in Canada: clinical syndrome, management, and outcome. Kidney Int. 1978;13(1):58.
Gökmen MR, Cosyns J-P, Arlt VM, Stiborová M, Phillips DH, Schmeiser HH, et al. The epidemiology, diagnosis, and management of aristolochic acid nephropathy: a narrative review. Ann Intern Med. 2013;158(6):469.
Goldfrank LR. Mushrooms. In: Hoffman RS, Howland MA, Lewin NA, Nelson LS, Goldfrank LR, editors. Goldfrank's toxicologic emergencies. 10th ed. New York: McGrawHill; 2014.
Grollman AP, Shibutani S, Moriya M, Miller F, Wu L, Moll U, et al. Aristolochic acid and the etiology of endemic (Balkan) nephropathy. Proc Natl Acad Sci USA. 2007;104(29):12129–34.
Han J, Xian Z, Zhang Y, Liu J, Liang A. Systematic overview of aristolochic acids: nephrotoxicity, carcinogenicity, and underlying mechanisms. Front Pharmacol. 2019;10:648.
Harari F, Sallsten G, Christensson A, et al. Blood lead levels and decreased kidney function in a population-based cohort. Am J Kidney Dis. 2018;72:381.
Holditch SJ, Brown CN, Lombardi AM, Nguyen KN, Edelstein CL. Recent advances in models, mechanisms, biomarkers, and interventions in cisplatin-induced acute kidney injury. Int J Mol Sci. 2019;20(12):3011.
Inglis JA, Henderson DA, Emmerson BT. The pathology and pathogenesis of chronic lead nephropathy occurring in Queensland. J Pathol. 1978a;124(2):65.
Inglis JA, Henderson DA, Emmerson BT. The pathology and pathogenesis of chronic lead nephropathy occurring in Queensland. J Pathol. 1978b;124(2):65–76.
Ivić M. Etiology of endemic nephropathy. Lijec Vjesn. 1969;91(12):1273–81.
Jelaković B, Dika Ž, Arlt VM, Stiborova M, Pavlović NM, Nikolić J, et al. Balkan endemic nephropathy and the causative role of aristolochic acid. Semin Nephrol. 2019;39(3):284–96.
Jha V, Garcia-Garcia G, Iseki K, et al. Chronic kidney disease: global dimension and perspectives. Lancet. 2013;382(9888):260–72.
Johri N, Jacquillet G, Unwin R. Heavy metal poisoning: the effects of cadmium on the kidney. Biometals. 2010;23(5):783–92.
Karaosmanoglu AD, Butros SR, Arellano R. Imaging findings of renal toxicity in patients on chronic lithium therapy. Diagn Interv Radiol. 2013;19(4):299.
Kim R, Rotnitsky A, Sparrow D, et al. A longitudinal study of low-level lead exposure and impairment of renal function. The normative aging study. AMA. 1996;275:1177.
Klotz K, Weistenhöfer W, Drexler H. Cadmium: from toxicity to essentiality. Metal Ions Life Sci. 2012;11:85–98.
Latcha S, Jaimes EA, Patil S, Glezerman IG, Mehta S, Flombaum CD. Long-term renal outcomes after cisplatin treatment. Clin J Am Soc Nephrol. 2016;11(7):1173. Epub 2016 Apr 12.
Launay-Vacher V, Oudard S, Janus N, Gligorov J, Pourrat X, Rixe O, Morere JF, Beuzeboc P, Deray G, Renal Insufficiency and Cancer Medications (IRMA) Study Group. Prevalence of renal insufficiency in cancer patients and implications for anticancer drug management: the renal insufficiency and anticancer medications (IRMA) study. Cancer. 2007;110(6):1376.
Lebeau C, Arlt VM, Schmeiser HH, Boom A, Verroust PJ, Devuyst O, et al. Aristolochic acid impedes endocytosis and induces DNA adducts in proximal tubule cells. Kidney Int. 2001;60(4):1332–42.
Li SJ, Zhang SH, Chen HP, Zeng CH, Zheng CX, Li LS, Liu ZH. Mercury-induced membranous nephropathy: clinical and pathological features. CJASN. 2010;5(3):439–44.

Loghman-Adham M. Aminoaciduria and glycosuria following severe childhood lead poisoning. Pediatr Nephrol. 1998;12(3):218.
Lunyera J, Mohottige D, Von Isenburg M, Jeuland M, Patel UD, Stanifer JW. CKD of uncertain etiology: a systematic review. Clin J Am Soc Nephrol. 2016;11(3):379–85.
Luxton RW. Radiation nephritis: a long term study of 54 patients. Lancet. 1961;2:1221–4.
MacFarland HN. The use of dimercaprol (BAL) in the treatment of cadmium oxide fume poisoning. Arch Environ Health. 1960;1(6):487–96.
Markowitz GS, Radhakrishnan J, Kambham N, Valeri AM, Hines WH, D'Agati VD. Lithium nephrotoxicity: a progressive combined glomerular and tubulointerstitial nephropathy. J Am Soc Nephrol. 2000;11(8):1439.
Motwani SS, McMahon GM, Humphreys BD, Partridge AH, Waikar SS, Curhan GC. Development and validation of a risk prediction model for acute kidney injury after the first course of cisplatin. J Clin Oncol. 2018;36(7):682. Epub 2018 Jan 10
Nordberg GF. Historical perspectives on cadmium toxicology. Toxicol Appl Pharm. 2009;238(3):192–200.
Nordberg M, Nordberg GF. Distribution of metallothionein-bound cadmium and cadmium chloride in mice: preliminary studies. Environ Health Perspect. 1975;12:103–8.
Occupational Safety and Health Administration Standards 1910. 1025 - Lead. https://www.osha.gov/laws-regs/regulations/standardnumber/1910/1910.1025. Accessed 18 May 2021.
Pappas RS, Fresquez MR, Martone N, Watson CH. Toxic metal concentrations in mainstream smoke from cigarettes available in the USA. J Anal Toxicol. 2014;38(4):204–11.
Prasad GVR, Rossi NF. Arsenic intoxication associated with tubulointerstitial nephritis. Am J Kidney Dis. 1995;26(2):373–6
Presne C, Fakhouri F, Noël LH, Stengel B, Even C, Kreis H, Mignon F, Grünfeld JP. Lithium-induced nephropathy: rate of progression and prognostic factors. Kidney Int. 2003;64(2):585.
Richter P, Faroon O, Pappas RS. Cadmium and cadmium/zinc ratios and tobacco-related morbidities. Int J Environ Res Public Health. 2017;14(10):1154.
Satarug S, Garrett SH, Sens MA, Sens DA. Cadmium, environmental exposure, and health outcomes. Environ Health Perspect. 2010;118(2):182–90.
Sera N, Hida A, Imaizumi M, Nakashima E, Akahoshi M. The association between chronic kidney disease and cardiovascular risk factors in atomic bomb survivors. Radiat Res. 2013;179:46–52.
Soderland P, Lovekar S, Weiner DE, Brooks DR, Kaufman JS. Chronic kidney disease associated with environmental toxins and exposures. Adv Chronic Kidney Dis. 2010;17(3):254–64.
Sommar JN, Svensson MK, Björ BM, et al. End-stage renal disease and low level exposure to lead, cadmium and mercury; a population-based, prospective nested case-referent study in Sweden. Environ Health. 2013;12:9.
Tankeu S, Vermaak I, Chen W, Sandasi M, Viljoen A. Differentiation between two "fang ji" herbal medicines, Stephania tetrandra and the nephrotoxic Aristolochia fangchi, using hyperspectral imaging. Phytochemistry. 2016;122:213–22.
Timmer RT, Sands JM. Lithium intoxication. JASN. 1999;10(3):666–74.
Tsai TL, Kuo CC, Pan WH, Chung YT, Chen CY, Wu TN, Wang SL. The decline in kidney function with chromium exposure is exacerbated with co-exposure to lead and cadmium. Kidney Int. 2017;92(3):710–20.
Tsaih SW, Korrick S, Schwartz J, et al. Lead, diabetes, hypertension, and renal function: the normative aging study. Environ Health Perspect. 2004;112:1178.
Tsuchiya K. Causation of ouch-ouch disease (itai-itai byo) - an introductory review. Keio J Med. 1969;18(4):181–94.
Vadivel N, Trikudanathan S, Singh AK. Analgesic nephropathy. Kidney Int. 2007;72(4):517–20.
Vanherweghem J-L, Tielemans C, Abramowicz D, Depierreux M, Vanhaelen-Fastre R, Vanhaelen M, et al. Rapidly progressive interstitial renal fibrosis in young women: association with slimming regimen including Chinese herbs. Lancet. 1993;341(8842):387–91.
Waalkes MP, Goering PL. Metallothionein and other cadmium-binding proteins: recent developments. Chem Res Toxicol. 1990;3(4):281–8.
Yang CW. Leptospirosis renal disease: emerging culprit of chronic kidney disease unknown Etiology. Nephron. 2018;138(2):129–36.

Reflux and Obstructive Nephropathy

J. Nelson Reed, Oana Nicoara, and Blaithin A. McMahon

1 Introduction

Reflux nephropathy (RN), a distinct pathological and radiological entity, previously known as chronic atrophic non-obstructive pyelonephritis in childhood, and accounts for end stage kidney disease (ESKD) in approximately 7–17% of the pediatric population worldwide and 10% of the adult population. In North America, RN accounts for approximately 5% of the pediatric ESKD population and is the fourth leading cause for dialysis and transplantation with 5.3% of transplant patients and 3.5% of dialysis patients having a diagnosis of RN, respectively. It is important to mention that the second and third leading causes for dialysis and transplantation in children are obstructive uropathy and aplasia/hypoplasia/dysplasia, respectively, both of which can be linked with RN. Reflux nephropathy is the second most common cause of chronic tubulointerstitial disease.

J. N. Reed
Department of Medicine, Medical University of South Carolina, Charleston, SC, USA
e-mail: reedjame@musc.edu

O. Nicoara
Department of Pediatrics, Division of Nephrology, MUSC Children's Hospital, Charleston, SC, USA
e-mail: nicoara@musc.edu

B. A. McMahon (✉)
Department of Medicine, Division of Nephrology, Medical University of South Carolina, Charleston, SC, USA

M. G. Atta, M. A. Perazella (eds.), *Tubulointerstitial Nephritis*, https://doi.org/10.1007/978-3-030-93438-5_15

2 Etiology

Vesico-ureteric reflux (VUR) of infected urine from the bladder into the kidney parenchyma is the most important factor in the development of pyelonephritis. VUR is a urinary tract defect in ureterovesical valves or mechanical obstruction in the lower urinary tract creating an abnormal uretero-vesical junction (UVJ) allowing the retrograde flow of urine from the bladder to the kidneys. An estimated 9–20% of patients with antenatal hydronephrosis have VUR when tested postnatally and while VUR is an important risk factor for pyelonephritis it is clear that the vast majority of patients with VUR do not develop ESKD.

Familial aggregation and twin studies support a hereditary basis. About 20% of infants with VUR have a parent with a family history of VUR, compared with a 1–2% frequency of VUR in the general population. The largest VUR pathogenic copy number variant analysis and genome-wide association study to date has identified five suggestive loci including WDPCP, OTX1, BMP5, WDPCP and WNT5 with large effects, the latter is implicated in urogenital development. In one study of 1395 VUR patients, 6% carried high-risk genotypes and have implications for VUR screening.

VUR is suspected in children with recurrent urinary tract infections. Though VUR is an important risk factor for pyelonephritis, up to 60% of young children with acute pyelonephritis do not have a history of VUR and factors unrelated to reflux, such as congenital factors can also contribute. Reflux nephropathy can lead to a chronic tubulointerstitial nephritis resulting in interstitial fibrosis, tubular atrophy, focal segmental glomerulosclerosis, kidney scarring, and chronic kidney disease (CKD) eventually culminating in end stage kidney disease (ESKD).

3 Clinical Presentation

Reflux nephropathy is often asymptomatic, and the diagnosis may not be suspected until late adolescent or early adulthood when an incidental rise in serum creatinine is noted on routine clinical assessment. A history of recurrent childhood UTIs may exist. Other signs and symptoms include hypertension, polyuria, nocturia, and mild-moderate proteinuria.

4 Diagnosis

Reflux nephropathy may be suspected antenatally or postnatally. Initial screening is done with ultrasonography, which is highly sensitive for the detection of hydronephrosis or urinary tract dilation (UTD). The careful clinical assessment of patients with suspected reflux nephropathy is outlined in Fig. 1. A detailed medical history

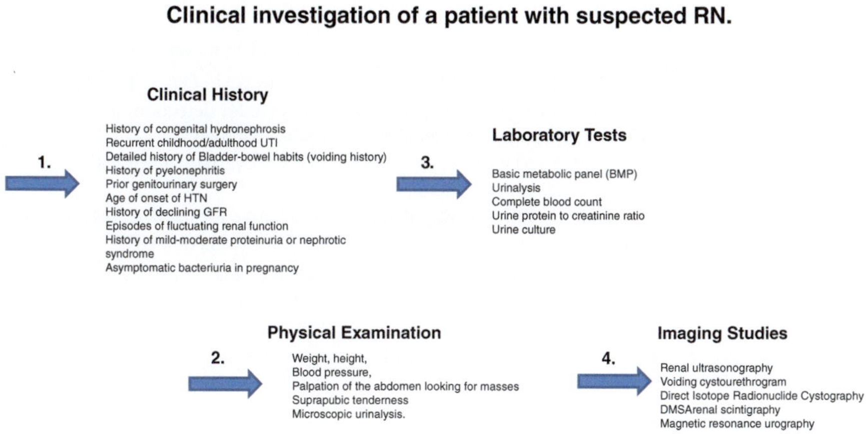

Fig. 1 Clinical evaluation of a patient with suspected reflux nephropathy

of prior UTIs, current voiding patterns, and a history of hypertension are important details to determine. Urinalysis and urine culture are performed as part of the initial assessment to detect infection. Many imaging modalities exist in the assessment of reflux nephropathy and the benefits and limitations of each are summarized in Table 1.

Kidney ultrasonography is used to evaluate kidney size and shape, hydronephrosis, and scarring. Ultrasonography can also identify the presence of congenital kidney malformations, which can contribute to VUR. The gold standard test for the diagnosis of VUR is a voiding cystourethrogram (VCUG), but it can be a challenging test for many young children as it requires catheterization of the urethra, followed by injection into the bladder with radio-opaque dye, and fluoroscopy imaging to view the urinary tract while the patient voids. The degree of VUR is graded on a scale (I-V) based on the extent of retrograde filling and ureteral dilatation observed from the VCUG (see below, Figs. 2 and 3). In the event the VCUG is not tolerated or there is a desire to avoid radiation exposure, a radionuclide cystogram may be performed; however, this study provides less anatomic detail and should not be performed for the initial evaluation of VUR but may be helpful in monitoring follow up assessments.

Tc-99m DMSA kidney scintigraphy is ideal for showing an active pyelonephritic lesion in the kidney as demonstrated by cortical defects of the involved kidneys. Tc-99m DMSA scan also estimate functional kidney mass and relative kidney function. Magnetic Resonance urography (MRU) has an emerging role in the evaluation of reflux nephropathy and can provide much higher contrast resolution than DMSA scan. MR urography is able to identify the acquired segmental scars associated with VUR and even in those children who have developed pyelonephritis in the absence of VUR. It can differentiate between pyelonephritis, scar, and dysplasia. MRU can provide information about the perfusion, concentration, and excretion of contrast media and can be used as a surrogate for the single nephron GFR (SNGFR) similar to DMSA scan.

Table 1 Imaging modalities used in the assessment of reflux nephropathy

Imaging modality	Study details	Benefit/Limitation of study
Renal ultrasonography	Provides information about structural kidney disease (presence of hydronephrosis (prenatally, postnatally) and kidney size. Can assess cortex thickness and post void residual volume. May detect cortical scarring	Non-invasive. Quick. Highly sensitive for detection of hydronephrosis Does not provide information on active reflux Insensitive for the detection of acute pyelonephritis or VUR
Voiding cystourethrogram (VCUG)	Uses iodine contrast medium. Requires catheterization of the urethra Primary diagnostic modality of choice for VUR	Provides anatomical detail (bladder, ureteral, kidneys) Provides a grading system for severity of VUR Radiation exposure with fluoroscopy
Direct Isotope Radionuclide Cystography (DIRC)	Radio-isotopic tracer (DTPA) is infused in the bladder after urethral catheterization and images are obtained during bladder filling and emptying	Prevents radiation exposure. Ideal for follow up assessment of VUR. Does not aid in the specific grading of VUR. Low definition of image. Does not allow the detection of other anatomic defects of the bladder or urethra
DMSA renal scintigraphy	Highly sensitive for the diagnosis of acute pyelonephritis and renal scarring Can estimate functional renal mass and relative renal function	Can take up to 3 h to complete
Magnetic resonance urography (MRU)	Provide information about the perfusion, concentration and excretion of contrast media and can be used as a surrogate for the single nephron GFR (SNGFR)	Does not employ ionizing radiation Less readily available Not practical for use in infants and children as may require sedation/ mechanical intubation More expensive

Abbreviations: *VUR* vesicoureteral reflux

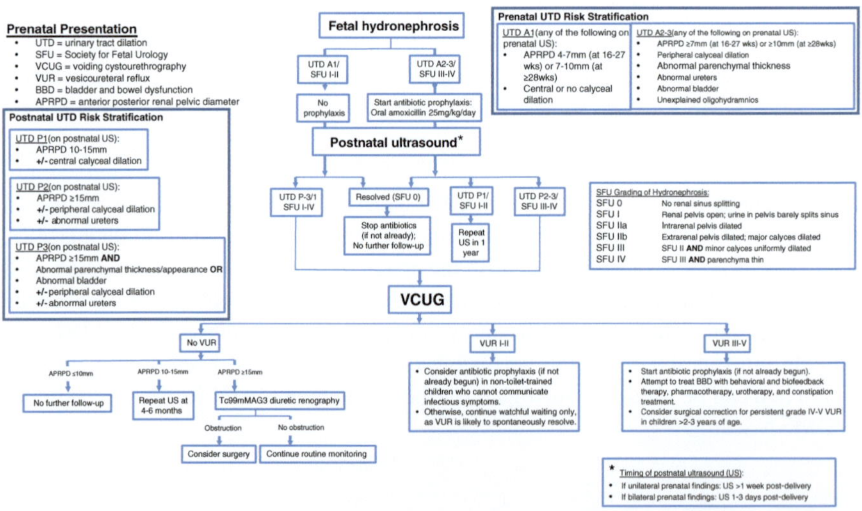

Fig. 2 Antenatal presentation, workup, and management of vesicoureteral reflux

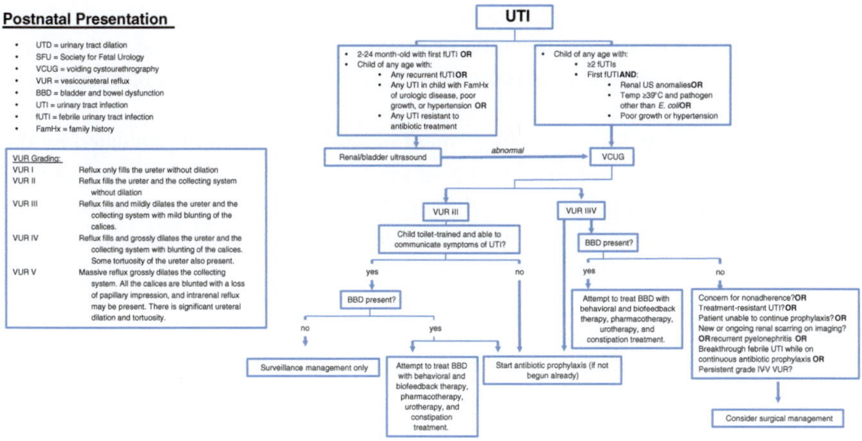

Fig. 3 Postnatal presentation, workup, and management of vesicoureteral reflux

In the right clinical setting when the diagnosis is not clear, kidney biopsy may be indicated and is most likely to show global glomerular hypertrophy and periglomerular fibrosis, patchy interstitial scarring, chronic interstitial nephritis, extensive tubular atrophy and secondary FSGS.

Figure 2 summarizes the approach to prenatal work up of fetal hydronephrosis and its management. Figure 3 describes the approach to work up of (postnatal) urinary tract infection, importance of the VCUG and its grading system and the approach to management of VUR.

5 Management

Spontaneous resolution of primary reflux is common, especially for low-grade VUR. 80% of cases typically resolves spontaneously over 5 years and many do not require any medical treatment except ongoing surveillance. Resolution of VUR depends on both initial grade of reflux, gender, age at initial diagnosis, voiding dysfunction, presence of kidney scarring, and occurrence of reflux during bladder filling or emptying. In general, VUR is less likely to resolve in younger children with a history of high-grade reflux with evidence of kidney scarring on ultrasound. In this setting surgery should be considered in the management of VUR.

Children with moderate symptomatic reflux are given medical management with long-term antimicrobial prophylaxis with a choice of agents (trimethoprim-sulfamethoxazole, trimethoprim alone, nitrofurantoin, and cephalexin that may need to be renally adjusted for patients GFR). Management of bladder and bowel dysfunction is crucial (stool softeners, timed voiding [2–3 h], pelvic floor exercises, and anticholinergic medications as needed). Figures 2 and 3 outline management of VUR antenatally and postnatally, respectively. Failed antimicrobial prophylaxis requires surgical correction and includes open, laparoscopic, and endoscopic techniques such as ureteral reimplantation or endoscopic injection of materials behind the ureter to prevent reflux (bladder contraction during voiding compresses the ureter).

Recommendations for surgical treatment of severe VUR were published by the International Reflux Study in Children in 2006. Relative indications for surgical correction are highlighted in Fig. 3. Surgery has no role in adolescents and adults with established kidney scarring and advanced chronic kidney disease. In patients with established RN and chronic kidney disease, it is very important to aggressively manage hypertension and proteinuria to delay progression to ESKD. Renin-angiotensin aldosterone system (RAAS) blockade remains the cornerstone of medical treatment in patients with glomerular hyperfiltration and patients with established proteinuria. RN patients should be evaluated for kidney transplantation once GFR drops below 20 ml/min/1.73 m^2 to improve overall life expectancy and quality of life. In the meantime, we must provide the best supportive care to patients to preserve kidney function and prevent ESKD in patients with vesicoureteral reflux and reflux nephropathy.

Suggested Reading

Austin JC, Cooper CS. Vesicoureteral reflux: who benefits from correction. Urol Clin N Am. 2010;37:243–52.

Brakeman P. Vesicoureteral reflux, reflux nephropathy, and end-stage renal disease. Adv Urol. 2008;2008:508949.

Damien Grattan-Smith J, Little SB, Jones RA. Evaluation of reflux nephropathy, pyelonephritis and renal dysplasia. Pediatr Radiol. 2008;38(Suppl 1):S83–S105.

Hodson EM, Wheeler DM, Vimalchandra D, Smith GH, Craig JC. Interventions for primary vesicoureteric reflux. Cochrane Database Syst Rev. 2007;3:CD001532.

International Reflux Study Committee. Medical versus surgical treatment of primary vesicoureteral reflux: report of the International Reflux Study Committee. Pediatrics. 1981;67:392–400.

Jakobsson B, Jacobson SH, Hjalmas K. Vesico-ureteric reflux and other risk factors for renal damage: identification of high- and low-risk children. Acta Paediatr Suppl. 1999;88:31–9.

Jodal U, Smellie JM, Lax H, Hoyer PF. Ten-year results of randomized treatment of children with severe vesicoureteral reflux. Final report of the International Reflux Study in Children. Pediatr Nephrol. 2006;21:785–92.

Kaefer M, Curran M, Treves ST, Bauer S, Hendren WH, Peters CA, Atala A, Diamond D, Retik A. Sibling vesicoureteral reflux in multiple gestation births. Pediatrics. 2000;105:800–4.

Knudson MJ, Austin JC, McMillan ZM, Hawtrey CE, Cooper CS. Predictive factors of early spontaneous resolution in children with primary vesicoureteral reflux. J Urol. 2007;178:1684–8.

Matsuoka H, Oshima K, Sakamoto K, Taguchi T, Takebayashi S. Renal pathology in patients with reflux nephropathy. The turning point in irreversible renal disease. Eur Urol. 1994;26(2):153–9.

Miyakita H, Hayashi Y, Mitsui T, et al. Guidelines for the medical management of pediatric vesicoureteral reflux. Int J Urol. 2020;27:480–90.

Nguyen HT, Benson CB, Bromley B, Campbell JB, et al. Multidisciplinary consensus on the classification of prenatal and postnatal urinary tract dilation (UTD classification system). J Pediatr Urol. 2014;10(6):982–98.

Onen A. Grading of hydronephrosis: an ongoing challenge. Front Pediatr. 2020;8:458.

RIVUR Trial Investigators, Hoberman A, Greenfield SP, Mattoo TK, Keren R, Mathews R, Pohl HG, Kropp BP, Skoog SJ, Nelson CP, Moxey-Mims M, Chesney RW, Carpenter MA. Antimicrobial prophylaxis for children with vesicoureteral reflux. N Engl J Med. 2014;370(25):2367.

Sargent MA. What is the normal prevalence of vesicoureteral reflux? Pediatr Radiol. 2000;30:587–93.

Scott JE, Swallow V, Coulthard MG, Lambert HJ, Lee RE. Screening of newborn babies for familial ureteric reflux. Lancet. 1997;350(9075):396–400.

Shaikh N, Craig JC, Rovers MM, et al. Identification of children and adolescents at risk for renal scarring after a first urinary tract infection: a meta-analysis with individual patient data. JAMA Pediatr. 2014;168(10):893–900.

Smellie JM, Prescod NP, Shaw PJ, Risdon RA, Bryant TN. Childhood reflux and urinary infection: a follow-up of 10-41 years in 226 adults. Pediatr Nephrol. 1998;12(9):727–36.

Subcommittee on Urinary Tract Infection, Steering Committee on Quality Improvement and Management, Roberts KB. Urinary tract infection: clinical practice guideline for the diagnosis and management of the initial UTI in febrile infants and children 2 to 24 months. Pediatrics. 2011;128(3):595–610.

Sung J, Skoog S. Surgical management of vesicoureteral reflux in children. Pediatr Nephrol. 2006;2012(27):551–61.

Verbitsky M, Krithivasan P, Batourina E, Khan A, Graham SE, Marasà M, Kim H, Lim TY, Weng PL, Sánchez-Rodríguez E, Mitrotti A, Ahram DF, et al. Copy number variant analysis and genome-wide association study identify loci with large effect for vesicoureteral reflux. JASN. 2021;32:805–20.

Williams G, Fletcher JT, Alexander SI, Craig JC. Vesicoureteral reflux. JASN. 2008;19(5):847–62.

Aristolochic Acid Nephropathy and Balkan Nephropathy

Joëlle L. Nortier, Jean-Louis Vanherweghem, and Bojan Jelakovic

1 Introduction

The term "aristolochic acid nephropathy" (AAN) is used to include any form of toxic interstitial nephropathy that is caused either by the ingestion of plants containing AA as part of traditional phytotherapies (formerly known as "Chinese herb nephropathy"), or by the environmental contaminants in food (BN).

It was initially reported in Belgium in 1993 as a rapidly progressive form of renal interstitial fibrosis in women after the intake of a weight loss diet including *Aristolochia fanchi,* a herb used in traditional Chinese medicine (Fig. 1a–d). Since then, AAN new cases are identified every year worldwide, particularly in Asian countries where *Aristolochia* species are still widely used in traditional medicine. Moreover, AA have been found to be the causative agent of the so-called Balkan Nephropathy (BN), a tubulointerstitial nephropathy described for more than 50 years in certain villages throughout the Danube Valley. It has been confirmed by

J. L. Nortier (✉)
Department of Nephrology-Dialysis, Brugmann University Hospital, Université libre de Bruxelles (ULB), Brussels, Belgium

Laboratory of Experimental Nephrology, Faculty of Medicine, Université libre de Bruxelles (ULB), Brussels, Belgium
e-mail: Joelle.Nortier@chu-brugmann.be; Joelle.Nortier@ulb.be

J.-L. Vanherweghem
Department of Nephrology, Erasme University Hospital, Université libre de Bruxelles (ULB), Brussels, Belgium
e-mail: jean-louis.vanherweghem@ulb.be

B. Jelakovic
Department of Nephrology, Hypertension, Dialysis and Transplantation, University Hospital Centre Zagreb, Zagreb, Croatia

School of Medicine, University of Zagreb, Zagreb, Croatia

M. G. Atta, M. A. Perazella (eds.), *Tubulointerstitial Nephritis*,
https://doi.org/10.1007/978-3-030-93438-5_16

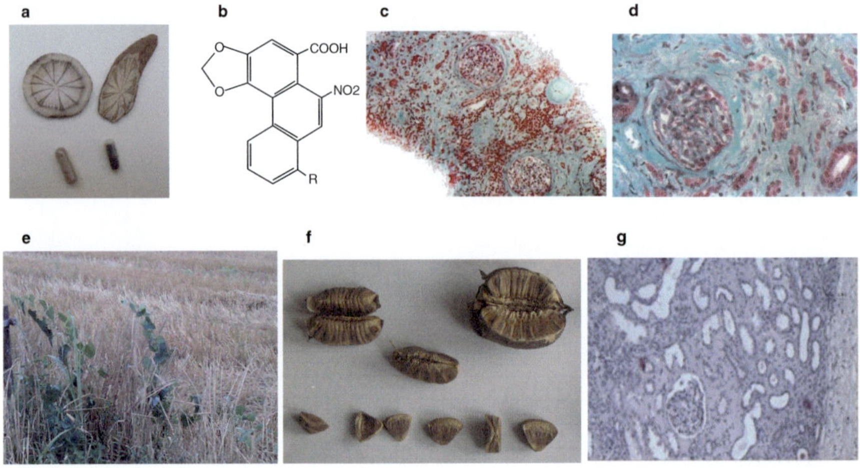

Fig. 1 (**a**) Transverse sections of the roots of *Aristolochia fangchi* (known as Guang Fang Ji in traditional Chinese medicine) and weight-loss capsules containing the powdered root, ingested by a Belgian patient who developed end-stage kidney disease. (**b**) Chemical structure of aristolochic acid I (AAI) and aristolochic acid II (AAII), nitrophenantrene derivatives present in all parts of *Aristolochia* plant (root, stem and leaves) and differing only by their radical R (OCH3 for AAI and H for AAII, respectively). (**c**) Microphotography of a renal biopsy performed in a Belgian AAN patient presenting with CKD stage 3b, showing extensive interstitial fibrosis, tubular atrophy, interstitial inflammatory infiltrate and glomeruli generally preserved. Goldner trichrome staining, magnification 200×. (Courtesy of Depierreux, MD, pathologist at Erasme Hospital, Brussels). (**d**) Same specimen as in C at higher magnification (400×), showing complete disappearance of the tubules and almost intact glomeruli. (**e**) *Aristolochia clematitis* growing in the wheat fields and having fruits in harvesting time. (Croatian endemic area near the endemic village of Kaniža, August 2013- photo by B. Jelaković). (**f**) Fruits and seeds of *Aristolochia clematitis* collected during the harvest of the wheat crop from fields in BN endemic areas. (Serbian endemic village of Vreoci, August 2015- photo by N. Pavlović). (**g**) Typical histopathological pattern observed in a renal tissue sample from a Croatian BN patient, showing severe interstitial fibrosis, tubular atrophy and spared glomeruli. Haematoxylin and eosin staining; magnification 100×; Nephrology dept., Zagreb University Hospital)

the discovery of specific DNA adducts formed by the metabolites of AA in the kidney tissue and the urothelial tumors of BN patients (Fig. 2). In endemic regions, AA from *Aristolochia clematis* proliferating in the wheat fields contaminate cereals either by a direct mixing of the plant's seeds or by diffusion in the soil either (Fig. 1e–g). Characteristics of BN and iatrogenic AAN are shown in Table 1.

In addition to its nephrotoxic effects, AA exposure has also been frequently associated with the development of urothelial malignancies and AA were classified has a human carcinogen class I by the World Health Organization (WHO) International Agency for Research of Cancer (IARC) in 2002. Despite warnings from the Food and Drug Administration (FDA), the European Medicines Agency (EMA) and IARC regarding the safety of products containing AA, AAN cases remain frequently

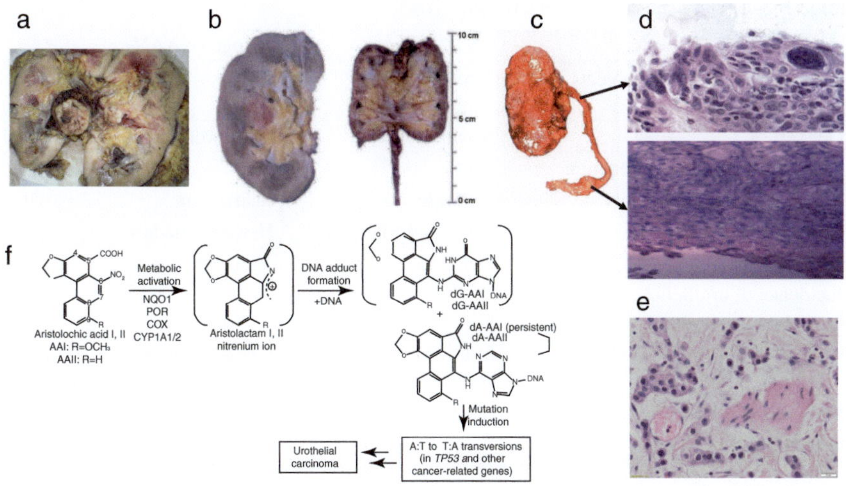

Fig. 2 (**a**) Macroscopic finding of a Croatian patient with pyelo cancer from endemic village of Slavonski Kobaš (data on positive aristolactam-DNA adducts and p53 signature mutation; courtesy by Karla Tomić, MD, PhD pathologist in General Hospital Slavonski Brod, Croatia. (**b**) Typical macroscopic aspect of a kidney removed from a Belgian ESRD patient who ingested pills containing *A. fangchi*; compared to a control, this kidney is characterized by a severe atrophy, a slightly wavy shape and a very thin cortex. (courtesy of M. Depierreux, MD, pathologist at Erasme Hospital, Brussels). (**c**) Right native kidney and ureter removed from a kidney recipient for end-stage AAN patient, showing a tumoral mass of the lower third of the ureter. (courtesy of M. Depierreux, MD, pathologist at Erasme Hospital, Brussels). (**d**) Upper panel: i*n situ* urothelial carcinoma detected in the upper third of the right ureter and pelvic cavity from the surgical material displayed in B. (courtesy of M. Depierreux, MD, pathologist at Erasme Hospital, Brussels). Lower panel: invasive urothelial carcinoma (pT2) of the lower third of the right ureter shown in B (courtesy of M. Depierreux, MD, pathologist at Erasme Hospital, Brussels). (**e**) Histological aspect of a nested variant of bladder carcinoma infiltrating the muscle wall in a Belgian kidney transplant recipient for end-stage AAN. Haematoxylin and eosin staining; magnification 400×. Photomicrograph kindly provided by S. Rorive, MD, PhD, pathologist at Erasme University Hospital, Brussels, Belgium. (**f**) Schematic representation of metabolic activation and DNA adduct formation by AA kindly provided by Volker M. Arlt and reproduced with his permission. R = OCH3 in AAI, and R = H in AAII. COX, cyclooxygenase; CYP, cytochrome P450; dA-AAI, 7-(deoxyadenosin-N^6-yl)aristolactam I; dA-AAII, 7-(deoxyadenosin-N^6-yl)aristolactam II; dG-AAI, 7-(deoxyguanosin-N^2-yl)aristolactam I; dG-AAII, 7-(deoxyguanosin-N^2-yl)aristolactam II; NQO1, NAD(P) H:quinone oxidoreductase; POR, NADPH: cytochrome P450 oxidoreductase

described worldwide. The history of this nephropathy demonstrates that it is mandatory to submit all « natural medicinal products » to the same controls of efficacy, toxicity, and conformity applied to the classical drugs derived from the pharmaceutical producers. Given the fact that the nephrotoxic effect of AA is irreversible and that their carcinogenic effects may be very slow in manifesting themselves after the patient's initial exposure, AAN and associated cancers should be considered as a major public health issue.

Table 1 Characteristics of BN and iatrogenic AAN

	BN	Iatrogenic AAN
Prevalence of affected subjects in exposed population	2–5%	3–5%
Gender[a]	No difference	More women
Familial/household aggregation	Yes	No
Awareness of plant toxicity	Unaware	Inadvertent
Route of ingestion	Home-baked bread	Herbal remedies
Pathology	Identical	Identical
Incidence of urothelial carcinoma of the upper urinary tract	30–50%	44%
Clinical course[b]	Insidious onset, slow progression	Rapidly progressive to ESKD, Fanconi syndrome

[a]More women than men in AAN due to high number of Belgium women who underwent slimming regime
[b]Clinical course is dose-dependent i.e. in Belgium and most of other AAN cases worldwide high dose of aristolochic acid was ingested in shorter period. *BN* Balkan nephropathy, *AAN* aristolochic acid nephropathy, *ESKD* end-stage kidney disease

1.1 Aristolochia Species

The *Aristolochia* species is a genus of herbaceous, perennial plants that include more than 500 species. They are widespread in the warm regions of the Mediterranean, Africa, and Asia. They grow mainly in limestone soil and can be found on roadsides, in coppices, vineyards, and other agricultural areas. Furthermore, *Aristolochia clematitis* is a parasitic plant that grows alongside wheat in the local wheat fields in the warm and humid regions of the Danube Valley.

In the past, *Aristolochia* were widely used in Western medicine. In fact, their first use, namely to stimulate the expulsion of the placenta during childbirth, was responsible for coining the name “Aristos lokos” or “excellent delivery”.

Regarding global public health issues, *Aristolochia* are considered an integral part of the herbology used in traditional Chinese medicine, Japanese Kampo, and Ayurvedic medicine. They are found within the same therapeutic family as the *Akebia*, *Asarum*, *Cocculus,* and *Stephania* plants. Referred to by common names such as Mu Tong, Mokutsu, and Fang ji, they are used in a multitude of herbal mixtures for therapeutic use. Due to the ambiguity surrounding the nomenclature of medicinal plants used in traditional medicine, the detection of AA by means of the phytochemical analysis of plant extracts is the only way to certify their potential toxicity.

2 The Toxicity of Aristolochic Acids

Under normal physiological conditions, AA are metabolised, by the reduction of nitro compounds, into active metabolites called “aristolactams”. These aristolactams are capable of forming covalent bonds with purine bases of DNA. However, the DNA adducts specific to aristolactams remain part of the body's cell structure for several years after the patients' initial exposure to AA. Consequently, their discovery in the kidney or cancerous tissues constitute a biomarker, which may be related to a previous exposure to AA, which possibly occurred much earlier (Fig. 2f).

AAN has been successfully reproduced in animals (rabbits, rats, mice) in various experimental models. Both experimental and clinical studies indicate that AA use the basolateral organic anion transporter as the main entrance into the epithelial cells of the proximal tubule, particularly in segment S3. After acute, non-regenerative tubular necrosis, the interstitium is infiltrated by activated macrophages, as well as B and T lymphocytes, resulting in tubular atrophy and interstitial fibrosis involving CD 8+ lymphocytes and TGF-β.

The carcinogenicity of AA can be explained by the fact that the DNA adducts formed in combination with aristolactams lead to a mutation of A:T to T:A in the tumor suppressor gene TP 53. This mutation has frequently been demonstrated in the urothelial tumors of cases described in Taiwan and in the Balkans, whereas this mutation rarely occurs in tumors that are not related to the exposure to AA (Fig. 2a–e). This mutation is very specific and considered as a marker of a previous exposure to AA.

Even though the severity of kidney failure as well as the frequency of cancers can each be correlated with an increased dose of plant extracts containing AA, there is no clear correlation between severe kidney failure and the development of urothelial cancers.

3 Natural History of the Disease

In the initial cohorts concerning iatrogenic nephropathy due to AA, the majority of patients were described as exhibiting a rapid and progressive evolution towards end-stage kidney disease (ESKD). A large series of patients described in China revealed a median GFR decline at –3.5 ml/min/year. The progression rate in environmental nephropathy due to AA is much slower, with ESKD occurring only after an evolution of 15–20 years.

Urine sediment is generally normal, while mild to moderate tubular proteinuria may be detected. Blood pressure is elevated in 50% of cases. Anemia is often more severe than what one would expect from the level of kidney failure, probably because of the premature destruction of peritubular cells that secrete erythropoietin. Kidney size is often reduced asymmetrically. A few cases of iatrogenic nephropathy due to AA took the form of Fanconi syndrome or acute kidney injury (AKI).

Whether iatrogenic or environmental, AAN is more frequently associated with urinary tract cancers. In cases where bilateral uretero-nephrectomies were performed on female patients from the initial cohorts treated by dialysis or transplantation, 40% of these women suffered from urothelial cancers, which were often diagnosed as multifocal (Fig. 2b–d). Cancers of the bladder appeared in female patients who had undergone transplants more than 15 years after the toxin had been stopped (Fig. 2e). Frequent iatrogenic exposure to AA in Taiwan explains why this region has the world's highest level of urothelial cancers.

4 Kidney Pathology

Examination of kidney biopsy is a key element in the diagnosis of AAN. From a macroscopic point of view, in advanced cases of nephropathy, the kidneys are small and the renal cortex is considerably thinned. Microscopically, the most characteristic type of lesion consists of pauci-cellular interstitial fibrosis associated with tubular atrophy. The severity of these lesions decreases when moving from the external to the internal cortex (Fig. 1c–d).

In the early stages of the disease, the glomeruli are spared. Due to the interstitial fibrosis, however, this is then followed by the fibrous thickening of the Bowman capsule and glomerular obsolescence (Fig. 1g). Finally, the dominant cortical fibrosis causes the medullary striae to collapse, resulting in tortuous and spiral-shaped interlobar arteries.

5 Diagnosis

The combination of interstitial nephropathy with cancer of the urinary tract should suggest the diagnostic of AAN. A consensus exists regarding the definition of diagnostic criteria. The diagnosis of AAN can be considered as certain in any person who suffers from kidney failure, in combination with any two of the following three criteria: kidney histology displaying interstitial fibrosis with a cortico-medullary gradient, a history of ingesting vegetal or herbal products whose phytochemical analysis has demonstrated the presence of AA, the demonstrated presence of DNA adducts formed with aristolactams (or the specific mutation A:T to T:A of the TP53 tumor suppressor gene) in a kidney tissue biopsy sample or a urothelial tumor. Nevertheless, if only one of these three criteria can be demonstrated, the diagnosis of AAN remains highly probable and examinations should be continued in this direction.

Whatever the case, the presence of either AA in plant extracts ingested by patients, or of DNA adducts formed with aristolactams in patients' kidney tissue, are central to a diagnosis and provides absolute certainty.

6 Prevention

In terms of health policy, the main goal is to prevent the exposure to AA. Legal provisions have already been taken in Europe, the USA, Taiwan, and mainland China. However, the use of herbs containing AA is still allowed in China under certain conditions. In addition, it is still possible, anywhere in the world, to obtain plant extracts that may contain AA, particularly via parallel markets such as the Internet.

7 Treatment

The treatment of AAN is similar to the treatment of any chronic kidney disease and includes controlling the patient's blood pressure, symptomatic treatment of metabolic complications, and preparing for replacement therapy by means of dialysis or kidney transplantation.

Based on a pilot study, treatment with steroids (1 mg/kg of prednisolone for a period of 4 weeks, which is then gradually decreased to a maintenance dose of 0.15 mg/kg) can be considered at the time of diagnosis, provided that kidney function has not been severely impaired (eGFR >20 ml/min/1.73 m^2) and with rapid evolution. If, however, there is no stabilization of the kidney function after 6 months, the treatment should be abandoned.

The major problem in monitoring patients suffering from AAN is that they regularly need to be screened for cancer of the urinary tract. Urinary cytology can be performed routinely in all patients, but this test is not very sensitive with regard to the detection of tumors of the upper urinary tract. Moreover, it cannot replace the more aggressive strategy. Indeed, annual monitoring by means of computed axial tomography or magnetic resonance, as well as by means of a cystoscopy is the recommended practice.

Patients with ESKD, who are treated with dialysis or kidney transplantation, should undergo a prophylactic bilateral uretero-nephrectomy and monitoring should continue with cystoscopies with planned bladder biopsies every 6 months.

In case of bladder cancer, treatment includes endoscopic resections supplemented by the endovesical instillation of mitomycin C. Endovesical therapy based on the Bacillus Calmette –Guerin (BCG) can also be performed, even in patients with a kidney transplant, provided that therapy is combined with modulation of immunosuppression and prophylactic anti-tuberculosis chemotherapy. Radical cystectomy with pyelostomy of the graft remains the ultimate measure in transplant patients with invasive bladder cancer.

Suggested Reading

Arlt VM, Stiborova M, Schmeiser HH. Aristolochic acid as a probable human cancer hazard in herbal remedies: a review. Mutagenesis. 2002;17:265–77.

Baudoux T, Pozdzik AA, Arlt VM, De Prez E, Quellard N, Goujon JM, Nortier JL. Probenecid prevents acute tubular necrosis in a mouse model of aristolochic acid nephropathy. Kidney Int. 2012;82:1105–13.

Baudoux T, Husson C, De Prez E, Jadot I, Antoine M-H, Nortier J, Hougardy J-M. CD4+ and CD8+ T cells exert regulatory properties during experimental acute aristolochic acid nephropathy. Sci Rep. 2018;8:5334. https://doi.org/10.1038/s41598-018-23565-2.

Bunel V, Souard F, Antoine M-H, Stevigny C, Nortier JL. Nephrotoxicity of natural products: aristolochic acid and fungal toxins. In: McQueen CA, editor. Comprehensive toxicology, vol. 14. 3rd ed. Oxford: Elsevier Ltd; 2018. p. 340–79.

Cosyns JP, Jadoul M, Squifflet JP, De Plaen JF, Ferluga D, van Ypersele de Strihou C. Chinese herbs nephropathy: a clue to Balkan endemic nephropathy ? Kidney Int. 1994;45:1680–8.

Cosyns JP, Jadoul M, Squifflet JP, Wese FX, van Ypersele de Strihou C. Urothelial lesions in Chinese-herb nephropathy. Am J Kidney Dis. 1999;33:1011–7.

Cosyns JP, Dehoux JP, Guiot Y, et al. Chronic aristolochic acid toxicity in rabbits: a model of Chinese herbs nephropathy? Kidney Int. 2001;59:2164–73.

Debelle FD, Nortier JL, De Prez EG, Vienne A, Garbar C, Salmon I, Deschodt-Lanckman M, Vanherweghem JL. Aristolochic acids induce chronic renal failure with interstitial fibrosis in salt-depleted rats. J Am Soc Nephrol. 2002;13:431–6.

Debelle FD, Vanherweghem JL, Nortier JL. Aristolochic acid nephropathy: a worldwide problem. Kidney Int. 2008;74:158–69.

De Broe ME. Chinese herbs nephropathy and Balkan endemic nephropathy: toward a single entity, aristolochic acid nephropathy. Kidney Int. 2012;81:513–5.

Depierreux M, Van Damme B, Vanden Houte K, Vanherweghem JL. Pathologic aspects of a newly described nephropathy related to the prolonged use of Chinese herbs. Am J Kidney Dis. 1994;24:172–80.

Duquesne M, Decleves AE, De Prez E, Nortier J, Colet JM. Interest of metabonomic approach in environmental nephrotoxicants: application to aristolochic acid exposure. Food Chem Toxicol. 2017;108:19–29.

El Dirdiri NI, Barakat SE, Adam SE. The combined toxicity of Aristolochia bracteata and Cadaba rotundifolia to goats. Vet Hum Toxicol. 1987;29:133–7.

Gökmen MR, Cosyns JP, Arlt VM, Stiborova M, Phillips DH, Schmeiser HH, Simmonds M, Cook HT, Vanherweghem JL, Nortier JL, Lord GM. The epidemiology, diagnosis, and management of aristolochic acid nephropathy: a narrative review. Ann Intern Med. 2013;158:469–77.

Grollman AP. Aristolochic acid nephropathy: harbinger of a global iatrogenic disease. Environ Mol Mutagen. 2013;54:1–7.

Hashimoto K, Higushi M, Makino B. Quantitative analysis of aristolochic acids, toxic compounds, contained in some medicinal plants. J Ethnopharmacol. 1999;64:185–9.

Heinrich M, Chan J, Wanke S, Neinhuis C, Simmonds MSJ. Local uses of aristolochia species and content of nephrotoxic aristolochic acid 1 and 2 - a global assessment based on bibliographic sources. J Ethnopharmacol. 2009;125:108–44.

Ivić M. Etiology of endemic nephropathy. Lijec Vjesn. 1969;91:1273–81.

Jadot I, Decleves AE, Nortier J, Caron N. An integrated view of aristolochic acid nephropathy: update of the literature. Int J Mol Sci. 2017a;18:297–319. https://doi.org/10.3390/ijms18020297.

Jadot I, Colombaro V, Martin B, Habsch I, Botton O, Nortier J, Decleves AE, Caron N. Restored nitric oxide bioavailability reduces the severity of acute-to-chronic transition in a mouse model of aristolochic acid nephropathy. PLoS One. 2017b;12:e0183604. https://doi.org/10.1371/journal.pone.0183604.

Jelaković B, Karanović S, Vuković-Lela I, Miller F, Edwards KL, Nikolić J, et al. Aristolactam-DNA adducts are a biomarker of environmental exposure to aristolochic acid. Kidney Int. 2012;81:559–67.

Jelakowic B, Dika Z, Arlt VM, Stiborova M, Pavlovic N, Nikolic J, Colet J-M, Vanherweghem JL, Nortier JL. Balkan endemic nephropathy and the causative role of aristolochic acid. Semin Nephrol. 2019;39:284–96.

Lemy A, Wissing KM, Rorive S, Zlotta A, Roumeguere T, Muniz-Martinez MC, Decaestecker C, Salmon I, Abramowicz D, Vanherweghem JL, Nortier JL. Late onset of bladder urothelial carcinoma after kidney transplantation for end-stage aristolochic acid nephropathy: a case series with 15-year follow-up. Am J Kidney Dis. 2008;51:471–7.

Lewis CJ, Alpert S. Letter to health care professionals on FDA concerned about botanical products, including dietary supplements containing aristolochic acid. Us Food and Drug Administration – Center for Food Safety and Applied Nutrition – Office of Nutritional Products. Labeling and Dietary supplements, 2000.

Martinez MC, Nortier J, Vereerstraeten P, Vanherweghem JL. Progression rate of Chinese herb nephropathy: impact of Aristolochia fangchi ingested dose. Nephrol Dial Transplant. 2002;17:408–12.

Nortier J, Muniz Martinez MC, Schmeiser HH, Arlt VM, Bieler CA, Petein M, Depierreux M, Simon J, De Pauw L, Kinnaert P, Abramowicz D, Vereerstraeten P, Vanherweghem J-L. Urothelial carcinoma associated with the use of a Chinese herb (Aristolochia fangchi). N Engl J Med. 2000;342:1686–92.

Nortier JL, Roumeguere T. Bladder cancer – a genotoxic causal agent recognized. In: Wild CP, Weiderpass E, Stewart BW, editors. World cancer report: cancer research for cancer prevention. Lyon: International Agency for Research on Cancer; 2020. http://publications.iarc.fr/586.

Pavlovic NM. Balkan endemic nephropathy – current status and future perspectives. Clin Kidney J. 2013;6:257–65.

Chan W, Pavlovic NM, Li W, Chan CK, Liu J, Deng K, Wang Y, Milosavljevic B, Kostic EN. Quantitation of aristolochic acids in corn, wheat grain, and soil samples collected in Serbia: identifying a novel exposure pathway in the etiology of Balkan endemic nephropathy. J Agric Food Chem. 2016;64:5928–34.

Pozdzik AA, Salmon IJ, Debelle FD, Decaestecker C, Van Den Branden C, Verbeelen D, Deschodt-Lanckman M, Vanherweghem JL, Nortier JL. Aristolochic acid induces proximal tubule apoptosis and epithelial to mesenchymal transformation. Kidney Int. 2008a;73:595–607.

Pozdzik AA, Salmon IJ, Husson C, Rogier E, Bourgeade MF, Deschodt-Lanckman M, Vanherweghem JL, Nortier JL. Patterns of interstitial inflammation during the evolution of renal injury in experimental aristolochic acid nephropathy. Nephrol Dial Transplant. 2008b;23:2480–91.

Pozdzik AA, Giordano L, Li G, Antoine M-L, Quellard N, Godet J, De Prez E, Husson C, Decleves AE, Arlt VM, Goujon JM, Brocheriou-Spelle I, Ledbetter SR, Caron N, Nortier JL. Blocking TGF-β signalling pathway preserves mitochondrial proteostasis and reduces early activation of PDGFRβ+ pericytes in aristolochic acid induced acute kidney injury in Wistar male rats. PLoS One. 2016;11:e0157288. https://doi.org/10.1371/journal.pone.0157288.

Roumeguere T, Broeders N, Jayaswal A, Rorive S, Quackels T, Pozdzik A, Arlt VM, Schmeiser HH, Nortier JL. BCG therapy in non-muscle-invasive bladder carcinoma after renal transplantation for end-stage aristolochic acid nephropathy. Transpl Int. 2015;28:199–205.

Sborchia M, De Prez E, Antoine M-H, Bienfait L, Indra R, Valbuena G, Phillips DH, Nortier JL, Stiborova M, Keun H, Arlt VM. The impact of p53 on aristolochic acid I-induced nephrotoxicity and DNA damage in vivo and in vitro. Arch Toxicol. 2019;93:3345–66.

Schmeiser HH, Nortier JL, Singh R, Gamboa Da Costa G, Sennesael J, Cassuto-Viguier E, Ambrosetti D, Rorive S, Pozdzik A, Phillips DH, Stiborova M, Arlt VM. Exceptionally long-term persistence of DNA adducts formed by carcinogenic aristolochic acid I in renal tissue from patients with aristolochic acid nephropathy. Int J Cancer. 2014;135:502–7.

Vanhaelen M, Vanhaelen-Fastre R, But P, Vanherweghem JL. Identification of aristolochic acid in Chinese herbs. Lancet. 1994;343:174.

Vanherweghem JL, Depierreux M, Tielemans C, Abramowicz D, Dratwa M, Jadoul M, Richard C, Vandervelde D, Verbeelen D, Vanhaelen-Fastre R, Vanhaelen M. Rapidly progressive interstitial renal fibrosis in young women: association with slimming regimen including Chinese herbs. Lancet. 1993;341:387–91.

Vanherweghem JL, Abramowicz D, Tielemans C, Depierreux M. Effects of steroids on the progression of renal failure in chronic interstitial renal fibrosis: a pilot study in Chinese herbs nephropathy. Am J Kidney Dis. 1996;27:209–15.

Vanherweghem JL. Aristolochia sp and chronic interstitial nephropathies in Indians. Lancet. 1997;349:1399.

Williamson EM, Chan K, Xu Q, Nachtergael A, Bunel V, Zhang L, Ouedrago M, Nortier J, Qu F, Liu X, Stevigny C, Kahumba J, Pelkonen O, Duez P. Evaluating the safety of herbal medicines: integrated toxicological approaches. Science. 2015;347:S47–9.

World Health Organization - International Agency for Research on Cancer. IARC monographs on the evaluation of carcinogenic risks to humans: some traditional herbal medicines, some mycotoxins, naphtalene and styrene. IARC Pub. 2002;82:118.

Yamani A, Bunel V, Antoine M-H, Husson C, Stevigny C, Duez P, Elachouri M, Nortier J. Substitution between *Aristolochia* and *Bryonia* genus in North-Eastern Morocco: toxicological implications. J Ethnopharmacol. 2015;166:250–60.

Yang L, Besschetnova TY, Brooks CR, Shah JV, Bonventre JV. Epithelial cell cycle arrest in G2/M mediates kidney fibrosis after injury. Nat Med. 2010;16:535–43.

Yang L, Su T, Li XM, et al. Aristolochic acid nephropathy: variation in presentation and prognosis. Nephrol Dial Transplant. 2012;27:292–8.

Yang HY, Wang JD, Lo TC, Chen PC. Occupational kidney disease among Chinese herbalists exposed to herbs containing aristolochic acids. Occup Environ Med. 2011;68:286–90.

Zlotta AR, Roumeguere T, Kuk C, Alkhateeb S, Rorive S, Lemy A, Van Der Kwast TH, Fleshner NE, Jewett MAS, Finelli A, Schulman C, Lotan Y, Shariat SF, Nortier J. Select screening in a specific high-risk population of patients suggests a stage migration toward detection of non-muscle-invasive bladder cancer. Eur Urol. 2011;59:1026–31.

Chronic Kidney Disease of Unknown Etiology

Marvin Gonzalez-Quiroz, Pablo Garcia, and Shuchi Anand

1 The Disease and Its Toll

Chronic kidney disease of unknown etiology (CKDu) is currently the world's most common tubulointerstitial kidney disease. It has also been labeled Mesoamerican nephropathy and chronic interstitial nephritis in agricultural communities (CINAC). A distinct profile of patients are affected: young-to-middle aged, predominantly men, working strenuously at high temperatures, applying pesticides without protection and drinking water from nearest available field sources. High rates of death that are completely out of the expected range given the demographics, and obesity and diabetes rates in the affected communities are being observed. In one seminal prospective study, nearly 10% of otherwise healthy men living in an endemic community experienced rapid decline in kidney function (Fig. 1).

Three regional epidemics of kidney disease have occurred in the twentieth century, all due to singular environmental exposures and all manifesting as a primary tubulointerstitial kidney disease.

M. Gonzalez-Quiroz
Research Centre on Health, Work and Environment (CISTA), National Autonomous University of Nicaragua, León, Nicaragua

Centre for Nephrology, University College London, London, UK

Facultad de Ciencias Médicas, Edificio C (CISTA), León, Nicaragua

P. Garcia
Stanford University School of Medicine, Division of Nephrology, Stanford, CA, USA
e-mail: pgarciah@stanford.edu

S. Anand (✉)
Center for Tubulointerstitial Kidney Disease, Stanford University School of Medicine, Palo Alto, CA, USA
e-mail: Sanand2@stanford.edu

M. G. Atta, M. A. Perazella (eds.), *Tubulointerstitial Nephritis*,
https://doi.org/10.1007/978-3-030-93438-5_17

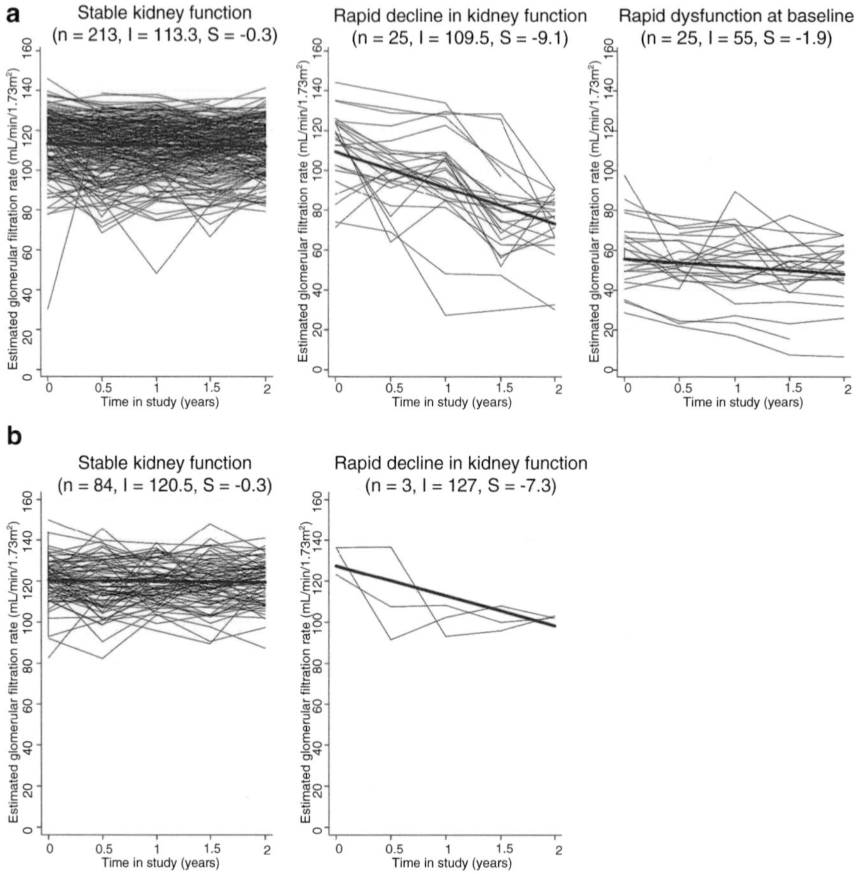

Fig. 1 (**a**) Men (**b**) Woman. Incident kidney function decline among 350 participants from a CKDu/MEN endemic community in Nicaragua: Although the study recruited people without prior history of CKD, 10% of men were diagnosed with baseline kidney dysfunction at the start of the study. An additional 10% of men and 3% of women experienced rapid decline from normal kidney function, with loss of nearly 10 ml/min/1.73 m^2 of eGFR per year. (Figure courtesy: Gonzalez-Quiroz, Marvin)

Most, similar to the current epidemic in agricultural communities; the Balkan nephropathy epidemic (see chapter "Aristolochic Acid Nephropathy and Balkan Nephropathy"), first described in the 1930s–1940s. Seeds of a local weed, *Aristolochia clematitis,* were admixing into the wheat harvest from select farms, slowly poisoning the kidney and bladder tissues of entire families with aristolochic acid. While pumping up production during World War II, Japanese mines leached cadmium into the Jintsu river basin; an astute physician servicing the area immediately caught the steep rise in painful bone lesions and kidney failure among residents of the area. Children playing in verandas with lead-laced paint on the railings were commonly hospitalized for acute lead poisoning in the early 1900s in Queensland, Australia. Decades later, the prevalence of "chronic nephritis" in adults

40 years or younger was three-fold higher in Queensland than in other Australian states.

Unfortunately, it took over five decades to uncover the cause of Balkan nephropathy. The current CKDu epidemic unfortunately seems to be following a similar arc. Despite its description in 2002, we have only managed to identify high-risk populations and characterize its basic pathology on kidney tissue. Key articles have highlighted the following potential causes: repeated kidney injury while working strenuously in hot temperatures, contamination of water or food chain with heavy metals, an infection with a new kidney-tropic pathogen, and a specific agrochemical exposure during application or via groundwater. The first hypothesis is the most prominent in the lay media, and has been linked to climate change, but none have been definitely proven or disproven. Unlike in acute-onset infections, the long lag between exposure and manifestation of symptomatic kidney disease has combined with the utter lack of resources for advanced methodological research to yield a frustrating medical mystery.

Meanwhile, CKDu is a terminal diagnosis in endemic regions. Dialysis is either unavailable or unaffordable. The death of a breadwinner reverberates through the entire household. In our qualitative work, a widow of a Sri Lankan farmer who died of kidney failure at age 47 reported that she could not afford to work due to lack of childcare. Her eldest daughter quit high school to work in a garment factory in the city to supply income for her two younger sisters. Kidney disease now consumes over 5% of Sri Lanka's overall health budget, and the Sri Lankan Ministry of Health hosts a Renal Disease Prevention Unit, conducting large-scale kidney disease surveillance in remote areas. A lowland coastal province in Nicaragua has been colloquially labeled 'La Isla de Las Viudas': The Isle of Widows. The CKDu epidemic has devastated individuals and communities.

While the two best described hotspots—Sri Lanka and Meso-America—are no doubt experiencing the worst toll of kidney disease, many experts suspect that other agricultural communities and workers may harbor higher rates of kidney dysfunction than evident in the general population. Systematic data on affected and unaffected regions would enable better evaluation of potential risk factors, and direct additional clinical resources to populations in need. The International Society of Nephrology recently generated a simple set of common data elements that could be integrated in population health studies, so as to enable a rigorous assessment of CKD prevalence, and its association with region of residence or occupation (Table 1).

2 Pathology Findings

The most common histopathological finding among patients with clinical characteristics of CKDu is tubulointerstitial nephritis, with accompanying glomerulosclerosis and ischemic injury. Despite the constraints on kidney biopsy in resource-settings, a few studies exist on pathological findings among people with CKDu, and show

Table 1 Minimum data set recommended by ISN to identify hotspots of CKDu

Age
Sex
Ethnicity/racial group
Occupation
Education and income
Address or geolocation
Average temperatures
Diabetes
Hypertension
IDMS calibrated creatinine
Quantified albuminuria, or dipstick proteinuria, as feasible

Abbreviations: *CKDu* chronic kidney disease of unknown etiology

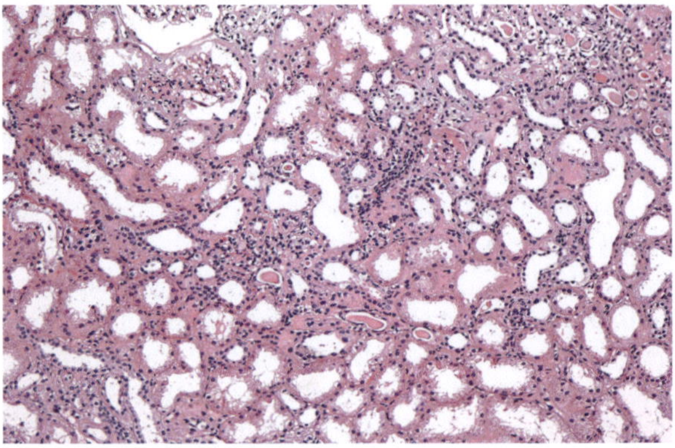

Fig. 2 Characteristic biopsy findings of CKDu in Sri Lanka: In a majority of biopsies, there is chronic tubular injury, with patchy areas of lymphocytic infiltration. (Figure courtesy Kambham, N, Ratnatunga N, and Nanayakkara N)

that the histopathological characteristics are similar among those affected with CKDu in Sri Lanka, Nicaragua, and El Salvador. In 2012, investigators in Sri Lanka looked at 57 kidney biopsies; the dominant histopathological lesion was interstitial fibrosis and tubular atrophy with or without nonspecific interstitial mononuclear cell infiltration followed by glomerular enlargement in 21 biopsies. Furthermore, Anand et al. reported that among 87 Sri Lankan patients who underwent a kidney biopsy due to abnormal urine sediment or kidney function, half of the patients had a biopsy diagnosis of primary tubulointerstitial kidney disease (Fig. 2).

In 2013, a group of investigators in El Salvador analyzed kidney tissue from eight male patients affected with Mesoamerican Nephropathy. The most common histopathological finding was glomerulosclerosis, chronic ischemic changes with tubular atrophy and interstitial fibrosis. A larger study in El Salvador including 46 patients with Mesoamerican nephropathy described interstitial fibrosis and tubular atrophy with or without inflammatory monocyte infiltration as the main histopathological lesion. Wijkstrom et al. compared kidney biopsies from both Sri Lanka and Meso-America, and found that in both regions most patients presented with mild to moderate interstitial fibrosis and glomerulosclerosis with signs of chronic glomerular ischemia.

In addition to chronic interstitial injury and glomerulosclerosis, a subset of individuals from both regions has been described to have acute interstitial nephritis, with active tubulitis and interstitial inflammation. Fischer et al. and Badurdeen et al. both described similar presentations—with back pain, fever, and pyuria present in varying degrees. In these cases, kidney biopsy findings were consistent with acute interstitial nephritis in studies performed via hospital surveillance.

Some authors have attempted to evaluate for 'signature' or pathognomonic lesions of CKDu. Vervaet et al. examined 34 kidney biopsies from Sri Lanka, El Salvador, India, and France of patients with CKD and clinical diagnosis of CKDu by light and electron microscopy. They described large dysmorphic lysosomes located in the proximal tubular cell . In addition, they described similar pathological findings (lysosomes) in kidney transplant biopsies exposed to calcineurin inhibitors. However subsequent studies have not confirmed these as pathognomonic lesions, but rather postulated that these are non-specific sign of tubular turn over.

3 Investigations into Cause: Major Hypotheses of Interest

The etiology and risk factors of CKDu remain unclear. In fact, researchers are still struggling to reconcile whether the disease occurring in Meso-America and Sri Lanka is the same entity (Fig. 3), since while several similarities exist, there are also several differences. Several possible causes have been suggested for CKDu in the last decade.

They include the following causes.

1. Occupational heat stress
2. Ground water contamination
3. Silica exposure through field burning
4. Genetic predisposition coupled with a common environmental exposure
5. New kidney tropic infection
6. Ad-mixed vegetation contaminating food
7. Ground water contaminating by agrochemicals

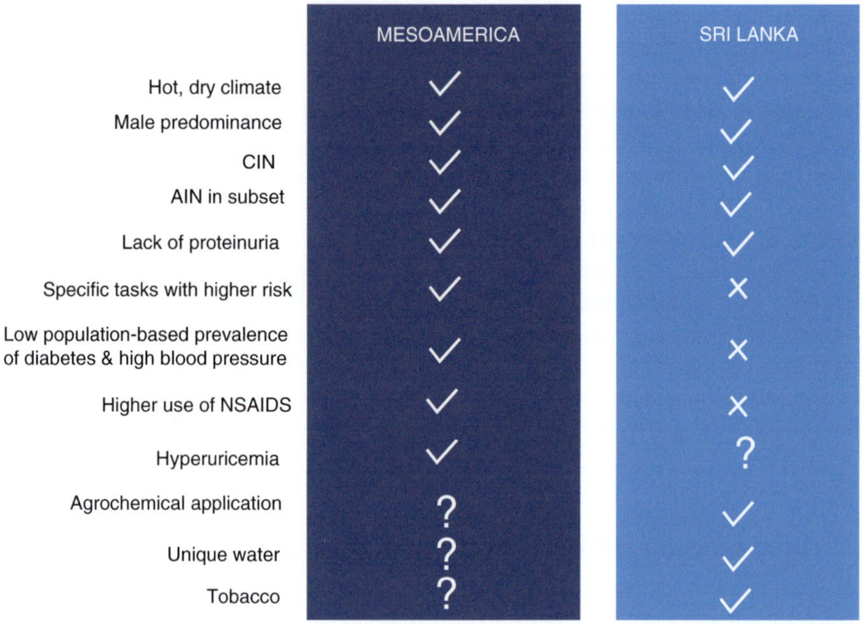

Fig. 3 Similarities and differences in presentation and described risk factors for kidney disease in Meso-America and Sri Lanka: While the timeline of the disease description (late 1990s and onwards) as well as the affected populations (predominantly, men working in agricultural fields) are similar between the two best described hotspots, important differences exist in the two populations as well

3.1 Social Determinants

CKDu is associated with a high mortality among young disadvantages population in rural areas in Mesoamerica and South Asia. Most studies have demonstrated that poverty is associated with CKDu. There are multiple potential causative or contributory pathways, including its impact on access to healthcare, access to education, and food security. People experiencing food insecurity may experience increased risk for incident CKDu or for progression with CKDu through multiple ways such as diet quality (unable to purchase healthful foods due to financial problems), dietary patterns, and via a direct contaminated food toxicity). In addition, disadvantaged groups experience limited access to medical healthcare and social security. This is thought to occur because workers are hired by subcontractors who evade their responsibility to pay the social security or insurance contribution for these workers. In Mesoamerican countries, when a worker is diagnosed with kidney disease because high serum creatinine level is detected, they are fired and lose access to medical care through the social security. This results in the inability of these workers to access the financial benefits of rightfully earned pensions. In addition, when men become too sick to work or die of CKDu, their sons are often forced to leave school and start working to support the family and medical expenses of their father. Ceron et al. also described a high incidence of CKD among children along the south coast of Guatemala, and Ramirez et al. found that Nicaraguan adolescents are having evidence of early kidney damage as assessed by biomarkers, thus increasing susceptibility for further kidney impairment in early adulthood.

3.2 Heat Stress and Dehydration

Heat stress and dehydration have become the most widely cited and studied causal hypotheses for CKDu in Mesoamerica, because groups with the highest prevalence—construction, agricultural and sugarcane workers—are performing strenuous labor and working outdoors exposed to high temperature during 8-hours a day. Ultimately, this puts them at increased of physical exertion and recurrent dehydration that can result in acute kidney injury (AKI).

Putative mechanisms for chronic dehydration contributing to or causing CKDu include repeated episodes associated with increased vasopressin secretion, cortical aldose reductase activation, and hyperuricemia. Increased vasopressin release induced by dehydration leads to glomerular hyperfiltration causing vasoconstriction in the short run but damages the glomerulus in long-term leading to reduced eGFR. Aldose reductase activation in cortical proximal tubular cells is induced by high serum osmolarity, which converts glucose to sorbitol and then to fructose, which is further metabolized, generating uric acid and consuming cellular ATP. This process leads to oxidative stress that results in the development of tubular injury and fibrosis.

Based on the above mechanisms, intervention studies have been implemented to mitigate the effects of heat stress and dehydration on the kidney by providing access to water, rest and shade among sugarcane farm workers in Nicaragua and Guatemala. The study from Nicaragua has shown a substantial decrease in incident kidney injury across the harvest (70%) in harvest 2 as compared with harvest 1 where there was less uptake of the mitigating intervention.

However, it is yet to be proven whether the reduction in incident (acute or subacute) kidney injury translates into a reduction in incident CKDu. Furthermore, workers living in other tropical regions exposed to heat have not, at least not yet, been reported to experience similar epidemics. The majority of the epidemiological studies have shown mild elevations in serum creatinine in cross-shift studies. There is also some concern that high water intake without assessment of water quality could be harmful as water sources may be contaminated with organic and inorganic contaminants (agrochemical and heavy metals). Also, high fructose (sugary beverages) or glucose (electrolyte solution) intake in the context of chronic dehydration can induce kidney injury by activating the polyol pathway and increase uric acid level that may damage the kidney tubules. Thus, while heat stress and dehydration remain the most studied hypotheses for a cause of CKDu, definitive causation is yet to be established.

3.3 Agrochemical and Metals

Agrochemicals have been used extensively and in an unregulated manner in Mesoamerica and South Asia. Farmers are highly exposed to them not only occupationally but also in daily life from food and water. Paraquat, 2,4-dichlorophenoxyacetic, glyphosate, and organophosphate (OP) are among the most used pesticides. Farm workers in these regions are using pesticides without protective gear. Up until recently, studies assessing pesticide use were based on self-reporting questionnaires, and while direct measurements of the bioburden of pesticides are now being pursued—mostly by urine measures—no definitive association with CKD has been established. Smpokou *et al* have measured serum level of twelve pesticides among healthy young adults in Nicaragua and did not find any association between these environmental toxins and incident decreased kidney function.

Exposure to metals such as lead, cadmium, mercury, arsenic, and other metals and toxins has also been suggested as potentially causative. However, several studies also reported that the exposure level, while higher than in Western regions, is insufficient to cause significant kidney injury. Recently, amorphous silica has been suggested to have a role in the development of CKDu. Rice and cane cutters are exposed to high concentration of amorphous silica due to the emissions from burning and harvesting sugarcane and rice husk ash. Silica nanoparticles (<40 nm) have localized in liver and kidney, where it can induce an inflammatory response, and these particles are phagocytosed by macrophages inducing cytotoxicity in different cell types in addition to activating inflammasomes in peripheral blood mononuclear cells. Nanoparticles can also potentially cross the basement membrane where they could be taken up by tubular cells causing chronic interstitial nephritis. Currently, promising work is being pursued in this area, especially using kidney biopsy tissue to evaluate for evidence of silica-related injury.

3.4 Genetics

Familial clustering of CKDu and geographical variation have been reported among men in hotspot regions. Family history of CKD and sex have been consistently associated with CKDu in Mesoamerica and South Asia. A whole-exome sequencing (GWAS) study was conducted in eight cases and controls respectively from Sri Lanka, and rs34970857 locus was identified at the KCNA10. This gene encodes a voltage-gated K channel and plays a role in stabilizing membrane voltage during sustained sodium entry at the apical membrane of proximal tubular cells. Also, four additional rare variants were revealed in the gene encoding for Laminin beta 2 (LAMB2), which drives to congenital nephrotic syndrome. Furthermore, a genetic study conducted in 334 CKDu cases and 334 controls matched by age and sex reported that participants carrying at least one mutant allele of CYP1A1*2A (TC, CC) and *2C (AG, GG) were highly associated with CKDu. These intriguing data point to the need for detailed genetic profiling of affected populations.

3.5 Use of Anti-inflammatory Drugs

Drug nephrotoxicity has been considered among the possible risk factors for CKD because the use of non-steroidal anti-inflammatory drugs (NSAIDs) or any other pain killers, diuretics, and antibiotics (gentamicin, and amikacin) is common in the population at risk for CKDu. Aminoglycosides and other antibiotics are used to treat dysuria (colloquioly termed 'Chistata') or urinary tract infections in hotspots regions. However, in Sri Lanka, use of NSAIDs is much less common.

3.6 Infectious Diseases

Infectious diseases have been suggested as additional risk factors for CKD. Dengue virus, Zika, leptospira, and hantavirus, which are diseases that are endemic in Mesoamerica and Asia regions (Sri Lanka and India), are thought to cause tubulointerstitial kidney injury. Case series from both Sri Lanka and Nicaragua have documented a small number of cases with a clinical syndrome of fever of unknown origin and kidney dysfunction, and biopsies in these patients show acute interstitial inflammation. However, a case-control study did not identify a higher prevalence of Leptospira or hantavirus exposure among cases with CKDu. Moreover, Araujo et al., reported that patients with a coinfection of dengue fever and Zika are more likely to develop a severe collapsing variant of focal segmental glomerulosclerosis. To date, while infectious causes remain a hypothesis of interest for CKDu, there hasn't been a single identified cause.

4 Ongoing Research Efforts

There are several groups employing a variety of epidemiological approaches to investigate the etiology of CKDu in Mesoamerica and Asia regions (Fig. 4). These approaches include community-based and occupational studies, cross-sectional, case control, prospective and interventional studies in Mesoamerica and Asia regions. As an example, Gonzalez-Quiroz et al. and Ruwanpathirana et al. have three community-based cohort studies in Nicaragua, India, and Sri-Lanka with the following aims: (1) investigate the evolution of, and risk factors for decrease in kidney function over time among young adults at risk of CKDu, and (2) compare the evolution and risk factors for kidney function decline in different population and regions at risk of CKDu. Each study site has recruited almost 1000 participants between 18 and 30 years old from different endemic communities and they have been followed-up annually over 2-years in Sri Lanka and India and over 7-years in Nicaragua. Moreover, there is one occupational prospective cohort study with the aim to identify occupational exposures associated with kidney injury and decrease

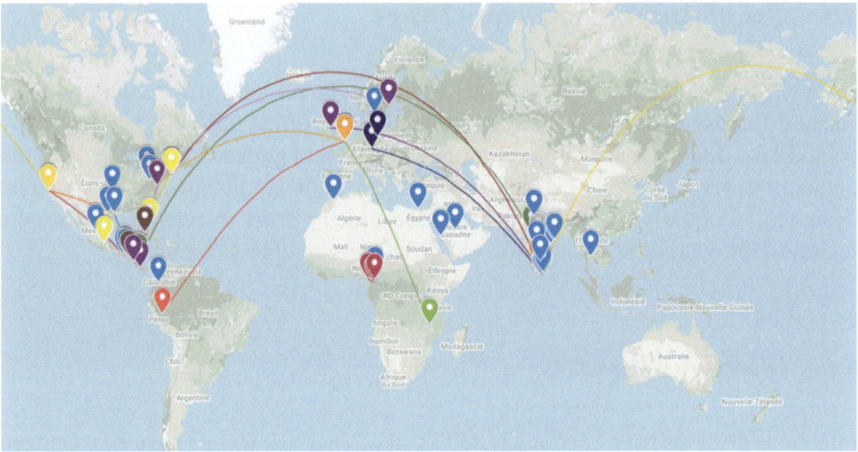

Fig. 4 Collaborations between institutions to investigate CKDu as reported to International Society of Nephrology Observatory on CKDu, as of January 2021: The mysterious kidney disease affecting a vulnerable population in low-resource settings has inspired global collaborations between academic centers throughout the world and across academic disciplines. These efforts will build capacity for kidney disease research and care

in kidney function over time. This study has recruited approximately 500 workers (sugarcane workers, agricultural workers, and brickmakers) in El Salvador and Nicaragua. Researchers have been collecting data and biological samples over 3 years and have measured cystatin c, serum creatinine and other kidney biomarkers. (https://www.bu.edu/sph/about/departments/epidemiology/research/researc)

A case-cohort study is ongoing in Sri Lanka where more than 300 participants with CKDu were recruited and followed for 2 years. The aims of this prospective study are to (1) describe the natural history of CKDu, (2) determine if a subset of participants experience more rapid progression, and (3) elucidate risk factors for rapid progression. This study is collecting a variety of environmental exposures and will analyze contaminants in drinking water. In addition, there is a historical and prospective case-cohort study in Nicaragua, El Salvador, Mexico India, and Sri Lanka, in which researchers will determine the silica nanoparticle content in kidney biopsy tissue from subjects with CKDu or from subjects from the same region who have different kidney diseases. This study is planning to recruit at 25 biopsies from each study site.

Finally, there two active intervention studies in Mesoamerica, (1) the first intervention is called We Adelante in Nicaragua, where researchers are examining the effectiveness of Water, Rest, and Shade program to reduce heat stress and dehydration and thus prevent or minimize kidney injury among sugarcane field workers. This study has found in its third phase a reduction of 70% of incidence kidney injury among cane cutter in Nicaragua by providing access to Water, Rest and Shade during the harvest. A similar intervention has been implemented by the University of Colorado and Pantaleon mill in Guatemala, where they recommend that electrolyte supplementation should be incorporated to standard workplace along with Water, Rest, and Shade programs for protecting workers.

5 Summary

A regional nephropathy of undetermined cause has led to a high rate of death and disability from kidney disease in otherwise healthy young-to-middle aged persons living in agricultural areas in Meso-America, Sri Lanka, and India. Due to the lack of systematic surveillance and diagnostics, it is not clear whether kidney health is suffering in other agricultural areas, but the long-described hotspots in Mesoamerica, Sri Lanka, and India offer an opportunity for collaborative, cross-disciplinary investigations integrating nephrology, pathology, occupational health, and environmental health. Several hypotheses are being tested, and as the field matures, many studies are accommodating evaluation of multiple potential exposures with additional resources being devoted to high-quality study design and exposure ascertainment.

Suggested Reading

Araujo SA, Cordeiro TME, Belisario AR, Araujo RFA, Marinho PES, Kroon EG, de Oliveira DB, Teixeira MM, Simoes ESAC. First report of collapsing variant of focal segmental glomerulosclerosis triggered by arbovirus: dengue and Zika virus infection. Clin Kidney J. 2019;12(3):355–61.

Badurdeen Z, Nanayakkara N, Ratnatunga NV, Wazil AW, Abeysekera TD, Rajakrishna PN, et al. Chronic kidney disease of uncertain etiology in Sri Lanka is a possible sequel of interstitial nephritis! Clin Nephrol. 2016;86(13):S106–S9.

Butler-Dawson J, Krisher L, Asensio C, et al. Risk factors for declines in kidney function in sugarcane workers in Guatemala. J Occup Environ Med. 2018;60:548–58.

Cerón A, Fort MP, Morine CM, Lou-Meda R. Chronic kidney disease among children in Guatemala. Rev Panam Salud Publica. 2014;36(6):376–82.

Chapman E, Haby MM, Illanes E, Sanchez-Viamonte J, Elias V, Reveiz L. Risk factors for chronic kidney disease of non-traditional causes: a systematic review. Rev Panam Salud Publica. 2019;43:e35. Published 2019 Mar 14. https://doi.org/10.26633/RPSP.2019.35.

Crowe J, Wesseling C, Solano BR, et al. Heat exposure in sugarcane harvesters in Costa Rica. Am J Ind Med. 2013;56:1157–64.

Fischer RSB, Vangala C, Truong L, Mandayam S, Chavarria D, Granera Llanes OM, et al. Early detection of acute tubulointerstitial nephritis in the genesis of Mesoamerican nephropathy. Kidney Int. 2018;93(3):681–90.

Fischer R, Unrine J, Vangala C, Sanderson W, Mandayam S, Murray K. Evidence of nickel and other trace elements and their relationship to clinical findings in acute Mesoamerican nephropathy: a case-control analysis. PLoS One. 2020;15(11):e0240988.

Friedman DJ. Genes and environment in chronic kidney disease hotspots. Curr Opin Nephrol Hypertens. 2019;28(1):87–96. https://doi.org/10.1097/MNH.0000000000000470.

Garcia-Garcia G, Jha V, World Kidney Day Steering Committee. Chronic kidney disease in disadvantaged populations. Braz J Med Biol Res. 2015;48(5):377–81. https://doi.org/10.1590/1414-431X20144519.

García-Trabanino R, Jarquín E, Wesseling C, Johnson RJ, González-Quiroz M, Weiss I, Glaser J, Vindell JJ, Stockfelt L, Roncal C, Harra T, Barregard L. Heat stress, dehydration, and kidney function in sugarcane cutters in El Salvador – a cross-shift study of workers at risk of Mesoamerican nephropathy. Environ Res. 2015. pii: S0013-9351(15)30028-1. https://doi.org/10.1016/j.envres.2015.07.007.

Ghosh R, Siddarth M, Singh N, et al. Organochlorine pesticide level in patients with chronic kidney disease of unknown etiology and its association with renal function. Environ Health Prev Med. 2017;22:49. https://doi.org/10.1186/s12199-017-0660-5.

Glaser J, Hansson E, Weiss I, et al. Preventing kidney injury among sugarcane workers: promising evidence from enhanced workplace interventions. Occup Environ Med. 2020;77:527–34.

Gomez Diana M, Silvio U-I, Hernandez JC. Silica nanoparticles induce NLRP3 inflammasome activation in human primary immune cells. Innate Immun. 2017;23(8):697–708.

González-Quiroz M, Camacho A, Faber D, Aragón A, Wesseling C, Glaser J, Le Blond J, Smeeth L, Nitsch D, Pearce N, Caplin B. Rationale, description and baseline findings of a community-based prospective cohort study of kidney function amongst the young rural population of Northwest Nicaragua. BMC Nephrol. 2017;18:16. https://doi.org/10.1186/s12882-016-0422-4.

Gonzalez-Quiroz M, Smpokou E-T, Silverwood RJ, Camacho A, Faber D, Garcia BLR, Oomatia A, Hill M, Glaser J, Le Blond J, Wesseling C, Aragon A, Smeeth L, Pearce N, Nitsch D, Caplin B. Decline in kidney function among apparently healthy young adults at risk of Mesoamerican nephropathy. J Am Soc Nephrol. 2018a;29:2200–12. https://doi.org/10.1681/ASN.2018020151.

Gonzalez-Quiroz M, Pearce N, Caplin B, Nitsch D. What do epidemiological studies tell us about chronic kidney disease of undetermined cause in Mesoamerica? A systematic review and meta-analysis. Clin Kidney J. 2018b;11(4):496–506. https://doi.org/10.1093/ckj/sfx136.

Gonzalez-Quiroz M, Nitsch D, Hamilton S, O'Callaghan-Gordo C, Saran R, Glaser J, Correa-Rotter R, Jakobsson K, Singh A, Gunawardena N, Levin A, Remuzzi G, Caplin B, Pearce N, on behalf of the DEGREE Study Steering Committee. Rationale and population-based prospective cohort protocol for the Disadvantaged Populations at Risk of Decline in eGFR (CO-DEGREE). BMJ Open. 2019;9(9):e031169. https://doi.org/10.1136/bmjopen-2019-031169.

Gracia-Trabanino R, Dominguez J, Jansa JM, et al. Proteinuria and chronic renal failure in the coast of El Salvador: detection with low cost methods and associated factors. Nefrologia. 2005;25:31–8.

Gunarathna S, Gunawardana B, Jayaweera M, et al. Glyphosate and AMPA of agricultural soil, surface water, groundwater and sediments in areas prevalent with chronic kidney disease of unknown etiology, Sri Lanka. J Environ Sci Health B. 2018;53:729–37.

Gutthann SP, Rodríguez LAG, Raiford DS, Oliart AD, Romeu JR. Nonsteroidal anti-inflammatory drugs and the risk of hospitalization for acute renal failure. Arch Intern Med. 1996;156(21):2433–9. https://doi.org/10.1001/archinte.1996.00440200041005.

Hansson E, Glaser J, Weiss I, et al. Workload and cross-harvest kidney injury in a Nicaraguan sugarcane worker cohort. Occup Environ Med. 2019;76:818–26.

Harari F, Sallsten G, Christensson A, Petkovic M, Hedblad B, Forsgard N, Melander O, Nilsson PM, Born Y, Engstr MG, et al. Blood lead levels and decreased kidney function in a population-based cohort. Am J Kidney Dis. 2018;72(3):381–9.

Herath C, Jayasumana C, De Silva P, De Silva PHC, Siribaddana S, De Broe ME. Kidney diseases in agricultural communities: a case against heat-stress nephropathy. Kidney Int Rep. 2018;3(2):271–80. [PubMed: 29725631]

Kulathunga MRDL, Ayanka Wijayawardena MA, Naidu R, et al. Chronic kidney disease of unknown aetiology in Sri Lanka and the exposure to environmental chemicals: a review of literature. Environ Geochem Health. 2019;41:2329–38. https://doi.org/10.1007/s10653-019-00264-z.

Laux TS, Bert PJ, Barreto Ruiz GM, et al. Nicaragua revisited: evidence of lower prevalence of chronic kidney disease in a highaltitude, coffee-growing village. J Nephrol. 2012;25:533–40.

Laws RL, Brooks DR, Amador JJ, Weiner DE, Kaufman JS, Ramírez-Rubio O, Riefkohl A, Scammell MK, López-Pilarte D, Sánchez JM, Parikh CR, McClean MD. Biomarkers of kidney injury among Nicaraguan sugarcane workers. Am J Kidney Dis. 2016;67(2):209–17. https://doi.org/10.1053/j.ajkd.2015.08.022. Epub 2015 Oct

Le Blond JS, Williamson BJ, Horwell CJ, Monro AK, Kirk CA, Oppenheimer C. Production of potentially hazardous respirable silica airborne particulate from the burning of sugarcane. Atmos Environ. 2008;42:5558–68.

Le Blond JS, Horwell CJ, Williamson BJ, Oppenheimer C. Generation of crystalline silica from sugarcane burning. J Environ Monit. 2010;12:1459–70.

Longmire M, Choyke PL, Kobayashi H. Clearance properties of nano-sized particles and molecules as imaging agents: considerations and caveats. Nanomedicine (Lond). 2008;3(5):703–17. https://doi.org/10.2217/17435889.3.5.703.

Lyndsay K, Jaime B-D, Hillary Y, Daniel P, Miranda D, Johnson Evan C, Diana J, Alex C, Claudia A, Newman Lee S. Electrolyte beverage intake to promote hydration and maintain kidney function in Guatemalan sugarcane workers laboring in hot conditions. J Occup Environ Med. 2020;62(12):e696–703. https://doi.org/10.1097/JOM.0000000000002033.

Michael FC, Elisabeth E, Per L, Fryzek Jon P, Dickman Paul W, Signorello Lisa B, Loren L, Carl-Gustaf E, Blot WJ, McLaughlin Joseph K, Zack Matthew M, Olof N. Acetaminophen, aspirin, and chronic renal failure. N Engl J Med. 2001;345:1801–8.

Nanayakkara S, Senevirathna ST, Parahitiyawa NB, Abeysekera T, Chandrajith R, Ratnatunga N, Hitomi T, Kobayashi H, Harada KH, Koizumi A. Whole-exome sequencing reveals genetic variants associated with chronic kidney disease characterized by tubulointerstitial damages in North Central Region, Sri Lanka. Environ Health Prev Med. 2015 Sep;20(5):354–9.

O'Donnell JK, Tobey M, Weiner DE, et al. Prevalence of and risk factors for chronic kidney disease in rural Nicaragua. Nephrol Dial Transplant. 2011;26:2798–805.

Orantes CM, Herrera R, Almaguer M, et al. Chronic kidney disease and associated risk factors in the Bajo Lempa region of El Salvador: Nefrolempa study, 2009. MEDICC Rev. 2011;13:14–22.

Orantes CM, Herrera R, Almaguer M, et al. Epidemiology of chronic kidney disease in adults of Salvadoran agricultural communities. MEDICC Rev. 2014;16:23–30.

Peiris-John R, Wanigasuriya J, Wickremasinghe A, Dissanayake W, Hittarage A. Exposure to acetylcholinesterase-inhibiting pesticides and chronic renal failure. Ceylon Med J. 2009;51(1):42–3. https://doi.org/10.4038/cmj.v51i1.1382.

Raines N, Gonzalez M, Wyatt C, et al. Risk factors for reduced glomerular filtration rate in a Nicaraguan community affected by Mesoamerican nephropathy. MEDICC Rev. 2014;16:16–22.

Ramirez-Rubio O, Scammell MK, et al. Chronic kidney disease in Nicaragua: a qualitative analysis of semi-structured interviews with physicians and pharmacists. 2011. http://www.cao-ombudsman.org/cases/document-links/documents/BUInterviewsReportFEB2012Eng.pdf.

Ramírez-Rubio O, Amador JJ, Kaufman JS, Weiner DE, Parikh CR, Khan U, McClean MD, Laws RL, López-Pilarte D, Friedman DJ, Kupferman J, Brooks DR. Urine biomarkers of kidney injury among adolescents in Nicaragua, a region affected by an epidemic of chronic kidney disease of unknown aetiology. Nephrol Dial Transplant. 2016;31(3):424–32. https://doi.org/10.1093/ndt/gfv292.

Riefkohl A, Ramirez-Rubio O, Laws R, McClean M, Weinar D, Kaufman J, Galloway R, Shadomy S, Guerra M, Amador J, Sanchez J, Lopez-Pilarte D, Parikh C, Leibler J, Brooks D. Leptospira seropositivity as a risk factor for Mesoamerican nephropathy. Int J Occup Environ Health. 2017;23(1):1–10. https://doi.org/10.1080/10773525.2016.1275462.

Roncal Jimenez CA, Ishimoto T, Lanaspa MA, Rivard CJ, Nakagawa T, Ejaz AA, Cicerchi C, Inaba S, Le M, Miyazaki M, Glaser J, Correa-Rotter R, González MA, Aragón A, Wesseling C, Sánchez-Lozada LG, Johnson RJ. Fructokinase activity mediates dehydration-induced renal injury. Kidney Int. 2014 Aug;86(2):294–302. https://doi.org/10.1038/ki.2013.492.

Roncal-Jimenez C, Lanaspa M, Jensen T, Sanchez-Lozada L, Johnson R. Mechanisms by which dehydration may lead to chronic kidney disease. Ann Nutr Metab. 2015;66(Suppl. 3):10–3.

Roncal-Jimenez C, García-Trabanino R, Barregard L, Lanaspa MA, Wesseling C, Harra T, Aragón A, Grases F, Jarquin ER, González MA, Weiss I, Glaser J, Sánchez-Lozada LG, Johnson RJ. Heat stress nephropathy from exercise-induced uric acid crystalluria: a perspective on Mesoamerican nephropathy. Am J Kidney Dis. 2016;67(1):20–30. https://doi.org/10.1053/j.ajkd.2015.08.021.

Ruwanpathirana T, Senanayake S, Gunawardana N, Munasinghe A, Ginige S, Gamage D, Amarasekara J, Lokuketagoda B, Chulasiri P, Amunugama S, Palihawasana P, Caplin B, Pearce

N. Prevalence and risk factors for impaired kidney function in the district of Anaradhapura, Sri Lanka. BMC Public Health. 2019;19:763.

SALTRA. Mesoamerican nephropathy: report from the first International Research Workshop on MeN. 2012. Salud Trabajo y Ambiente, No 10.

Sanoff SL, Callejas L, Alonso CD, et al. Positive association of renal insufficiency with agriculture employment and unregulated alcohol consumption in Nicaragua. Ren Fail. 2010;32:766–77.

Schaeffer JW, et al. A pilot study to assess inhalation exposures among sugarcane workers in Guatemala: implications for chronic kidney disease of unknown origin. Int J Environ Res Public Health. 2020;17(16):5708.

Siddarth M, Datta SK, Ahmed RS, Banerjee BD, Kalra OP, Tripathi AK. Association of CYP1A1 gene polymorphism with chronic kidney disease: a case control study. Environ Toxicol Pharmacol. 2013;36(1):164–70. https://doi.org/10.1016/j.etap.2013.03.008.

Smpokou E-T, González-Quiroz M, Martins C, Alvito P, Le Blond J, Glaser J, Aragón A, Wesseling C, Nitsch D, Pearce N, Norman J, Lindh C, Morton J, Caplin B. Environmental exposures in young adults with declining kidney function in a population at risk of Mesoamerican nephropathy. Occup Environ Med. 2019;76:920–6.

Torres C, Aragón A, González M, López I, Jakobsson K, Elinder CG, Lundberg I, Wesseling C. Decreased kidney function of unknown cause in Nicaragua: a community-based survey. Am J Kidney Dis. 2010;55(3):485–96. Epub 2010, Feb 8.

Valcke M, Levasseur ME, Soares da Silva A, Wesseling C. Pesticide exposures and chronic kidney disease of unknown etiology: an epidemiologic review. Environ Health. 2017;16:49.

Vela XF, Henriquez DO, Zelaya SM, et al. Chronic kidney disease and associated risk factors in two Salvadoran farming communities, 2012. MEDICC Rev. 2014;16:55–60.

Vlahos P, Schensul SL, Nanayakkara N, Chandrajith R, Haider L, Anand S, Silva KT, Schensul JJ. Kidney progression project (KiPP): protocol for a longitudinal cohort study of progression in chronic kidney disease of unknown etiology in Sri Lanka. Glob Public Health. 2018;14:1–13. https://doi.org/10.1080/17441692.2018.1508480.

Wesseling C, Aragón A, González M, Weiss I, Glaser J, Rivard CJ, Roncal-Jiménez C, Correa-Rotter R, Johnson RJ. Heat stress, hydration and uric acid: a cross-sectional study in workers of three occupations in a hotspot of Mesoamerican nephropathy in Nicaragua. BMJ Open. 2016;6:e011034. https://doi.org/10.1136/bmjopen-2016-011034.

Wijkstrom J, Jayasumana C, Dassanayake R, Priyawardane N, Godakanda N, Siribaddana S, Ring A, Hultenby K, Soderberg M, Elinder CG, Wernerson A. Morphological and clinical findings in Sri Lankan patients with chronic kidney disease of unknown cause (CKDu): similarities and differences with Mesoamerican nephropathy. PLoS One. 2018;13(3):e0193056.

Yih WK, Kulldorff M, Friedman DJ, Leibler JH, Amador JJ, López-Pilarte D, Galloway RL, Ramírez-Rubio O, Riefkohl A, Brooks DR. Investigating possible infectious causes of chronic kidney disease of unknown Etiology in a Nicaraguan mining community. Am J Trop Med Hyg. 2019;101(3):676–83.

Infiltrative Disease of the Tubulointerstitium

Abinet M. Aklilu and Randy L. Luciano

1 Infiltrative Diseases of the Tubulointerstitium

Acute kidney injury (AKI) in malignancy contributes to significant morbidity in the form of hospital admissions and increased length of stay, and perhaps more importantly, treatment delay and potentially suboptimal dosing of chemotherapeutic agents. Furthermore, AKI is an independent determinant of 6-month remission for newly diagnosed high-grade hematologic malignancies. The incidence and etiology of AKI in cancer varies depending on the type and extent of malignancy, concomitant comorbidities, and treatment. The most common causes of kidney injury in malignancies are pre-renal azotemia and acute tubular injury (ATI), although obstruction, glomerular injury, and tubulointerstitial infiltration may also occur to a lesser degree. Tubulointerstitial diseases in malignancy, can result from infiltration of the interstitial space by the cancer cells or a secondary inflammation caused by cancer targeted therapy such as immune check point inhibitors. In this chapter, we will discuss non-immune mediated infiltrative tubulointerstitial diseases of the kidney in the context of both solid organ and hematologic malignancies (Table 1).

Infiltrative lesions expand the interstitium, leading to a distortion of the normal kidney micro-structures. Histology will show an influx of cells (either pleomorphic or monomorphic, depending on the underlying cause), leading to compression of tubular lumen, inflammation, invasion of renal tubular epithelial cells (tubulitis), and the presence of white blood cell casts that can cause further tubular damage or obstruction (Fig. 1). These lesions are unique in that they may be entirely clinically silent depending on the extent of parenchymal involvement but when clinically significant, can present an indication for treatment particularly in cases of indolent

A. M. Aklilu · R. L. Luciano (✉)
Yale University School of Medicine, Section of Nephrology, Department of Internal Medicine, New Haven, CT, USA
e-mail: abinet.aklilu@yale.edu; randy.luciano@yale.edu

M. G. Atta, M. A. Perazella (eds.), *Tubulointerstitial Nephritis*,
https://doi.org/10.1007/978-3-030-93438-5_18

Table 1 Tubulointerstitial disease from various cancer

Malignancies with tubulointerstitial manifestations			
Hematologic		Solid	
Lymphoproliferative diseases	Lymphomatous infiltrates – rarely primary	Primary	Secondary (Metastatic)
	Leukemia	**Adult** • Renal cell carcinoma • RCC with sarcomatous features • Urothelial carcinoma • Primary renal sarcoma (rarest) • Most common - Leiomyosarcoma • Most likely to be infiltrative - Rhabdomyosarcoma and Angiosarcoma **Pediatric** • Wilm's tumor • Rhabdoid tumor • PNET • Diffuse type nephroblastomatosis	Most commonly bronchogenic carcinoma, followed by breast cancer, and GI malignancies
	Lymphoplasmacytic lymphoma		
	Immunodeficiency-related lymphoproliferative disorders (e.g. PTLD, HIV)		
Paraneoplastic or paraprotein-related cancers	• Light chain deposition disease • Crystal storing histiocytosis • Infiltration by plasma cells		

Abbreviations: *RCC* renal cell carcinoma, *PTLD* post-transplant lymphoproliferative disorder, *HIV* human immunodeficiency virus, *PNET* primary neuro-ectodermal tumors, *GI* gastrointestinal

hematologic dyscrasias that otherwise do not meet criteria for treatment based on standard hematology guidelines. The kidney injury that results from infiltrative lesions is believed to be due to increased interstitial pressure and the severity depends on the extent of involvement by the infiltrative cells. Kidney biopsy may also show other structural lesions coexisting with the infiltrative cells as well as bowman capsule thickening as a result of chronic ischemia from chronic infiltration.

2 Lymphoproliferative Disorders

Lymphoproliferative disorders may originate from lymphoid tissues as in lymphomas, or the bone marrow, as in leukemia and multiple myeloma. These disorders can present with a myriad of kidney manifestations ranging from pre-renal to obstructive to intrarenal, the latter of which can include glomerular, tubular and tubulointerstitial injuries. Leukemias, lymphomas, and even benign clonal disorders may present with infiltrative kidney lesions alone or in combination with other kidney-related manifestations. As evidenced by their higher incidence on autopsy, these infiltrates are usually silent and may only be detected when the disease is

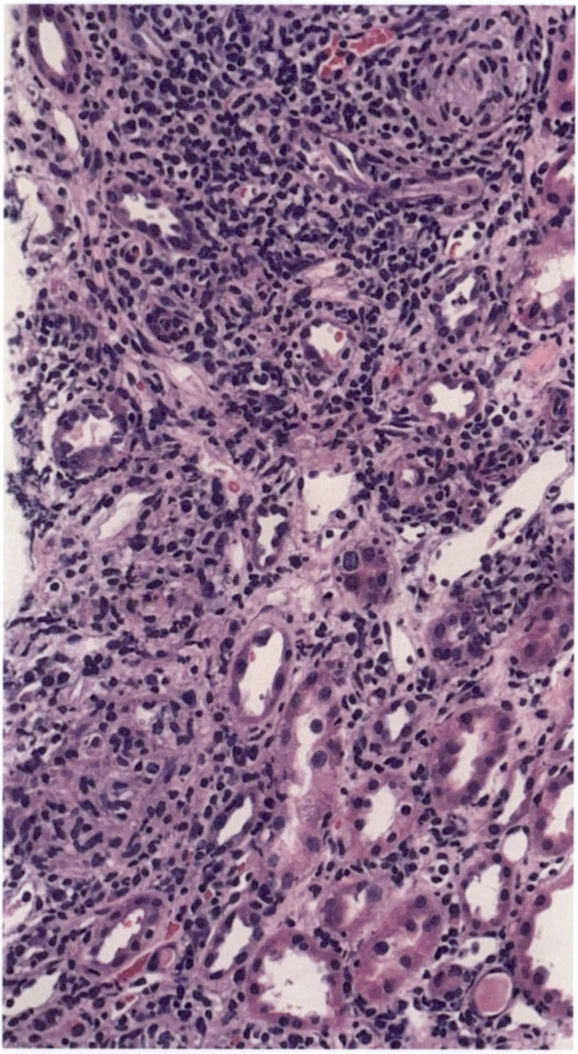

Fig. 1 Kidney biopsy from a patient with acute interstitial nephritis. 160× light microscopy image stained with hematoxylin and eosin showing extensive interstitial inflammation and renal tubular compression

advanced. Clinically significant infiltrative diseases are even more rare. AKI is believed to occur as a result of increased interstitial pressure leading to reduced renal blood flow and tubular injury. Symptoms include abdominal or flank pain from the enlarged kidneys and hypertension, and urine analysis may reveal hematuria and often mild sub-nephrotic proteinuria. Computed tomography (CT) scan is the preferred imaging modality which may show solitary lesions, perirenal lesions and/or direct invasion from contiguous retroperitoneal disease where the lesions would show as areas of decreased enhancement. However, imaging is nondiagnostic as it often misses histologically evident lesions. Once pre-renal and obstructive etiologies are excluded, kidney biopsy is absolutely essential in making an accurate diagnosis for persistent AKI as the management will differ based on the type of lesion. Immunohistochemistry is a helpful diagnostic tool in identifying the infiltrative cell type and guiding therapy.

2.1 *Lymphomatous Infiltrates*

Since the first cases of lymphomatous infiltrates on 9 autopsies presented to the Pathological Society of London by Sutton and Turner in 1878, several reports have come out showing kidneys as the most common site of involvement in extranodal metastatic lymphoma, with an incidence of 6–60% in autopsy reports. Infiltration of the kidneys has been reported on autopsy in up to 50% of patients with non-Hodgkin lymphoma (NHL) and in one in three patients in the case of diffuse large B cell lymphoma. AKI can rarely be the initial presenting symptom of non-Hodgkin lymphoma. Primary renal lymphoma isolated to the parenchyma on the other hand is highly uncommon, accounting for <1% of cases of extranodal lymphoma. Imaging may show bilateral symmetric kidney enlargement. However, imaging finding is only reported in 3–8% of patients with lymphoma as opposed to the high frequency seen on autopsy which highlights not only the poor correlation between imaging and histologic findings but also that infiltration is clinically silent in most cases. Kidney biopsy may be required to distinguish lymphomatous infiltration from non-neoplastic infiltration caused by medications or infections. In disease due to lymphoma, biopsy will demonstrate a dense interstitial infiltrate with a predominance of lymphocytes (Fig. 2). Prognostically, AKI associated with infiltration of aggressive NHL is often highly responsive to tumor directed therapy but kidney function recovery does not necessarily correlate with overall disease remission or disease-free survival.

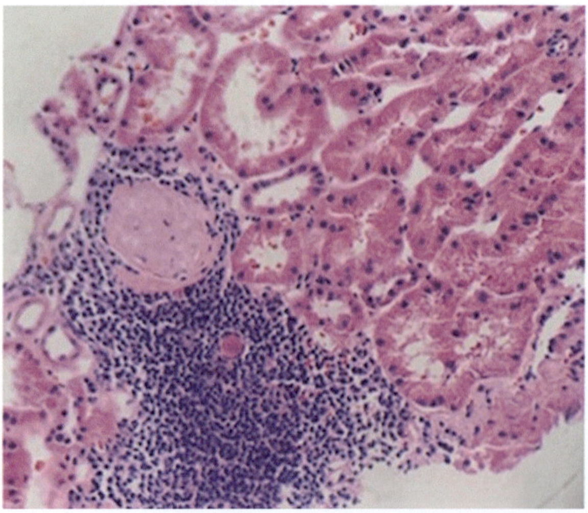

Fig. 2 160× light microscopy image from a kidney biopsy stained with hematoxylin and eosin from a patient with Non-Hodgkin's Lymphoma. Biopsy shows focal lymphocytic infiltration

2.2 Lymphoplasmacytic Lymphomas

Lymphoplasmacytic lymphomas are rare indolent Non Hodgkin Lymphoma which are a variable mixture of three types of cells (B cells, plasmacytoid lymphocytes, and plasma cells), the majority of which are Waldenstrom's macroglobulinemia occurring in 3–4 cases per million per year. In a French cohort of 35 patients with IgM monoclonal gammopathy, interstitial infiltration with B cells was the most common manifestation in 51% of the patients. This may be the only systemic manifestation of the disease in some cases and in 15% of cases, it represented an indication for treatment in what was thought to be an otherwise indolent Waldenstrom's macroglobulinemia.

Waldenstrom's macroglobulinemia, which is rare with an incidence of 2% of hematologic malignancies, has diverse kidney manifestations. It is an IgM associated B cell lymphoproliferative disorder characterized by the presence of an IgM monoclonal protein >1 g/dl with 10% lymphoplasmacytic infiltrate in the bone marrow. Diffuse infiltration by clonal B-cells has been reported in about 74% of patients with Waldenstrom's macroglobulinemia that have tubulointerstitial manifestation. Of 1363 patients with IgM-secreting B cell lymphoproliferative disorders including Waldenström macroglobulinemia evaluated at the Mayo Clinic between 1996 and 2015, 57 had both bone marrow and kidney biopsies of which 14% ($n = 8$) had tubulointerstitial nephritis. Lymphomatous infiltrate alone was the most common tubulointerstitial lesion in 4% of all lesions, the rest being light-chain cast nephropathy ($n = 2$), one with both light-chain cast nephropathy and lymphoma infiltration, and one with lymphoma infiltration along with ANCA-associated glomerulonephritis.

2.3 Leukemic Infiltrates

Leukemic tubulointerstitial infiltration is commonly reported in literature. The prevalence of kidney infiltration by leukemic cells in CLL has been reported in 63 to 90% of autopsy reports but similar to lymphomatous infiltrative disease, AKI as a result of leukemic infiltration is rare. In a study of 668 consecutive patients with lymphoproliferative disease, bilateral kidney enlargement was the most common imaging finding. Biopsy will reveal extent of infiltration and fibrosis, both of which can influence prognosis (Fig. 3a). Biopsy can also reveal leukemic subtypes that may alter treatment (Fig. 3b).

2.4 Plasma Cell Dyscrasia Associated Infiltrative Diseases

Multiple myeloma is the hematologic malignancy that is most commonly associated with direct tumor related kidney injury. AKI secondary to cast nephropathy is the most common manifestation and considered a myeloma defining event. An

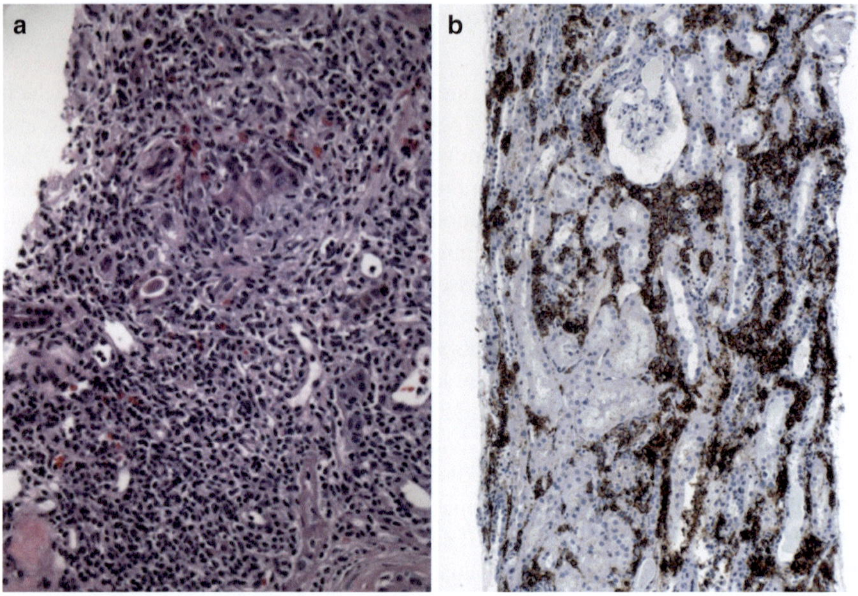

Fig. 3 Kidney biopsy from a patient with chronic lymphocytic leukemia. (**a**) 160× light microscopy image of kidney biopsy specimen stained with hematoxylin and eosin showing extensive interstitial inflammation and renal tubule compression. (**b**) 160× light microscopy image of kidney biopsy specimen stained with anti-CD3 T-cell marker showing a significant infiltrate of CD3 positive T-cells

extremely rare presentation of multiple myeloma is interstitial infiltration by plasma cells and has been reported in up to 3.8% of autopsy findings of patients with multiple myeloma. Infiltrating plasma cells are diagnosed by IHC staining for CD138. It may present along with other more common myeloma manifestations such as light chain cast nephropathy, monoclonal immunoglobulin deposition disease, and nodular glomerulosclerosis.

Crystal storing histiocytosis (also known as pseudo-Gaucher cells) is another rare manifestation of dysproteinemias that presents with infiltration of the bone marrow or other organs by histiocytes containing eosinophilic, lysosomal immunoglobulinemic crystalline inclusions, which can also infiltrate the tubulointerstitium of the kidneys.

2.5 *Immunodeficiency Related Lymphoproliferative Disorders of the Kidney*

Immunodeficiency related lymphoproliferative disorders are seen with prior EBV, CMV or HHV8 infection in those with HIV or in individuals who are on immunosuppression post-transplant. Post-transplant lymphoproliferative disorder (PTLD) has been reported in about 1–5% of kidney transplant patients of which 50–80% are associated with EBV infection. Kidney transplant patients overall have the lowest risk of PTLD compared to other solid organ transplants. EBV negative recipients who receive an EBV positive organ have a 10–75-fold risk of PTLD than EBV seropositive recipients. The risk is highest in the early post-transplant period (<2 years) but continues for approximately 10–14 years out from transplant. Immunosuppression with tacrolimus and cyclosporin are believed to increase the likelihood of PTLD due to impaired apoptosis of infected cells. Patients may be asymptomatic or present with B-symptoms such as weight loss, fatigue, night sweats and fevers. It is treated with reduction of immunosuppression along with chemotherapy plus rituximab in some cases.

3 Solid Cancers

The most common presentation of solid malignancies in the kidney is as focal space occupying lesions that are well circumscribed and distort the kidney architecture. Rarely, solid cancers can also present as infiltrative lesions that respect the architecture of the kidney. Renal cell carcinoma, urothelial carcinoma, and primary renal sarcomas can all present as infiltrative lesions. Metastases to the kidneys manifesting as infiltrative lesions are very rare. Radiographically on CT scan, they can be identified as poorly circumscribed lesions that are poorly enhancing during the venous phase compared to the normal renal parenchyma.

3.1 Renal Cell Carcinoma

Renal cell carcinomas (RCC) are a group of cancers that originate from renal tubular epithelial cells. They are adenocarcinomas that arise from the cortex and constitute about 3% of all cancers and 90% of all cancers of the renal parenchyma. The majority of RCC present as focal lesions except for about 6%, which present as infiltrating lesions (Fig. 4). However, because they are relatively more common than the other kidney cancers, they still constitute a significant proportion of infiltrative cancers. There are over 15 subtypes of RCC according to the newest 2016 WHO classification of urogenital cancers of which ~75–80% are clear cell type, ~15% are papillary, and chromophobe RCCs make about 5%. An RCC of any subtype can present with the high-grade transformation type, which is an RCC with sarcomatous features. This has an incidence of about 8% and can present with infiltrating lesions. On H&E, sarcomatous RCC presents as densely packed spindle-shaped cells with a high nuclear to cytoplasmic (N/C) ratio and often has areas of fibrosis and necrosis.

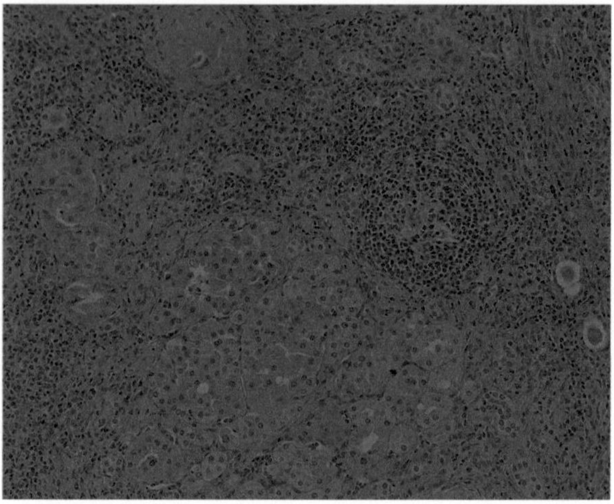

Fig. 4 Kidney biopsy from a patient with renal papillary carcinoma. 160× light microscopy image of kidney biopsy specimen stained with hematoxylin and eosin showing well-circumscribed area of neoplasm with adjacent interstitial inflammation

3.2 Urothelial Carcinomas

Urothelial carcinomas make up about 10% of all upper urinary tract neoplasms and can involve the renal pelvis or the infundibulum. About 90% are transitional cell carcinomas, 9% are squamous cell carcinomas and 1% are mucinous. They can be confused with infiltrating RCC when it extends out from the pelvis invading the renal parenchyma (Fig. 5).

3.3 Primary Renal Sarcoma

Primary renal sarcomas originate from mesenchymal cells and are the most rare of the three making up about 1% of all parenchymal neoplasms of the kidneys. There are several subtypes of primary renal sarcoma including leiomyosarcoma, which is the most common subtype, as well as rhabdomyosarcoma, angiosarcoma, hemangiosarcoma, fibrosarcoma and osteosarcoma. Of these subtypes, rhabdomyosarcoma and angiosarcoma can present as infiltrative lesions.

3.4 Metastases to the Kidneys

Metastases to the kidneys are found in 7–13% of autopsies of patients with cancer. The most common primary malignancy to metastasize to the kidney is bronchogenic carcinoma, followed by breast cancer, and gastrointestinal malignancies. These tend to be indolent and are usually noted on surveillance imaging where they appear as multiple bilateral discrete lesions. They commonly present as expansile or

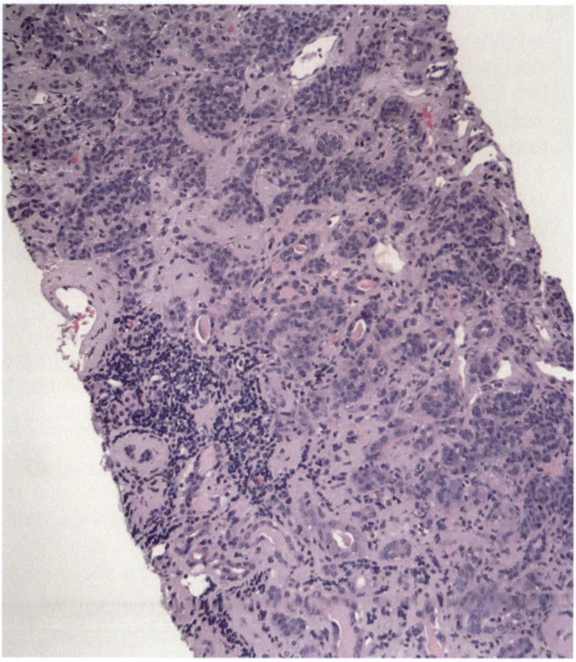

Fig. 5 Kidney biopsy from a patient with metastatic urothelial cancer. 160× light microscopy image of kidney biopsy specimen stained with hematoxylin and eosin showing areas of urothelial cell infiltration with focal and adjacent interstitial inflammation

exophytic mass rather than infiltrative and can pose a diagnostic challenge if solitary as they may be confused as a separate primary renal tumor.

3.5 Pediatric Kidney Tumors

The most common pediatric kidney tumor is Wilm's tumor, which often presents as discrete expansile lesion but can also present as infiltrative lesion. Other primary kidney tumors of childhood include the benign mesoblastic nephroma which occurs in the first 3 months of life, the rarest and most aggressive rhabdoid tumor, diffuse-type nephroblastomatosis that may become Wilm's tumor, and primitive neuroectodermal tumor (PNET) which is seen in older children and young adults, all characteristically present as infiltrative lesions.

Suggested Reading

Agarwal G, Mannon RB. Post-transplant lymphoproliferative disorder in a kidney transplant recipient. Clin J Am Soc Nephrol. 2019;14(5):751–3. https://doi.org/10.2215/CJN.00180119.

Ambos M, Bosniak M, Madayag M, Lefleur R. Infiltrating neoplasms of the kidney. Am J Roentgenol. 1977;129(5):859–64. https://doi.org/10.2214/ajr.129.5.859.

Bach AG, Behrmann C, Holzhausen HJ, et al. Prevalence and patterns of renal involvement in imaging of malignant lymphoproliferative diseases. Acta Radiol. 2012;53(3):343–8. https://doi.org/10.1258/ar.2011.110523.

Baldus M, Klooker P, Kress S, Waldherr R, Mollwe P, Brass H. Primary bilateral renal centrocytic non-Hodgkin's lymphoma as a cause of renal failure. Nephron. 1996;73(1):86–90.

Ballard DH, De Alba L, Migliaro M, Previgliano CH, Sangster GP. CT imaging spectrum of infiltrative renal diseases. Abdom Radiol (NY). 2017;42(11):2700–9. https://doi.org/10.1007/s00261-017-1193-5.

Campbell GA, Hu D, Okusa MD. Acute kidney injury in the cancer patient. Adv Chronic Kidney Dis. 2014;21(1):64–71. https://doi.org/10.1053/j.ackd.2013.08.002.

Canet E, Zafrani L, Lambert J, et al. Acute kidney injury in patients with newly diagnosed high-grade hematological malignancies: impact on remission and survival. Glod JW, ed. PLoS One. 2013;8(2):e55870. https://doi.org/10.1371/journal.pone.0055870.

Chauvet S, Bridoux F, Ecotière L, et al. Kidney diseases associated with monoclonal immunoglobulin M–secreting B-cell lymphoproliferative disorders: a case series of 35 patients. Am J Kidney Dis. 2015;66(5):756–67. https://doi.org/10.1053/j.ajkd.2015.03.035.

Coggins CH. Renal failure in lymphoma. Kidney Int. 1980;17(6):847–55. https://doi.org/10.1038/ki.1980.97.

Dharnidharka VR, Webster AC, Martinez OM, Preiksaitis JK, Leblond V, Choquet S. Post-transplant lymphoproliferative disorders. Nat Rev Dis Primer. 2016;2(1):15088. https://doi.org/10.1038/nrdp.2015.88.

El Hamel C, Thierry A, Trouillas P, et al. Crystal-storing histiocytosis with renal Fanconi syndrome: pathological and molecular characteristics compared with classical myeloma-associated Fanconi syndrome. Nephrol Dial Transplant. 2010;25(9):2982–90. https://doi.org/10.1093/ndt/gfq129.

Hanawa S, Akimoto T, Uehara E, et al. Renal failure caused by plasma cell infiltration in multiple myeloma. Clin Exp Nephrol. 2011;15(4):586–90. https://doi.org/10.1007/s10157-011-0437-x.

Herrera GA, Joseph L, Gu X, Hough A, Barlogie B. Renal pathologic spectrum in an autopsy series of patients with plasma cell dyscrasia. Arch Pathol Lab Med. 2004;128(8):875–9. https://doi.org/10.1043/1543-2165(2004)128<875:RPSIAA>2.0.CO;2.

Higgins L, Nasr SH, Said SM, et al. Kidney involvement of patients with Waldenström macroglobulinemia and other IgM-producing B cell lymphoproliferative disorders. Clin J Am Soc Nephrol. 2018;13(7):1037–46. https://doi.org/10.2215/CJN.13041117.

Kapoor P, Ansell SM, Fonseca R, et al. Diagnosis and management of Waldenström macroglobulinemia: mayo stratification of macroglobulinemia and risk-adapted therapy (mSMART) guidelines 2016. JAMA Oncol. 2017;3(9):1257. https://doi.org/10.1001/jamaoncol.2016.5763.

Kaur T, Krishnaprasad S, Shankar R, Kumar R, Gowrishankar S, Padua MD. Plasma cell infiltration of the kidney as a manifestation of myeloma: a report of three cases. Indian J Nephrol. 2017;27(5):395–8. https://doi.org/10.4103/ijn.IJN_215_16.

Luciano RL, Brewster UC. Kidney involvement in leukemia and lymphoma. Adv Chronic Kidney Dis. 2014;21(1):27–35. https://doi.org/10.1053/j.ackd.2013.07.004.

Mills NE, Goldenberg AS, Liu D, et al. B-cell lymphoma presenting as infiltrative renal disease. Am J Kidney Dis. 1992;19(2):181–4. https://doi.org/10.1016/S0272-6386(12)70131-2.

Moch H, Cubilla AL, Humphrey PA, Reuter VE, Ulbright TM. The 2016 WHO classification of tumours of the urinary system and male genital organs—part a: renal, penile, and testicular tumours. Eur Urol. 2016;70(1):93–105. https://doi.org/10.1016/j.eururo.2016.02.029.

Monfared A, Orangpoor R, Fakheri T, Falahatkar S. Acute renal failure and bilateral kidney infiltration as the first presentation of non-Hodgkin lymphoma. Iran J Kidney Dis. 2009;3(1):4.

Morel P, Dupriez B, et al. Aggressive lymphomas with renal involvement: a study of 48 patients treated with the LNH-84 and LNH-87 regimens. Groupe d'Etude des Lymphomes de l'Adulte. Br J Cancer. 1994;70(1):154–9. https://doi.org/10.1038/bjc.1994.267.

Obrador GT, Price B, O'Meara Y, Salant DJ. Acute renal failure due to lymphomatous infiltration of the kidneys. J Am Soc Nephrol. 1997;8(8):1348–54. https://doi.org/10.1681/ASN.V881348.

Okubo T, Hirashio S, Shimizu M, Kuroda Y, Doi S, Masaki T. Diffuse large B-cell lymphoma presenting as bilateral renal infiltration leading to acute kidney injury. CEN Case Rep. 2017;6(2):140–7. https://doi.org/10.1007/s13730-017-0261-6.

Pickhardt PJ, Lonergan GJ, Davis CJ, Kashitani N, Wagner BJ. From the archives of the AFIP: infiltrative renal lesions: radiologic-pathologic correlation. Radiographics. 2000;20(1):215–43. https://doi.org/10.1148/radiographics.20.1.g00ja08215.

Richmond J, Sherman RS, Diamond HD, Craver LF. Renal lesions associated with malignant lymphomas. Am J Med. 1962;32(2):184–207. https://doi.org/10.1016/0002-9343(62)90289-9.

Sakhuja V, Jha V, Varma S, et al. Renal involvement in multiple myeloma: a 10-year study. Ren Fail. 2000;22(4):465–77. https://doi.org/10.1081/jdi-100100888.

Sheth S, Ali S, Fishman E. Imaging of renal lymphoma: patterns of disease with pathologic correlation. Radiographics. 2006;26(4):1151–68. https://doi.org/10.1148/rg.264055125.

Stallone G, Infante B, Manno C, Campobasso N, Pannarale G, Schena FP. Primary renal lymphoma does exist: case report and review of the literature. J Nephrol. 2000;13(5):367–72.

Törnroth T, Heiro M, Marcussen N, Franssila K. Lymphomas diagnosed by percutaneous kidney biopsy. Am J Kidney Dis. 2003;42(5):960–71. https://doi.org/10.1016/j.ajkd.2003.08.004.

Uppal NN, Monga D, Vernace MA, et al. Kidney diseases associated with Waldenström macroglobulinemia. Nephrol Dial Transplant. 2019;34(10):1644–52. https://doi.org/10.1093/ndt/gfy320.

Uprety D, Peterson A, Shah BK. Renal failure secondary to leukemic infiltration of kidneys in CLL—a case report and review of literature. Ann Hematol. 2013;92(2):271–3. https://doi.org/10.1007/s00277-012-1547-6.

Wang W, Lin P. Lymphoplasmacytic lymphoma and Waldenström macroglobulinaemia: clinicopathological features and differential diagnosis. Pathology (Phila). 2020;52(1):6–14. https://doi.org/10.1016/j.pathol.2019.09.009.

Part V
Diagnosis

Clinical Features and Laboratory Findings in Acute Tubulointerstitial Nephritis

Ravi Kodali and Dennis G. Moledina

1 Introduction

Acute tubulointerstitial nephritis (ATIN) is a histological diagnosis characterized by the presence of mononuclear infiltrate in the renal interstitium, which is often accompanied by tubulitis and interstitial eosinophils. There are numerous causes of ATIN including medications, infections, and autoimmune diseases (Table 1). In a majority of patients, ATIN is triggered by various medication classes, which are associated with varying clinical presentations. ATIN can also occur in association of various autoimmune diseases with characteristic features consistent with the underlying disease. Clinical care of patients with ATIN is challenging due to its uncharacteristic and often atypical presentation in many patients. This is particularly true for drug-induced ATIN where most patients do not manifest allergic symptoms, signs or laboratory findings. Here we will review the accuracy of conventional and novel clinical tests for ATIN.

R. Kodali
Section of Nephrology, Department of Internal Medicine, Yale School of Medicine, New Haven, CT, USA
e-mail: ravi.kodali@yale.edu

D. G. Moledina (✉)
Section of Nephrology, Department of Internal Medicine, Yale School of Medicine, New Haven, CT, USA

Clincal and Translational Research Accelerator, Department of Internal Medicine, Yale School of Medicine, New Haven, CT, USA
e-mail: dennis.moledina@yale.edu

M. G. Atta, M. A. Perazella (eds.), *Tubulointerstitial Nephritis*,
https://doi.org/10.1007/978-3-030-93438-5_19

Table 1 Typical features of drug and autoimmune causes of acute tubulointerstitial nephritis

Etiology of ATIN	Clinical and laboratory features	Typical histopathologic features
Drug-induced	**Most common etiology (70% in developed countries)**	**Mixed inflammatory cell infiltrate with eosinophils +/−granuloma**
Proton pump inhibitors and H2-blockers	Few typical clinical features; long latent period (weeks to months)	Mononuclear infiltrate: plasma cells, T-lymphocytes
Non-steroidal anti-inflammatory drugs	Multitude of kidney manifestations: Reversible pre-renal azotemia, ATN, hyperkalemia; ATIN is often associated with massive proteinuria; long latent period; rarely present with typical allergic manifestations	Interstitial eosinophilia may be absent. Glomerular lesions of minimal change disease and membranous sometimes present
Beta-lactams (Penicillin and its derivatives, cephalosporins); Sulfonamides	More likely to present with systemic allergic manifestations of rash, eosinophilia, and fever (particularly with methicillin and penicillin); short latent period (days)	Interstitial eosinophilia is common and sometimes granuloma is present
Immune checkpoint inhibitors (PD-1, CTLA4, PD-L1 inhibitors)	Extra-renal immune-related adverse effects in 40–50%, poor sensitivity and specificity of serum and urine tests; long latent period (weeks-months)	Mononuclear infiltrate: plasma cells, T-lymphocytes, eosinophils and sometimes granuloma are present
Immune-mediated diseases	**More common in younger individuals**	**Mononuclear cell infiltration +/−granuloma**
SLE nephritis	Systemic features of SLE. Hematuria, proteinuria, pyuria, white cell casts and AKI. Positive SLE serologies, evidence of complement activation	Usually seen with other kidney manifestations of SLE: focal or diffuse proliferative GN with "full house" IF staining. Rarely seen without glomerular disease
Sarcoidosis	Hypercalcemia, normocalcemic hypercalciuria, concentrating defects, nephrocalcinosis/ nephrolithiasis, and CKD	Focal lymphocytic infiltrate and interstitial noncaseating granulomas composed of giant cells, histiocytes, and lymphocytes
Sjögren's syndrome	Characterized by dry eyes and mouth. Serologies often positive	Lymphoplasmocytic infiltrate
IgG4-related disease	Systemic disorder with elevated serum IgG4 level involving salivary glands, pancreas, retroperitoneum and kidneys. Affects middle aged men	Lymphoplasmocytic interstitial infiltrate with a predominance of IgG4 positive plasma cells and interstitial fibrosis in a "storiform" pattern
Tubulointerstitial nephritis and uveitis syndrome (TINU)	Uveitis: painful red eyes, photophobia; renal failure; common in young women	Mixed inflammatory infiltrate with granuloma formation

Abbreviations: *ATIN* acute tubulointerstitial nephritis, *ATN* acute tubular necrosis, *AKI* acute kidney injury, *CKD* chronic kidney disease, *GN* glomerulonephritis, *SLE* systemic lupus erythematosus, *PD-1* programmed death-1, *CTLA-4* cytotoxic T-lymphocyte associated protein-4, *PD-L1* programmed death ligand-1, *IF* immunofluorescence

2 Clinical Features

Most patients with ATIN are asymptomatic and are identified due to evidence of kidney dysfunction (rise in serum creatinine concentration). Therefore it is important to maintain a high index of suspicion for ATIN as it may be overlooked. Clinical history can often give clues to the possibility and etiology of ATIN. In all patients with loss of kidney function, it is important to obtain a detailed history focused on recent prescription and over-the-counter medication exposures. Common drugs implicated in ATIN include antibiotics, proton pump inhibitors (PPIs), non-steroidal anti-inflammatory drugs (NSAIDs), and immune checkpoint inhibitors. Any recent exposure to these drugs should raise suspicion for ATIN. The time from drug initiation to development of ATIN can vary from a few days for antibiotics to weeks for NSAIDs and immune checkpoint inhibitors to months for PPIs.

Specific symptoms and signs of ATIN can include fever and rash but only about 5–10% of patients have the classic "triad" of fever, skin rash, and eosinophilia. The rash is typically described as morbilliform and involves the trunk. Skin rash is reported in 15–50% of cases of ATIN in various studies and is most common with β-lactam antibiotics. Allergic features are more common in patients with β-lactams or sulfa drugs-related ATIN but absent in those with PPI-related and NSAID-associated ATIN. Some patients can present with symptoms associated with progressive kidney dysfunction such as nausea, vomiting, malaise, or weakness due to accompanying anemia. Only about half of the patients have oliguria.

ATIN can also occur due to autoimmune conditions such as Sjogren's syndrome, sarcoidosis, IgG4-related disease, SLE, or other forms of vasculitis. In these cases, patients may have systemic symptoms specific to the autoimmune disease, such as sicca symptoms (dry eyes and/ dry mouth) in patients with Sjogren's syndrome; pulmonary manifestations such as cough in sarcoidosis; and symptoms of pancreatitis and obstructive uropathy in IgG4-related disease. Patients with drug rash (Fig. 1) with eosinophilia and systemic symptoms (DRESS) associated ATIN will typically have skin rash associated with other extra-renal manifestations. In tubulointerstitial nephritis with uveitis (TINU), uveitis presents with painful red eye with photophobia and can precede the onset of ATIN by several weeks to months.

3 Serum Tests

While there are no specific serum tests that can confirm the diagnosis of ATIN, some tests can offer a clue.

Serum Creatinine

The initial presentation for most patients with ATIN is an incidental finding of rise in serum creatinine often accompanied by abnormalities on urinalysis. The decline in glomerular filtration rate (GFR) in patients with ATIN can be acute to sub-acute. Rapid decline in GFR satisfying KDIGO acute kidney injury (AKI) definition

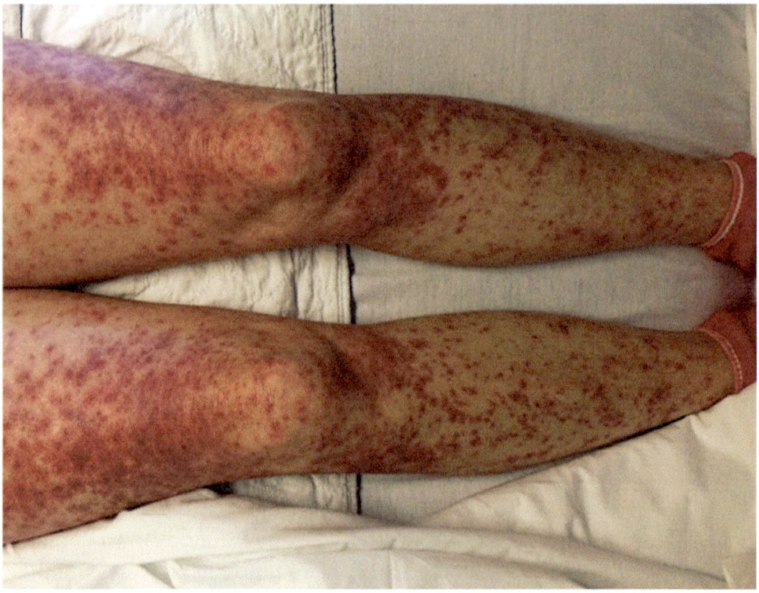

Fig. 1 Severe erythematous rash in a patient with DRESS. The culprit medication causing this skin reaction was vancomycin

criteria is seen in about half of ATIN cases, with the rest consistent with acute kidney disease. Given the subacute decline in GFR with ATIN, the diagnosis can be delayed leading to fibrosis and development of CKD.

Blood Eosinophil Testing
Peripheral eosinophilia can be present in 20–25% of cases of ATIN. Eosinophilia (along with skin rash) is more common in patients with antibiotic-associated ATIN than in those with ATIN from PPIs and NSAIDs. When present, this can offer an additional clue in diagnosis of ATIN, especially that associated with antibiotics. However, peripheral eosinophilia is not a specific marker of ATIN. It can also be seen in other conditions that can also result in AKI including atheroembolic disease, vasculitis, malignancies, and parasite infections.

C-Reactive Protein (CRP) and Erythrocyte Sedimentation Rate (ESR)
ESR and CRP are markers of inflammation and could theoretically be used to differentiate ATIN from other causes of AKI. However, these markers are non-specific and are elevated in a wide variety of conditions including infections, vasculitis, trauma, infarction, and malignancies. Moreover, these markers have not been systematically been evaluated in ATIN. Small, uncontrolled studies have show that ESR and CRP are elevated in ATIN and correlated with higher degrees of interstitial inflammation and lower degree of fibrosis on histology. Thus, further research is needed to determine if these clinically available tests can differentiate between ATIN and other causes of AKI.

4 Urine Findings

A summary of urinary abnormalities in patients with ATIN is noted in Table 2.

Urinalysis
Urinalysis is an essential test for workup of patients with kidney dysfunction. Urinalysis abnormalities are often noted in patients with ATIN. While many of these changes are neither sensitive nor specific for diagnosis of ATIN, they provide clues to rule out other causes of AKI. Notably, as many as 20% of patients with ATIN can have a "normal" or "bland" urinalysis.

Pyuria
The presence of white blood cells (WBCs) in the urine, particularly in the absence of a urinary traction infection i.e., sterile pyuria, should raise suspicion for ATIN. However, pyuria can be seen in conditions other than ATIN such as glomerulonephritis, pyelonephritis, and papillary necrosis. Moreover, pyuria may be absent in as many as 40% of patients with biopsy-proven ATIN.

Proteinuria
ATIN is accompanied by tubular injury, and its related urinary abnormalities may be seen with ATIN. For example, some degree of tubular proteinuria, often described as <1 g/day, is commonly present in ATIN. Almost 90% of patients with ATIN have at least low grade proteinuria (0.3 g or higher). . Nephrotic range proteinuria is generally not seen except with NSAID-associated ATIN, where concomitant glomerular lesions are often seen.

Hematuria
Microscopic hematuria is common in patients with ATIN and is reported in almost half of the cases. While the presence of RBC casts is generally considered to be pathognomonic of glomerular origin of disease, some studies have reported RBC casts even in patients with ATIN. The mechanism or reproducibility of this finding remains unclear, however, the erythrocyte casts may develop due to the leak of RBCs from the inflamed/injured interstitium into the tubular lumens.

Urinary Casts
WBC casts (Fig. 2) are thought to be more specific for diagnosis of ATIN than pyuria albeit with low sensitivity. Proliferative glomerulonephritis can have WBC

Table 2 Summary of urine abnormalities in acute tubulointerstitial nephritis

Urinalysis	Often abnormal, but can be normal in as many as 20% of cases of ATIN
Urine WBCs	About 50–60% of patients and WBC casts can be indicative of ATIN, but low sensitivity
Urine eosinophils	Neither sensitive, nor specific for diagnosis of ATIN; generally not recommended
Urine protein	Present in 90% of cases; usually <1 g/day
Hematuria	Is often present but not specific

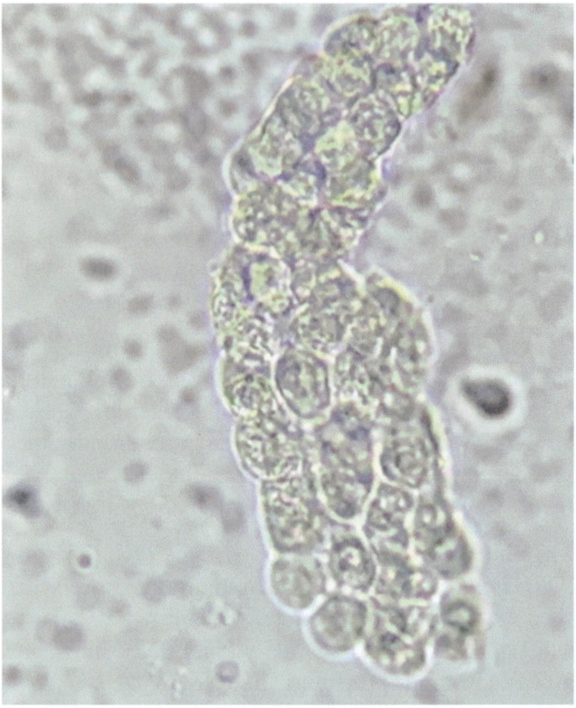

Fig. 2 White blood cell cast. A patient with piperacillin-tazobactam-related ATIN had sterile pyuria and WBC casts present in the urine sediment

casts, but they are often accompanied by dysmorphic RBCs and sometimes RBC casts. In a study of ATIN patients with carefully examined urine sediments, only 14% had WBC casts. Since tubular injury often occurs with ATIN, granular casts and renal tubular epithelial cells and casts can also be seen in patients with ATIN.

Eosinophiluria

Given the diagnostic utility of eosinophils in the kidney tubulointerstitium noted in ATIN, the presence of urine eosinophils has long been considered a non-invasive biomarker for ATIN. The use of eosinophiluria as a marker for ATIN was based on several studies in the late 1980's showing the test's association with ATIN. However, the findings of these studies were disputed due to two main limitations; first, many patients in these studies did not undergo kidney biopsy to confirm the diagnosis, which could have led to misclassification of the diagnosis; and second, the studies overrepresented ATIN due to antibiotics, which tend to have far greater number of interstitial eosinophils on biopsy than other causes of ATIN. A more recent retrospective study by Muriithi et al., showed lower accuracy of urine eosinophils in a large cohort of patients with biopsy-proven ATIN and controls. Urine eosinophils (both at 1% and 5% cutoff thresholds) were present across all diagnoses of AKI (such as ATN, glomerulonephritis, diabetic nephropathy, and others). Furthermore, at 1% cutoff, sensitivity of urine eosinophils was 31% while specificity was 68%. At a higher cutoff of 5%, sensitivity was only 20%, while specificity increased to 91%. One major limitation of this study is that it might have missed patients who did not undergo a biopsy based on the results of their urine eosinophil results; for example, a very high level of urine eosinophils in those with suggestive clinical scenario may be have been managed without a biopsy and not included in this study. Despite this limitation, this study suggests that urine eosinophils may not be helpful in most clinical scenarios where the diagnosis is unclear and a biopsy is being considered.

5 Imaging Tests

Imaging studies (also see Chapter "Imaging Modalities for Acute Tubulointerstitial Nephritis") such as renal ultrasound and computed tomography (CT) of abdomen are often obtained in patients with AKI to rule out urinary tract obstruction, but do not show any typical features of ATIN. However, these tests can reveal associated conditions such as retroperitoneal fibrosis in IgG4 related disease.

Gallium-67 is used as a radiotracer to detect inflammation as it has affinity to certain inflammatory proteins such as lactoferrin and may be able to detect kidney inflammation occurring in patients with ATIN. After injection with gallium-67, images with gamma camera are obtained to identify the pooling of this tracer thereby identifying sites of infection or inflammation. Given inflammation is restricted mostly to the kidneys in ATIN, an increased uptake of the tracer restricted to the kidneys could indicate ATIN. However, studies have shown widely differing accuracies of this test for ATIN diagnosis. A recent retrospective study showed that Gallium scan had an AUC of 0.75 for ATIN diagnosis. However, this was a single center study and many patients did not have biopsy confirmation of the diagnosis. Thus, further prospective evaluation is needed to determine the clinical utility of gallium scintigraphy scan and other imaging studies in ATIN.

6 Novel Serum and Urine Biomarkers

Given the lack of a reliable non-invasive biomarker and need to obtain a kidney biopsy, several studies have attempted to identify a diagnostic biomarker for ATIN. Finding a biomarker that can detect ATIN with high sensitivity and specificity is important in certain cases where biopsy could be potentially risky due to high bleeding risks such as in patients with severe thrombocytopenia or AKI.

Urine Tumor Necrosis Factor (TNF)-α and Interleukin (IL)-9

In a study by Moledina et al., 265 patients who underwent kidney biopsy for loss of kidney function were evaluated. Three pathologists identified presence or absence of ATIN. Twelve urinary and ten plasma cytokines involved in CD4+ T cells (thought to be predominant mediators of pathogenesis in ATIN) as well as general inflammatory mediators were studied. Of the biomarkers studied, two urine cytokines, urine interleukin (IL)-9 and tumor necrosis factor (TNF)-α were independently associated with ATIN. None of the ten plasma cytokines were different between ATIN and other causes of AKI. When various causes of acute kidney disease (AKD) were compared, patients with ATIN had higher urine TNF-α and IL-9 compared to any other cause of AKD including glomerular lesions, acute tubular injury, diabetic kidney disease, or other causes of CKD. Both these biomarkers also correlated with histological degree of severity such as percentage of biopsy tissue with lymphocytic infiltration, tubulitis and number of eosinophils in interstitium per high power field. Addition of biomarker information to clinicians' pre-biopsy diagnosis of ATIN improved the AUC from 0.62 (0.53, 0.71) to 0.84 (0.78, 0.91) (Fig. 3). In addition, the performance of IL-9 at two different cutoff values was evaluated to understand its practical use. If a patient had a pre-test probability of 50% of having ATIN based on clinical information and is found to be positive for IL-9 at high specificity cut off which corresponds to top 15% of patients in the study, the post-test probability increased to 0.94. On the other hand, if the same patient tests negative for high sensitivity cutoff which corresponds to median of the cohort, the post-test probability reduced to 0.17. In both cases, kidney biopsy may be avoided.

Other Tests

In one of the first studies of ATIN biomarkers, Wu et al. studied a cohort of 40 patients with drug induced ATIN and 20 healthy controls. They found that urinary monocyte chemotactic protein (MCP)-1 and neutrophil gelatinase associated

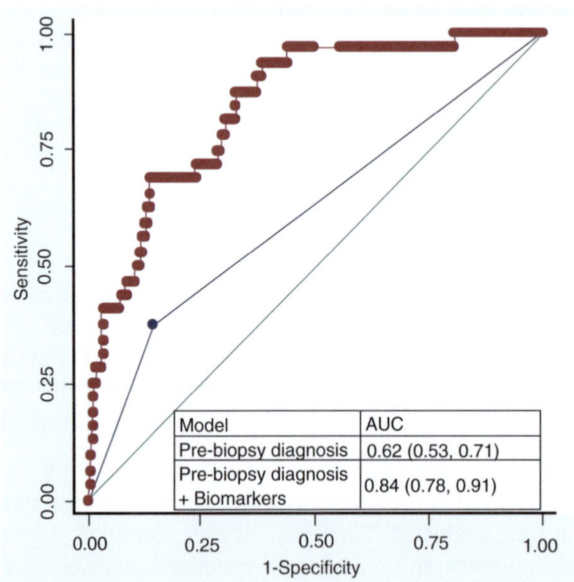

Fig. 3 Urine biomarkers impact on area under receiver operating characteristics (AUC) curve. The addition of urine biomarkers improved the AUC from 0.62 to 0.84 when added to clinicians' pre-biopsy diagnosis of ATIN

lipocalin (NGAL) levels were higher in patients with ATIN compared to controls. A subsequent study evaluated kidney injury molecule (KIM)-1 and complement factors (C5b-9) and found similar results. However, these studies either compared patients within various forms of ATIN (acute vs chronic or drug induced vs non-drug induced) or compared patients with ATIN to healthy controls. Since ATIN is often accompanied by acute tubular injury (ATI), it is not surprising that markers of ATI such as NGAL are elevated in ATIN as compared to healthy controls. However, in a patient with AKI, it is critical to differentiate between ATI and ATI, rather than ATIN from healthy controls limiting the real word applicability of these findings.

Sun et al. evaluated macrophages in the urine sediment to determine correlation with ATIN. Macrophages being important cells of inflammation are thought to play an active role in AKI. By determining the ratio of M1 (pro-inflammatory) macrophages to M2 (pro-reparative) macrophages in urine sediment, the authors found that a high M1/M2 ratio was significantly associated with ATIN. This ratio could differentiate ATIN from other causes of AKI. At a cutoff of M1/M2 ratio of more than 2.35, sensitivity was 98%, specificity was 100% with area under ROC of 0.99 for diagnosis of ATIN.

Lymphocyte transformation test (LTT) is a novel test is based on direct activation of lymphocytes in presence of culprit drug. One study showed that lymphocytes from peripheral blood from a small subset of patients with ATIN reacted in presence of culprit drug. However, the findings of this study have not been reproduced.

In conclusion, patients with ATIN come to clinical attention with loss of kidney function but without other specific symptoms or signs. To establish the diagnosis, the clinician must keep a high index of suspicion for this disease in all patients with acute or sub-acute loss of kidney function and piece together information from history as well as blood and urine testing. A kidney biopsy is often required to establish the diagnosis and characteristic kidney biopsy findings are described elsewhere in this textbook. Many novel tests are currently being evaluated and may be available for use in the near future.

Suggested Reading

Baker RJ, Pusey CD. The changing profile of acute tubulointerstitial nephritis. Nephrol Dial Transplant. 2004;19(1):8–11.

Buysen JGM, Houthoff HJ, Krediet RT, Arisz L. Acute interstitial nephritis: a clinical and morphological study in 27 patients. Nephrol Dial Transplant. 1990;5(2):94–9.

Clarkson MR, Giblin L, O'Connell FP, O'Kelly P, Walshe JJ, Conlon P, et al. Acute interstitial nephritis: clinical features and response to corticosteroid therapy. Nephrol Dial Transplant. 2004;19(11):2778–83.

Cortazar FB, Kibbelaar ZA, Glezerman IG, Abudayyeh A, Mamlouk O, Motwani SS, et al. Clinical features and outcomes of immune checkpoint inhibitor–associated AKI: a multicenter study. J Am Soc Nephrol. 2020;31(2):435–46.

Corwin HL, Bray RA, Haber MH. The detection and interpretation of urinary eosinophils. Arch Pathol Lab Med. 1989;113(11):1256–8.

Corwin HL, Korbet SM, Schwartz MM. Clinical correlates of eosinophiluria. Arch Intern Med. 1985;145(6):1097–9.
Davison AM, Jones CH. Acute interstitial nephritis in the elderly: a report from the UK MRC glomerulonephritis register and a review of the literature. Nephrol Dial Ttransplant. 1998;13(Suppl 7):12–6.
Farrington K, Levison DA, Greenwood RN, Cattell WR, Baker LRI. Renal biopsy in patients with unexplained renal impairment and normal kidney size. Q J Med. 1989;70(3):221–33.
Ferrari B, Fogazzi GB, Garigali G, Messa P. Acute interstitial nephritis after amoxycillin with hematuria, red blood cell casts and hematuriainduced acute tubular injury. Clin Nephrol. 2013;80(2):156–60.
Fogazzi GB, Ferrari B, Garigali G, Simonini P, Consonni D. Urinary sediment findings in acute interstitial nephritis. Am J Kidney Dis. 2012;60(2):330–2.
Goicoechea M, Rivera F, López-Gómez JM. Increased prevalence of acute tubulointerstitial nephritis. Nephrol Dial Transplant. 2013;28(1):112–5.
Graham GD, Lundy MM, Moreno AJ. Failure of gallium-67 scintigraphy to identify reliably noninfectious interstitial nephritis: concise communication. J Nucl Med. 1983;24(7):568–70.
Korbet SM, Gashti CN, Evans JK, Whittier WL. Risk of percutaneous renal biopsy of native kidneys in the evaluation of acute kidney injury. Clin Kidney J. 2018;11(5):610–5.
Linton AL, Richmond JM, Clark WF, Lindsay RM, Driedger AA, Lamki LM. Gallium67 scintigraphy in the diagnosis of acute renal disease. Clin Nephrol. 1985;24(2):84–7.
Moledina DG, Luciano RL, Kukova L, Chan L, Saha A, Nadkarni G, et al. Kidney biopsy-related complications in hospitalized patients with acute kidney disease. Clin J Am Soc Nephrol. 2018;13(11):1633–40.
Moledina DG, Wilson FP, Pober JS, Perazella MA, Singh N, Luciano RL, et al. Urine TNF-α and IL-9 for clinical diagnosis of acute interstitial nephritis. JCI Insight. 2019;4(10):e127456.
Muriithi AK, Leung N, Valeri AM, Cornell LD, Sethi S, Fidler ME, et al. Biopsy-proven acute interstitial nephritis, 1993-2011: a case series. Am J Kidney Dis. 2014;64(4):558–66.
Muriithi AK, Leung N, Valeri AM, Cornell LD, Sethi S, Fidler ME, et al. Clinical characteristics, causes and outcomes of acute interstitial nephritis in the elderly. Kidney Int. 2015;87(2):458–64.
Muriithi AK, Nasr SH, Leung N. Utility of urine eosinophils in the diagnosis of acute interstitial nephritis. Clin J Am Soc Nephrol. 2013;8(11):1857–62.
Nolan CR, Anger MS, Kelleher SP. Eosinophiluria — a new method of detection and definition of the clinical. Spectrum. 1986;315(24):1516–9.
Pusey CD, Saltissi D, Bloodworth L, Rainford DJ, Christie JL. Drug associated acute interstitial nephritis: clinical and pathological features and the response to high dose steroid therapy. Q J Med. 1983;52(2):194–211.
Ruffing KA, Hoppes P, Blend D, Cugino A, Jarjoura D, Whittier FC. Eosinophils in urine revisited. Clin Nephrol. 1994;41(3):163–6.
Shi Y, Su T, Qu L, Li X, Yang L, Wang C. Evaluation of urinary biomarkers for the prognosis of drug-associated chronic tubulointerstitial nephritis. Am J Med Sci. 2013;346(4):283–8.
Simpson IJ, Marshall MR, Pilmore H, Manley P, Williams L, Thein H, et al. Proton pump inhibitors and acute interstitial nephritis: report and analysis of 15 cases. Nephrology (Carlton). 2006;11(5):381–5.
Spanou Z, Keller M, Britschgi M, Yawalkar N, Fehr T, Neuweiler J, et al. Involvement of drug-specific T cells in acute drug-induced interstitial nephritis. J Am Soc Nephrol. 2006;17(10):2919–27.
Sun P-p, Zhou X-j, Su J-q, Wang C, Yu X-j, Su T, et al. Urine macrophages reflect kidney macrophage content during acute tubular interstitial and glomerular injury. Clin Immunol. 2019;205:65–74.
Wood BC, Sharma JN, Germann DR, Wood WG, Crouch TT. Gallium citrate Ga 67 imaging in noninfectious interstitial nephritis. Arch Intern Med. 1978;138(11):1665–6.

Wu Y, Yang L, Su T, Wang C, Liu G, Li X-M. Pathological significance of a panel of urinary biomarkers in patients with drug-induced tubulointerstitial nephritis. Clin J Am Soc Nephrol. 2010;5(11):1954–9.

Zhao WT, Huang JW, Sun PP, Su T, Tang JW, Wang SX, et al. Diagnostic roles of urinary kidney injury molecule 1 and soluble C5b-9 in acute tubulointerstitial nephritis. Am J Physiol Renal Physiol. 2019;317(3):F584–F92.

Zheng X-z, Gu Y-H, Su T, Zhou X-J, Huang J-W, Sun P-P, et al. Elevation of erythrocyte sedimentation rate and C-reactive protein levels reflects renal interstitial inflammation in drug-induced acute tubulointerstitial nephritis. BMC Nephrol. 2020;21(1):514.

Imaging Modalities for Acute Tubulointerstitial Nephritis

Megan L. Baker and Mark A. Perazella

1 Introduction

Acute tubulointerstitial nephritis (ATIN) is a relatively common cause of acute and chronic kidney disease (CKD) and is associated with progression to end-stage kidney disease (ESKD). As such, it is an important problem for clinicians caring for these patients. ATIN is primarily an immune-mediated kidney injury triggered by use of certain medications, autoimmune diseases, or infections. Diagnosing ATIN clinically is often quite challenging, and delayed or missed diagnosis promotes ongoing inflammation with resulting interstitial fibrosis, tubular atrophy, and permanent kidney damage. This likely explains the observation that CKD develops in 40–60% of patients after an episode of ATIN. In fact, ATIN is the primary cause of ESKD in 3–4% incident patients. Accordingly, it is one of the few potentially treatable causes of acute kidney injury (AKI) if identified and treated early.

Clinically diagnosing ATIN is difficult as most patients do not have any characteristic signs or symptoms such as rash, fever, or flank pain. Most often, they manifest nonspecific constitutional symptoms, symptoms of kidney failure, or no symptoms at all. Serum and urine laboratory tests also lack sensitivity and specificity. Establishing the diagnosis of ATIN based primarily on current imaging modalities is also challenging, however several may have potential roles in the workup of ATIN (Table 1). They can serve both as tools to help rule out other causes of AKI, and to help inform clinicians of the need for additional workup with biopsy. Radiographic findings can be particularly helpful in cases where kidney biopsy is not an option.

M. L. Baker · M. A. Perazella (✉)
Section of Nephrology, Department of Internal Medicine, Yale University, New Haven, CT, USA
e-mail: megan.baker@yale.edu; mark.perazella@yale.edu

M. G. Atta, M. A. Perazella (eds.), *Tubulointerstitial Nephritis*,
https://doi.org/10.1007/978-3-030-93438-5_20

Table 1 Imaging modalities employed in the diagnostic workup of ATIN and their test characteristics in this setting

Imaging study	Advantages	Disadvantages	ATIN features on imaging	Clinical use in ATIN
Ultrasound	Easily accessible Cost effective Bedside procedure Rapid results	No findings specific to ATIN Often limited by body habitus	Bilateral kidney enlargement, diffuse cortical hyper-echogenicity	Starting point in basic workup of AKI; rule out obstruction, other causes of AKI
CT imaging	Rapid results Widely available across institutions	No findings specific to ATIN Risk of CIN to vulnerable cohort with AKI	Bilateral kidney enlargement, diffuse cortical hyper-echogenicity	No role for CT imaging in workup of ATIN
^{67}Gallium scintigraphy	Best studied imaging modality for ATIN Higher specificity at upper levels of tracer uptake	Up to 72 h delay from tracer injection to test Intermediate uptake neither sensitive nor specific	Uptake of ^{67}gallium in the kidneys, ideally to a degree greater than or equal to that of the liver or spine	Useful tool where biopsy must be avoided; may be helpful in distinguishing ATIN from ATI
PET-CT	Rapid tracer uptake and rapid results Likely more specific tracer to identify ATIN than ^{67}gallium Higher spatial resolution than ^{67}gallium scintigraphy Uptake corresponds to disease activity	Not well studied; no published test performance characteristics Interpretation more challenging in non-oliguric patients	Uptake of FDG in the kidneys; uptake may in more discrete pattern than ^{67}gallium scintigraphy	May be useful tool where biopsy must be avoided; interpretation remains challenging given lack of data on test performance characteristics. May also have a future role in monitoring response to treatment
MRI	Rapid tracer uptake provides for rapid results High spatial resolution	Poorly characterized Likely negligible risk of NSF with newer contrast agents	Heterogeneous, striated enhancement of cortex; restricted water diffusion on DW-MRI	No current role in workup given paucity of data

Abbreviations: *ATIN* acute tubulointerstitial nephritis, *CT* computed tomography, *CIN* contrast-induced nephropathy, *ATI* acute tubular injury, *PET* positron emission tomography, *FDG* fluorodeoxyglucose, *MRI* magnetic resonance imaging, *NSF* nephrogenic systemic fibrosis, *DW* diffusion-weighted

2 Ultrasonography

The role of ultrasonography in the evaluation for ATIN is primarily as a tool to characterize the etiology of undifferentiated AKI early in the diagnostic workup. In drug-induced ATIN, kidney ultrasonography may often demonstrate bilateral kidney enlargement and diffuse cortical hyper-echogenicity, thought to be due to cellular infiltration and edema. However, these findings are neither sensitive nor specific, and may also be present to a lesser degree in ATIN caused by non-pharmacologic processes or other inflammatory causes of AKI (glomerulonephritis, acute tubular injury, lymphoma, leukemia, acute pyelonephritis, etc.). However, kidney ultrasonography should be employed in even the most convincing cases of ATIN as a non-invasive and cost-effective modality to easily rule out other more basic causes of AKI such as urinary obstruction.

3 Computed Tomography Imaging

Similar to ultrasonography, computed tomography (CT) findings in ATIN are non-specific and not present in all cases, but include bilateral kidney enlargement and diffuse cortical hyper-echogenicity (Fig. 1). In contrast to ultrasonography, there are the risks associated with iodinated contrast administration employed with CT scan to provide an optimal study, particularly in this vulnerable cohort of patients with apparent kidney injury prior to administration. Even if obtained without contrast, CT imaging should not be routinely employed in the workup of ATIN, given its limited diagnostic value which can be more readily and safely obtained via ultrasonography.

4 ^{67}Gallium Scintigraphy

^{67}Gallium imaging of the kidney has been employed to evaluate for ATIN since the 1980s. However, the utility of ^{67}gallium scintigraphy in the workup of ATIN remains poorly defined and controversial, with the extremes of uptake potentially providing helpful information, and intermediate results being of indeterminate value. The uptake of ^{67}gallium tracer into the kidneys is measured 48–72 h following its injection, and the intensity of uptake is measured in comparison to surrounding tissues, such as the spine and liver (Fig. 2). Gallium binds lactoferrin, which is both expressed on leukocyte cell surfaces and released from these cells into surrounding tissues, and hence was considered a rational marker to evaluate for the inflammatory interstitial infiltrate seen in ATIN. Based on this, an investigation in rats demonstrated that ^{67}gallium scanning was highly accurate in differentiating experimentally induced ATIN from both drug-induced acute tubular injury/necrosis (ATI/ATN) and

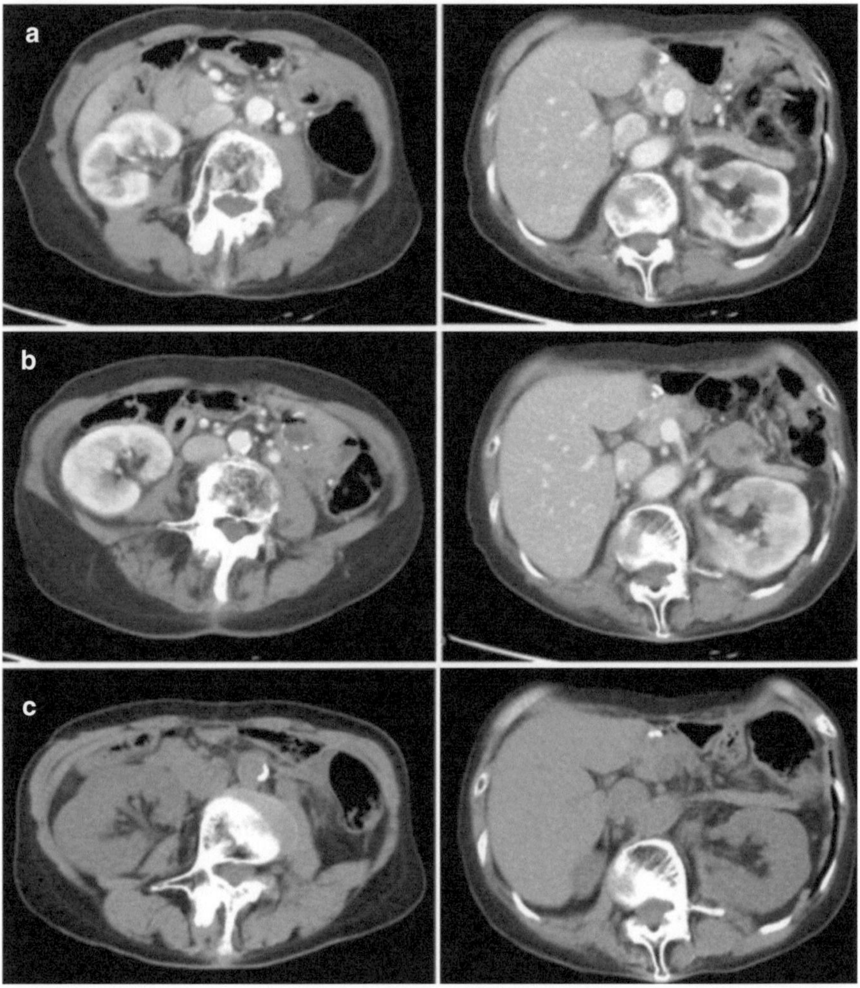

Fig. 1 Computed tomography images of kidneys in patient with acute tubulointerstitial nephritis associated with immune checkpoint inhibitor therapy. Three rows display images after 34 cycles of therapy (**a**), 37 cycles of therapy (**b**), and 1 week after completion of 38 cycles of therapy (**c**). With continued therapy, the bilateral kidneys show progressive enlargement in size. (Reference: Nakatani Y, Kawakami H, Ichikawa M, Yamamoto S, Otsuka Y, Mashiko A, Takashima Y, Ito A, Nakagawa K, Arima S. Nivolumab-induced acute granulomatous tubulointerstitial nephritis in a patient with gastric cancer. Invest New Drugs. 2018;36:726–31. Springer Nature publication – agreement submitted and receipt available on request)

normal rat kidneys. Historically, human studies evaluating the sensitivity and specificity of this modality have been flawed by inconsistent or poorly defined scoring methods, which resulted in incompatible conclusions. For example, an early study demonstrated excellent sensitivity (11/11, 100%) in patients with biopsy-proven ATIN. Subsequent studies, however, have noted lower sensitivities of 58% and 69%

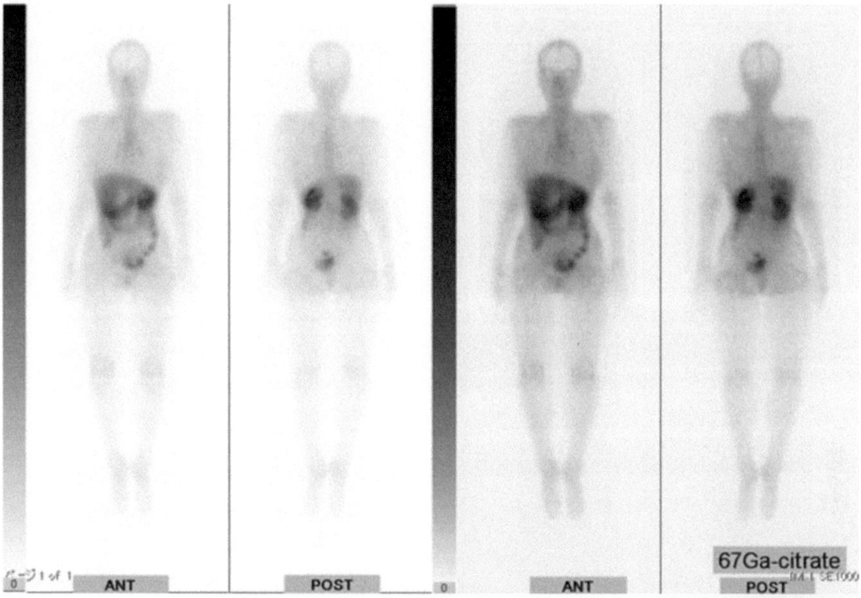

Fig. 2 ^{67}Gallium uptake in a patient with acute tubulointerstitial nephritis associated with immune checkpoint inhibitor therapy. (Reference: Nakatani Y, Kawakami H, Ichikawa M, Yamamoto S, Otsuka Y, Mashiko A, Takashima Y, Ito A, Nakagawa K, Arima S. Nivolumab-induced acute granulomatous tubulointerstitial nephritis in a patient with gastric cancer. Invest New Drugs. 2018;36:726–31. Springer Nature publication – agreement submitted and receipt available on request)

with a test specificity of only 50–60%. In fact, positive ^{67}gallium scan results have been observed with other inflammatory conditions such as glomerulonephritis, pyelonephritis, renal atheroemboli, and ATI/ATN as well as normal kidney tissue on biopsy.

Graham and colleagues used a well-defined scoring scale (Fig. 3) to retrospectively grade patients who had undergone ^{67}gallium scintigraphy and had a biopsy-proven diagnosis or in whom ATIN could be excluded with high certainty. Different scoring cutoffs for the diagnosis of ATIN were then evaluated for their test performance. Very low uptake, in which the kidneys show no uptake (grade 0) or uptake lower than the spine (grade 1), offered a high negative predictive value of 0.89, which would allow for the exclusion of ATIN with a reasonably high probability. High uptake, with kidney uptake equal to (grade 4) or greater than (grade 5) the uptake in the liver, conferred a high specificity (0.86 and 1, respectively). These results suggest that grade 4 or 5 gallium uptake can be used to reasonably establish the diagnosis of ATIN, but using this high uptake as the threshold for diagnosis also has a poor sensitivity of <0.5. Between these two extremes of uptake lies a gray area which provides inadequate positive or negative predictive values for clinicians to draw strong conclusions from. In cases of intermediate ^{67}gallium uptake, establishment of the diagnosis will rely more heavily on pre-test probability, and ultimately on alternate methods of diagnosis such as biopsy. Weaknesses associated with this

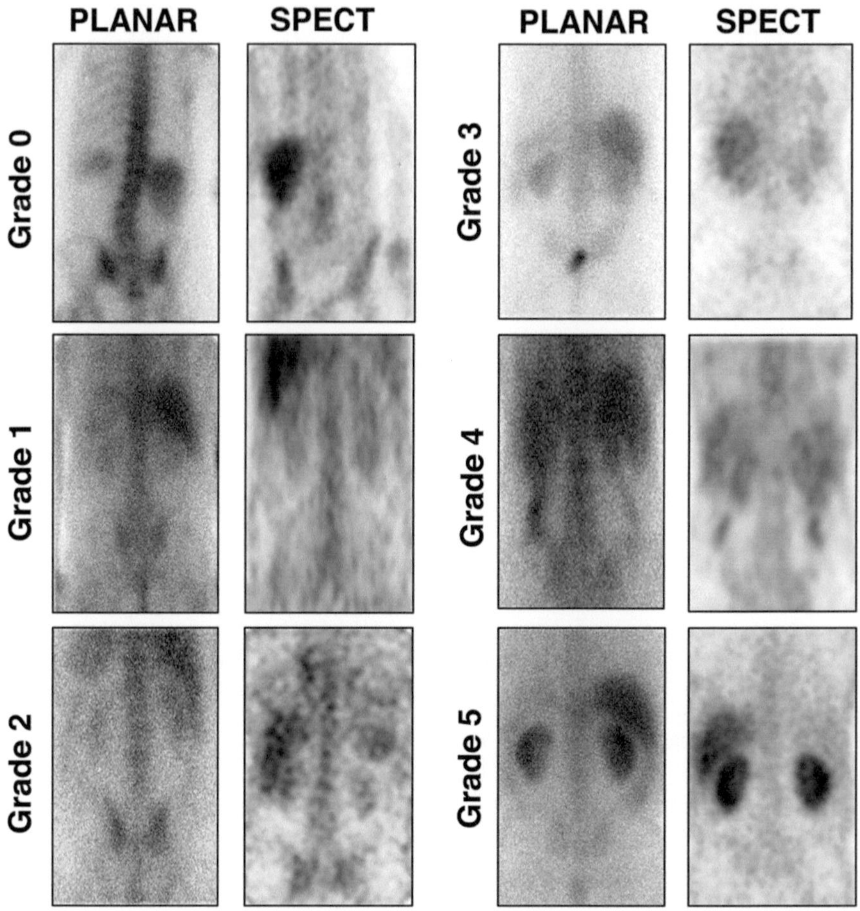

Fig. 3 Examples of different grades of ^{67}gallium uptake in the kidneys, in both SPECT (coronal view) and planar scintigraphy. Grading scheme — Grade 0: no kidney uptake; 1: kidney uptake lower than spine; 2: kidney uptake equal to spine; 3: kidney uptake higher than spine but lower than liver; 4: kidney uptake equal to liver; and 5: kidney uptake higher than liver. (Reference: Graham F, Lord M, Froment D, Cardinal H, Bollée G. The use of gallium-67 scintigraphy in the diagnosis of acute interstitial nephritis. Clin Kidney J. 2015;9:76–81. This is an Open Access article distributed under the terms of the Creative Commons Attribution Non-Commercial License (http://creativecommons.org/licenses/by-nc/4.0/), which permits non-commercial re-use, distribution, and reproduction in any medium, provided the original work is properly cited)

study include that it was a retrospective analysis, only 20 out of 76 patients underwent kidney biopsy to confirm or exclude ATIN, and those who determined the diagnostic outcome were likely not blinded to ^{67}gallium results.

In practice, ^{67}gallium scintigraphy may serve as a tool to avoid kidney biopsy in patients with undifferentiated AKI in which there is a low pretest probability for ATIN, and minimal uptake on ^{67}gallium scintigraphy would help add information to exclude the diagnosis. Alternatively, in patients with a contraindication to kidney biopsy or with a very uncertain etiology of AKI in whom the diagnosis of ATIN is being considered, ^{67}gallium scintigraphy can provide additional data to support or refute the diagnosis within the clinical context and may aid in distinguishing ATIN from ATI/ATN, which is often not associated with ^{67}gallium uptake. In patients with a high pretest probability for ATIN, ^{67}gallium scintigraphy may be deferred with a preference toward kidney biopsy to definitively establish diagnosis and avoid delays in treatment than an intermediate scan result may cause.

Outside of its possible contribution to the establishment of the diagnosis of ATIN, the degree of ^{67}gallium uptake is of uncertain additional clinical significance. In patients with biopsy-proven ATIN, it is unknown whether those with intermediate uptake represent a cohort with a reduced degree of interstitial inflammation compared to those with higher uptake. As previously noted, ^{67}gallium uptake can be present in many other disease processes, and as such these should be considered when other potential causes of AKI exist.

5 Positron Emission Tomography-CT Imaging

Positron emission tomography (PET)-CT imaging is primarily used to evaluate malignant disease, but several small case reports have suggested it to be a more specific and more rapid indicator of ATIN than ^{67}gallium scintigraphy. In addition, PET-CT imaging is able to distinguish drug-induced and immune checkpoint inhibitor-associated ATIN from ATI/ATN, prerenal azotemia, cardiorenal syndrome, and glomerulonephritis.

The physiologic basis for the use of PET in ATIN relies on the premise that the tracer fluorodeoxyglucose (FDG) accumulates in metabolically active lymphocytes, neutrophils, and activated macrophages infiltrating the interstitium, similarly to its accumulation in tumor cells. FDG-positivity appears to correlate to disease process activity, as follow up scans post-treatment and at recovery from ATIN showed interval resolution of tracer uptake.

Unlike ^{67}gallium tracer, which requires a delay of up to 72 h after administration prior to scanning for adequate uptake into tissues, FDG uptake is rapid, and PET-CT can be done within hours. Additionally, PET imaging provides far higher spatial resolution on imaging than other conventional imaging techniques, and much greater resolution than ^{67}gallium scintigraphy (Fig. 4). This characteristic has allowed for its utility in the detection of smaller, more discrete areas of inflammation, such as in granulomatous interstitial nephritis associated with sarcoidosis.

However, no studies to date have examined the sensitivity and specificity of PET in the diagnosis of ATIN. Additionally, the utility of PET-CT is at least theoretically limited to oliguric or anuric patients undergoing workup for ATIN, as it can be challenging to distinguish FDG excreted in the urine from that accumulating in inflammatory lesions in patients with normal kidney function. In patients with prior PET-CT scans for comparison, increased uptake even in the absence of declining urine output may be interpreted as suggestive of ATIN in the appropriate context.

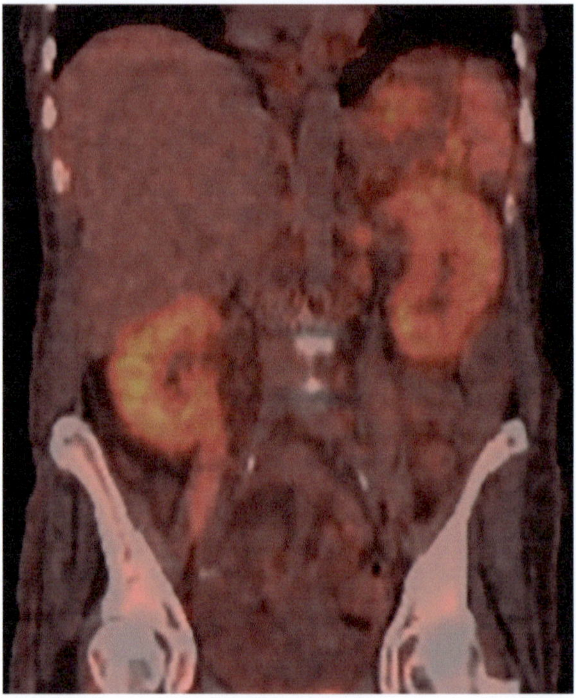

Fig. 4 Merged PET/CT scan in a patient with ATIN, demonstrating brisk uptake of ^{18}F-FDG in the kidneys bilaterally. (Reference: Krishnan N, Perazella MA. The role of PET scanning in the evaluation of patients with kidney disease. Adv Chronic Kidney Dis. 2017;24:154–61. Elsevier Publication – agreement submitted and receipt available on request)

Given the promise of its potential as outlined in the few number of case reports to date, significant further investigation is needed to clarify whether PET-CT could be a reliable diagnostic tool to evaluate for different types of ATIN.

6 Magnetic Resonance Imaging

Gadolinium-based imaging with magnetic resonance imaging (MRI) has in recent history been avoided in patients with acute or chronic kidney disease due to the concern for nephrogenic systemic fibrosis (NSF). NSF was discovered with the use of older, primarily linear chelate gadolinium-based contrast agents. While NSF is generally an infrequent complication of gadolinium exposure in patients with kidney disease, the morbidity and mortality associated with the disease prohibited its use in these patients.

Since the advent of the newer macrocyclic chelate gadolinium-based contrast agents, NSF is considered exceedingly rare and for several of these agents no cases have been reported. Hence, MRI is not absolutely contraindicated in these patients. However, its diagnostic role for ATIN is very poorly defined due to lack of data from years of avoided use. In fact, only case reports of specific MRI findings in patients with ATIN currently exist in the literature.

In the handful of case reports to date, ATIN has been reported to appear as a heterogeneous enhancement of the renal cortex with a striated appearance on MRI. In one case report, diffusion-weighted MRI led to the diagnosis of IgG4-related ATIN after a targeted biopsy of an area of restricted water diffusion was performed within previously identified kidney lesions. Much further data are needed to determine whether MRI can serve a diagnostic role in ATIN as clinicians become more comfortable with using gadolinium-based contrast agents in patients with kidney disease again.

7 Conclusion

Acute tubulointerstitial nephritis remains a challenging diagnosis, which often requires kidney biopsy to definitively establish. While ^{67}gallium scintigraphy remains the most widely employed imaging modality to evaluate for ATIN, interpretation of its results is often challenging given its limited sensitivity and specificity. PET-CT imaging has shown promise as a potential new non-invasive modality to evaluate for ATIN, but to date our experience is based largely on case series, and its performance characteristics remain unestablished. However, when employed judiciously with considerations given to a patient's pre-test probability for ATIN, likelihood of alternative diagnoses, and appropriateness for kidney biopsy, these imaging studies can serve as valuable tools in the workup of ATIN.

Suggested Reading

Fogazzi GB, Ferrari B, Garigali G, Simonini P, Consonni D. Urinary sediment findings in acute interstitial nephritis. Am J Kidney Dis. 2012;60:330–2.

Graham F, Lord M, Froment D, Cardinal H, Bollée G. The use of gallium-67 scintigraphy in the diagnosis of acute interstitial nephritis. Clin Kidney J. 2015;9:76–81.

Graham GD, Lundy MM, Moreno JJ. Failure of 67Gallium scintigraphy to identify reliably noninfectious interstitial nephritis. J Nucl Med. 1983;24:568–70.

Haas M, Spargo BH, Wit EJ, Meehan SM. Etiologies and outcome of acute renal insufficiency in older adults: a renal biopsy study of 259 cases. Am J Kidney Dis. 2000;35:433–47.

Horino T, Matsumoto T, Inoue K, Ichii O, Terada Y. A case of acute kidney injury caused by granulomatous interstitial nephritis associated with sarcoidosis. CEN Case Rep. 2018;7:34–8.

Joaquim AI, Mendes GEF, Ribeiro PFF, Baptista MAF, Burdmann EA. Ga-67 scintigraphy in the differential diagnosis between acute interstitial nephritis and acute tubular necrosis: an experimental study. Nephrol Dial Transplant. 2010;25:3277–82.

Katagiri D, Masumoto S, Katsuma A, Minami E, Hoshino T, Inoue T, et al. Positron emission tomography combined with computed tomography (PET-CT) as a new diagnostic tool for acute tubulointerstitial nephritis (AIN) in oliguric or haemodialysed patients. NDT Plus. 2010;3:155–9.

Kimura Y, Kawamura M, Owada M, Fujiwara T, Maesawa C, Hiramori K. Successful steroid therapy for cefdinir-induced acute tubulointerstitial nephritis with progressive renal failure. Intern Med. 2001;40(2):114–7.

Koselj M, Kveder R, Bren AF, Rott T. Acute renal failure in patients with drug-induced acute interstitial nephritis. Ren Fail. 1993;15(1):69–72.

Krishnan N, Perazella MA. The role of PET scanning in the evaluation of patients with kidney disease. Adv Chronic Kidney Dis. 2017;24:154–61.

Linton AL, Richmond JM, Clark WF, Lindsay RM, Driedger AA, Lamki LM. Gallium67 scintigraphy in the diagnosis of acute renal disease. Clin Nephrol. 1985;24:84–7.

Moinuddin I, Bracamonte E, Thajudeen B, Sussman A, Madhrira M, Costello J. Allergic interstitial nephritis manifesting as a striated nephrogram. Case Rep Med. 2015;2015:250530.

Moledina DG, Perazella MA. Drug-induced acute interstitial nephritis. Clin J Am Soc Nephrol. 2017;12:2046–9.

Moledina DG, Perazella MA. PPIs and kidney disease: from AIN to CKD. J Nephrol. 2016;29:611–6.

Moledina DG, Perazella MA. Treatment of drug-induced acute tubulointerstitial nephritis: the search for better evidence. Clin J Am Soc Nephrol. 2018;13:1785–7.

Muriithi AK, Leung N, Valeri AM, et al. Biopsy-proven acute interstitial nephritis, 1993-2011: a case series. Am J Kidney Dis. 2014;64:558–66.

Nakatani Y, Kawakami H, Ichikawa M, Yamamoto S, Otsuka Y, Mashiko A, Takashima Y, Ito A, Nakagawa K, Arima S. Nivolumab-induced acute granulomatous tubulointerstitial nephritis in a patient with gastric cancer. Investig New Drugs. 2018;36:726–31.

Nochaiwong S, Ruengorn C, Awiphan R, et al. The association between proton pump inhibitor use and the risk of adverse kidney outcomes: a systematic review and meta-analysis. Nephrol Dial Transplant. 2018;33:331–42.

Perazella MA, Markowitz GS. Drug-induced acute interstitial nephritis. Nat Rev Nephrol. 2010;6:461–70.

Perazella MA. Diagnosing drug-induced AIN in the hospitalized patient: a challenge for the clinician. Clin Nephrol. 2014;81:381–8.

Pozdzik AA, Matos C, Rorive S, Brocheriou I, Van Gansbeke D, Delhaye M, Nortier JL, Neild GH. Diffusion-weighted magnetic resonance imaging as a new diagnostic tool of subclinical IgG4-related acute tubulointerstitial nephritis. Clin Kidney J. 2013;6:235–7.

Qualls D, Seethapathy H, Bates H, Tajmir S, Heidari P, Endres P, et al. Positron emission tomography as an adjuvant diagnostic test in the evaluation of checkpoint inhibitor-associated acute interstitial nephritis. J Immunother Cancer. 2019;7:356.

Sharma K, Geagan N, Tengsupakul S. Severe acute interstitial nephritis secondary to minocycline use in an adolescent girl. SAGE Open Med Case Rep. 2020;8:2050313X20943069.

Shima H, Tashiro M, Yamada S, Matsuura M, Okada K, Doi T, et al. Cilostazol-induced acute tubulointerstitial nephritis accompanied by IgA nephropathy: a case report. BMC Nephrol. 2018;19:52.

Simpson IJ, Marshall MR, Pilmore H, et al. Proton pump inhibitors and acute interstitial nephritis: report and analysis of 15 cases. Nephrology (Carlton). 2006;11:381–5.

Saran R, Robinson B, Abbott KC, et al. US renal data system 2019 annual data report: epidemiology of kidney disease in the United States. Am J Kidney Dis. 2020;75:A4.

Wilkinson SP, Stewart WK, Spiers EM, Pears J. Protracted systemic illness and interstitial nephritis due to minocycline. Postgrad Med J. 1989;65:53–6.

Pathology of Tubulointerstitial Nephritis

Jean Hou, Lynn D. Cornell, and Cynthia C. Nast

1 Introduction

Interstitial nephritis (IN) is characterized by inflammatory cells in the interstitium often with associated acute tubular cell injury of varying severity. When inflammation extends into tubular walls and/or lumens, it is termed tubulointerstitial nephritis (TIN). IN most often involves the kidney cortex, may occur at the corticomedullary junction particularly with drug-induced injury and infrequently involves the medulla in specific settings such as bacterial pyelonephritis and polyomavirus nephropathy. In contrast to some other organs where mononuclear leukocytes are considered chronic inflammation, in the kidney these cell types can be part of an acute/active or chronic interstitial or tubulointerstitial process while neutrophils are exclusively involved in acute/active injury. Acute and active are not synonymous; acute refers to a process of sudden onset or short duration occurring over days to weeks while an active process is one in which there may be acute or ongoing disease which may co-occur with chronic injury. As mononuclear leukocytes are found in both active and chronic IN, it is the interstitial edema that identifies an active process and interstitial fibrosis, typically with tubular atrophy, that defines chronic injury (Fig. 1).

The type and intrarenal distribution of inflammation may provide clues to the etiology of IN. Most types of IN are characterized by interstitial infiltration with lymphocytes, macrophages, and plasma cells, with varying numbers of eosinophils or neutrophils in specific situations. Chronic parenchymal injury due to glomerular or vascular disease has associated tubulointerstitial scarring usually with mild

J. Hou · C. C. Nast (✉)
Department of Pathology, Cedars-Sinai Medical Center, Los Angeles, CA, USA
e-mail: Jean.Hou@cshs.org; Cynthia.Nast@cshs.org

L. D. Cornell
Division of Anatomic Pathology, Department of Laboratory Medicine and Pathology, Mayo Clinic, Rochester, MN, USA
e-mail: Cornell.Lynn@mayo.edu

M. G. Atta, M. A. Perazella (eds.), *Tubulointerstitial Nephritis*,
https://doi.org/10.1007/978-3-030-93438-5_21

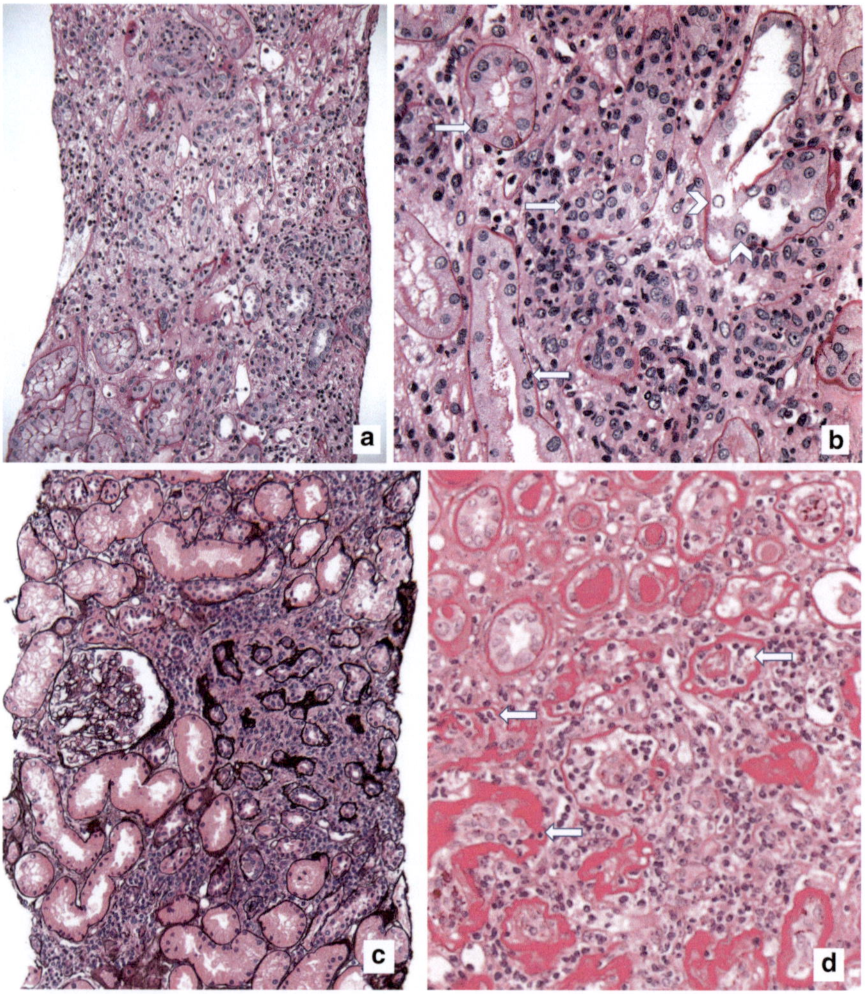

Fig. 1 Tubulointerstitial nephritis. (**a**, **b**) Acute tubulointerstitial nephritis. There are interstitial edema causing separation of tubules and interstitial inflammation predominantly composed of mononuclear cells including lymphocytes and macrophages with few eosinophils. (**a**, Periodic-acid Schiff ×200). Inflammation is in tubular walls (arrows) with acute tubular cell injury and foci of denuded tubular basement membranes due to epithelial cell sloughing (arrowheads). (**b**, Periodic-acid Schiff ×400). (**c**, **d**) Chronic interstitial nephritis. There is cortical inflammation in areas of tubular atrophy and interstitial fibrosis. Note the adjacent well preserved tubulointerstitium does not have inflammation. (**c**, Jones methenamine silver ×200; **d**, Periodic-acid Schiff ×400)

mononuclear inflammation representing an innate immune response. In chronic IN however, the tubulointerstitial scarring and amount of inflammation are in excess of what is expected in the above setting. It has been suggested that mast cells are important in progressive kidney injury. In glomerulonephritis-associated tubulointerstitial inflammation, mast cells have been identified in the cortical tubulointerstitium and medullary interstitium. Hiromura et al. demonstrated a correlation of mast cell infiltration with serum creatinine levels for most glomerular lesions and with the extent of tubulointerstitial injury overall, but not with the degree of proteinuria. It is now recognized that mast cells play an important role in the progression of chronic tubulointerstitial injury by regulating immunity and modulating inflammation through release of growth factors, proteases, chemokines, cytokines, and leukotrienes regardless of the initial intrarenal disease process.

TIN may be associated with nonspecific histopathologic changes secondary to, and possibly altering, the primary inflammatory injury. In the setting of tubular inflammation, tubular basement membranes (TBMs) may rupture with luminal contents such as Tamm-Horsfall protein (THP), also known as uromodulin, spilling into the adjacent interstitium. THP may be antigenic and elicit an eosinophilic or macrophage and granulomatous response; therefore, when granulomas are present it is important to look for associated ruptured tubules or extra-tubular THP (Fig. 2). Tubules also may rupture into thin-walled veins (tubulovenous herniation), resulting in venous thrombi containing inflammatory cells and THP (Fig. 3). This process also allows venous blood to enter the tubular lumen causing microscopic, and in severe cases gross hematuria.

A caveat to the identification of IN or TIN in native kidney, biopsies is the lack of definitive criteria for how much interstitial or tubular inflammation is required to make the diagnosis. This differs from transplant kidney biopsies, where specific amounts of tubular and interstitial inflammation are delineated (Banff criteria) for a diagnosis of cell-mediated rejection, which is a form of TIN. This lack of diagnostic histopathologic criteria in TIN results in poor reproducibility and inter-rater agreement among pathologists. Interstitial inflammation occurs in other types of kidney disease such as active glomerulonephritis and acute tubular injury, and it is uncertain when this indicates an additional diagnosis of IN due to an independent process. As in all areas of kidney pathology, clinical pathologic correlation is necessary for correct interpretation of the biopsy findings.

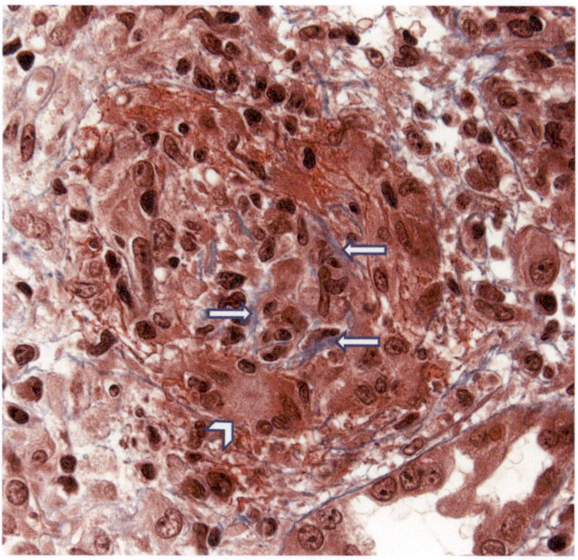

Fig. 2 Non-necrotizing interstitial granuloma surrounding extra-tubular Tamm-Horsfall protein, which is blue on Masson's trichrome stain (arrows). Note the foreign body multinucleated giant cell (arrowhead). (Masson's trichrome ×600)

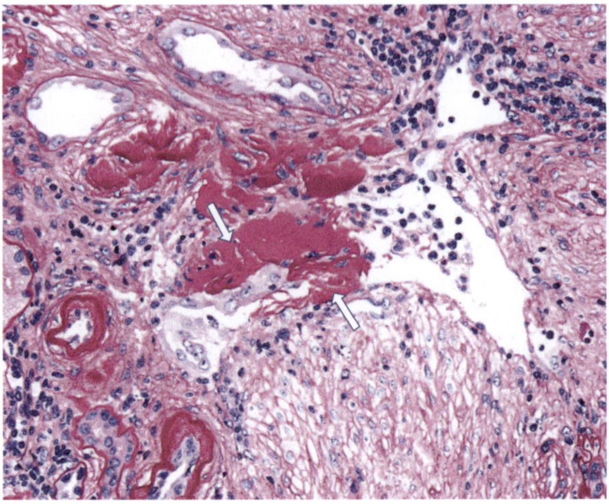

Fig. 3 Tubular rupture into a vein (tubulovenous herniation). There is periodic-acid Schiff positive Tamm-Horsfall protein in the interstitium and extending into a vein (arrow). (Periodic-acid Schiff ×400)

2 Allergic/Drug-Induced Interstitial Nephritis

The most common IN in developed countries is caused by medications, with antibiotics, nonsteroidal anti-inflammatory agents (NSAIDs), and proton pump inhibitors (PPIs) as the top offenders. Drug-induced IN often begins with inflammation at the corticomedullary junction including the deep cortex and superficial medulla (Fig. 4). With more severe active disease there is interstitial edema with lymphocytes more diffusely in the cortical interstitium and often migrating into the walls of tubules with associated acute tubular cell injury or necrosis. There are varying numbers of macrophages and usually no to a modest number of plasma cells. With progression to chronic IN, there is moderate to dense inflammation in areas of interstitial fibrosis, often with lymphocytes in the walls of atrophic tubules. Chronic interstitial nephritis may be found alone or concurrently with features of active disease (Fig. 5). Histologic features portending a worse prognosis in drug-induced TIN include diffuse interstitial inflammation and the presence of granulomas.

In drug-induced TIN the inflammatory infiltrate usually is composed of T-cells, primarily CD4+ cells without or with lesser numbers of CD8+ cells, CD20+ B cells, and macrophages. Neutrophils are occasionally present as a reaction to tissue injury, but their presence raises the specter of active infection. Certain drugs may evoke more specific inflammatory responses. Berney-Meyer et al. found that omeprazole-induced acute TIN is associated predominantly with CD4+ cells with frequent lymphocytic aggregates in kidney biopsies. Th17+ lymphocytes were present in 20/23 biopsies, of which 13 also had Foxp3+ tubulointerstitial lymphocytes. Th17+ Foxp3- biopsies contained interstitial macrophages positive for the Th1 related transcription factor T-bet, suggesting a role for a Th1-Th17 inflammatory process. Several studies have shown no increase in perforin, granzyme or CD56+ cells, suggesting that cytotoxic T

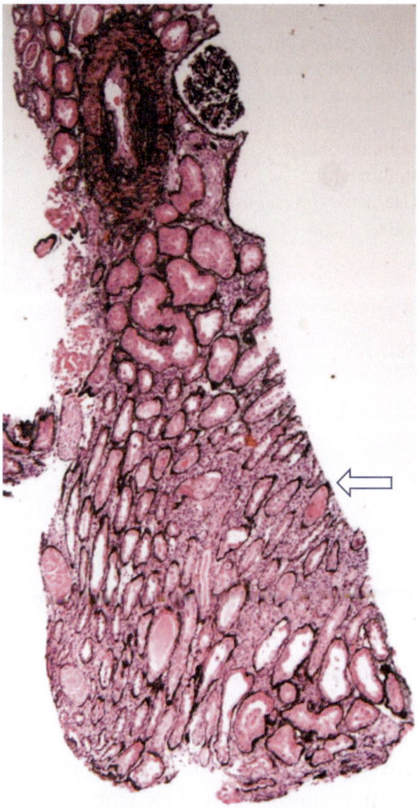

Fig. 4 There is localized interstitial inflammation near the corticomedullary junction (arrow). (Jones methenamine silver ×100)

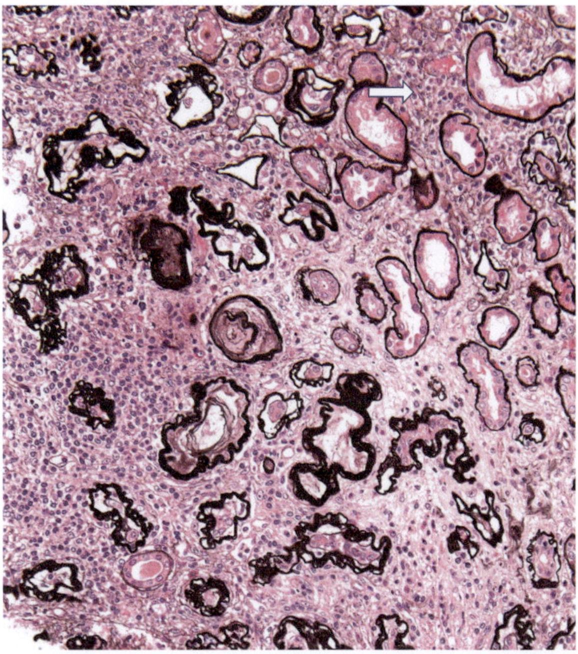

Fig. 5 Chronic active interstitial nephritis. There are tubular atrophy with interstitial fibrosis, interstitial inflammation and scattered lymphocytes in the walls of atrophic tubules. The interstitium also is edematous and associated with inflammation in areas of preserved tubulointerstitium (arrow). (Jones methenamine silver ×200)

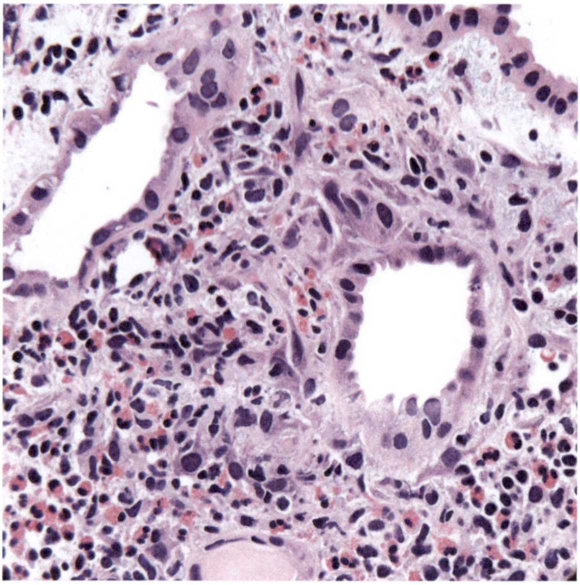

Fig. 6 Interstitial inflammation composed of many eosinophils in addition to lymphocytes and scattered macrophages without tubular inflammation. (Hematoxylin and eosin ×600)

cells have no significant role in drug-induced inflammatory kidney injury. Eosinophils historically have been a hallmark of drug-induced IN, initially identified related to the penicillin class of antibiotics (Fig. 6). However, in the last few decades, IN related to medications such as NSAIDs and PPIs often contains few eosinophils. Notably, the presence of urine eosinophils is not helpful in distinguishing acute TIN from other causes of kidney disease, including acute tubular necrosis, when using kidney biopsies as the gold standard for diagnosis. In a study of IN associated with three different drugs, Spanou et al. demonstrated that the extent of infiltrating eosinophils was related to the expression of IL-5 by CD4+ cells. TIN with prominent eosinophils also may occur in drug rash with eosinophilia and systemic symptoms (DRESS) syndrome and idiopathic hypereosinophilic syndrome, is rarely observed in Kimura's disease and Ascaris lumbricoides infection and has been reported in interstitial aggregates in diabetic kidney disease without exposure to nephrotoxic medications.

3 Infectious Interstitial Nephritis

The kidney may be directly infected by viruses, bacteria, fungal organisms, and parasites (Table 1). The latter two are not frequent in developed countries, even in immunosuppressed patients and in areas of endemic fungal infection such as the California Central Valley. The type of inflammatory infiltrate and tubular cell features may help identify the class of organism involved.

Table 1 Infection-associated interstitial nephritis

Pathogen		Histologic features		Ancillary studies		
		Inflammatory infiltrate	*Other features*	*Special stains*	*IF findings*	*EM findings*
Bacterial	Non-mycobacterial	Mixed inflammation, neutrophils and neutrophilic casts (microabscesses) in acute infection, variable plasma cell component in chronic infection	Infrequent granulomas, chronic infection with tubular thyroidization	Gram stain	Non-contributory	Non-contributory
	XGP	Collections of foamy histiocytes, mixed inflammation with variable neutrophils	Frequent granulomas with foamy histiocytes and MNGCs	CD68 to highlight macrophages	Non-contributory	Non-contributory
	Malakoplakia, MIN	Enlarged histiocytes with finely granular PAS positive cytoplasm	Michaelis-Gutman bodies in malakoplakia	CD68 to highlight macrophages	Non-contributory	Identification of intracellular Michaelis-Gutman bodies
	Mycobacterial	Mixed inflammation	Granulomas with necrotizing features	Ziehl-Neelson or Kinyoun stains	Auramine-rhodamine stain	Non-contributory
Fungal		Mixed inflammation, variable plasma cells	May be granulomas	Routine PAS and JMS, GMS	Non-contributory	Non-contributory
Viral	Polyomavirus	Mixed inflammation, can be plasma cell rich, viral cytopathic effect in infected tubular epithelial cells	"Ground glass" nuclear inclusions	SV40 IHC	Variable granular TBM staining for IgG and complement	May be TBM deposits, viral particles sometimes in paracrystalline arrays
	Adenovirus		Nuclear inclusions, may be necrosis, granulomas	Adenovirus IHC		
	Cytomegalovirus		Nuclear ("owl's eye") and cytoplasmic inclusions	CMV IHC	Non-contributory	Round to pleomorphic 120–200 nm virions

Abbreviations: *IF* immunofluorescence, *EM* electron microscopy, *XGP* xanthogranulomatous pyelonephritis, *MIN* megalocytic interstitial nephritis, *MNGC* multinulcleated giant cell, *PAS* Periodic acid Schiff, *JMS* Jones methenamine silver, *GMS* Gomori methenamine silver, *IHC* immunohistochemistry, *TBM* tubular basement membrane, *CMV* cytomegalovirus

3.1 Viral Infections

Intrarenal productive viral infections have a prominent IN characteristic, which is often plasma cell rich, defined as plasma cells accounting for more than 10% of the infiltrating leukocytes. Lymphocytic tubular inflammation is common. Tubular cells may have viral cytopathic changes including nuclear enlargement and hyperchromasia, prominent nucleoli, smudgy "ground glass" inclusions composed of viral particles, and sloughing of necrotic cells into tubular lumens. As viral cytopathic changes are not specific, definitive virus identification requires immunohistochemistry (polyomavirus, CMV, adenovirus, others), in situ hybridization (EBV) and/or identifying viral particles by electron microscopy (EM).

Polyomavirus preferentially infects collecting duct and distal tubular epithelium with more medullary than cortical involvement. The inflammation, associated progressive tubular atrophy, and interstitial fibrosis are focal and geographic being localized to areas of infected tubules (Fig. 7). In transplant kidney biopsies with polyomavirus infection, Buettner et al. showed increased plasma cells, more T-cells than B-cells and a predominance of Th2 cells, suggesting a possible role for humoral immunity. Interestingly, tubular basement membrane (TBM) deposits occur in approximately half the cases of polyomavirus nephropathy. They

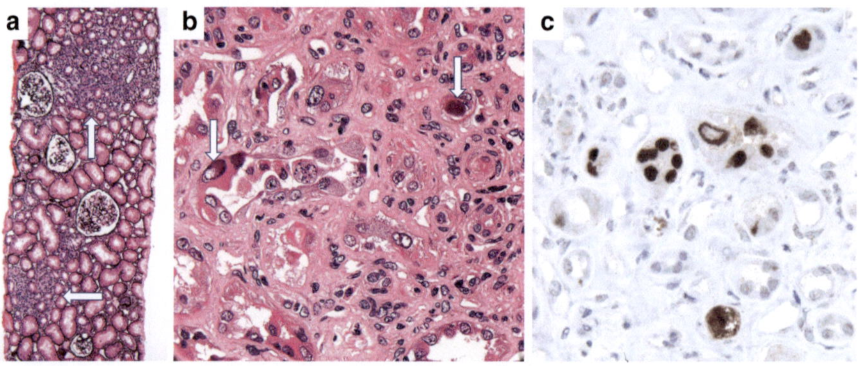

Fig. 7 Polyomavirus infection. (**a**) Kidney cortex with zonal geographic areas of tubulointerstitial inflammation (arrows). (Jones methenamine silver ×100). (**b**) Tubular cells show viral cytopathic change with enlarged nuclei, smudgy intranuclear ("ground glass") inclusions (arrows) and sloughing of necrotic cells into tubular lumens. (Hematoxylin and eosin ×600). (**c**) Immunohistochemical stain for SV40 showing positive staining in tubular cell nuclei. (×600). (**d**) Immunofluorescence staining showing granular to confluent granular IgG in tubular basement membranes. (×200). (**e**) Electron microscopy showing many discrete electron dense deposits (arrows) circumferentially in the thickened basement membrane of an atrophic tubule (×1500). (**f**) Electron microscopy showing viral particles within an infected tubular epithelial cell nucleus. Viral particles can be randomly dispersed (right) or can spontaneously aggregate into tightly packed paracrystalline arrays (left, arrows) (×40,000)

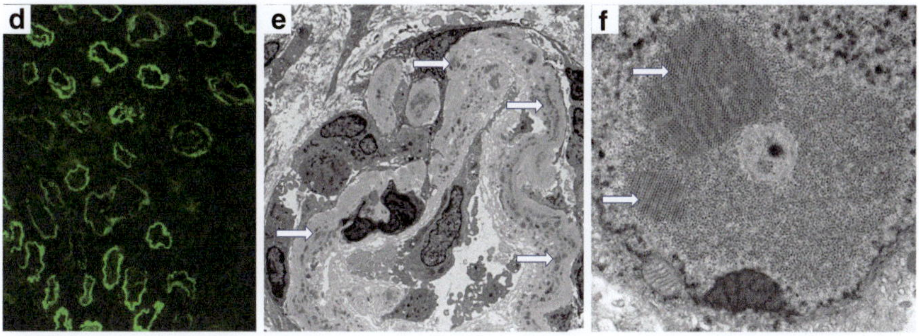

Fig. 7 (continued)

typically are composed of IgG and/or C3 seen on immunofluorescence (IF), contain the SV40 antigen, appear as electron dense deposits by EM, and are associated with more severe tubulointerstitial injury and extensive infection. There are two species of polyomavirus, BK virus (BKV) and JC virus (JCV). The simian virus 40 (SV40) immunohistochemical stain is used most often to identify polyomavirus; however, does not differentiate BKV from JCV. This may cause confusion when strongly positive SV40 staining occurs in a biopsy but BKV serologic titers are negative. In-situ hybridization can be used to detect polyomavirus but does not reliably distinguish between BKV and JCV inclusions, although the former stain more strongly. In these cases, serologic testing for JCV should be performed. In productive polyomavirus infection, infected tubular cell nuclei contain virus visualized by EM as non-enveloped particles measuring 30–50 nm in diameter and randomly dispersed or organized into paracrystalline arrays. These ultrastructural features are characteristic of the family polyomaviridae but cannot differentiate BKV from JCV.

CMV infection results in tubular cell, macrophage and/or endothelial cell viral cytopathic change with nuclear and/or cytoplasmic inclusions (Fig. 8). Adenovirus also causes tubular cell cytopathic change but with more pronounced tubular cell and even interstitial necrosis and a reactive neutrophilic infiltrate, sometime with associated granulomatous inflammation or TBM immune complex deposits (Fig. 9). Epstein Barr virus infection tends to have a more mixed inflammatory infiltrate, which varies depending on the stage of infection. In acute disease, CD8+ cells predominate due to antigen-directed cell cytotoxicity with fewer CD20+ cells, macrophages, and plasma cells; few eosinophils and neutrophils may be present. With chronic infection, there are reactive CD8+ cells with pronounced proinflammatory and profibrotic signaling. There is no cytopathic change; therefore, EBV infection needs to be suspected clinically, diagnosed with serologic findings and virus identification in using special staining. In a transplant kidney, lymphoproliferative disorder is also in the differential diagnosis particularly in patients with EBV infection.

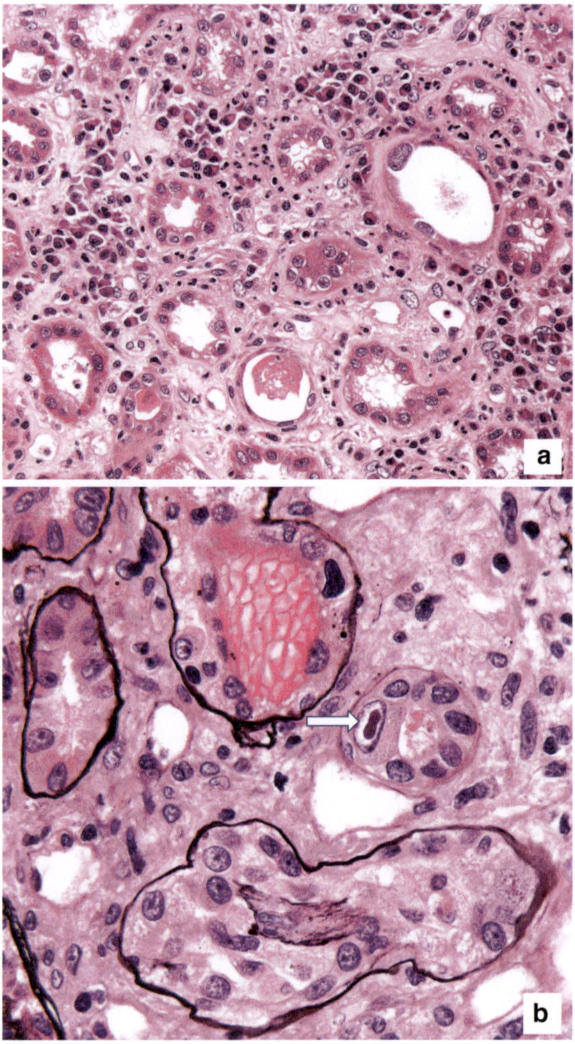

Fig. 8 Cytomegalovirus infection. (**a**) There is a plasma cell rich interstitial inflammatory infiltrate with interstitial edema and acute tubular cell injury. (Hematoxylin and eosin ×400). (**b**) Enlarged tubular cell with a single nuclear ("owl's eye") viral inclusion (arrow). (Jones methenamine silver ×800)

3.2 Bacterial Infections (Pyelonephritis)

Neutrophilic infiltration is most often associated with an ascending acute bacterial or rarely fungal infection (pyelonephritis). Neutrophils migrate from the peritubular capillaries through the interstitium into the tubular lumens, where the bacteria are ascending from the lower urinary tract (Fig. 10). Therefore, the process may begin in the medulla and spread to the cortex, typically with glomerular sparing. There is often marked peritubular inflammation with interstitial edema. Tubular cells show injury or necrosis and tubular lumens focally have neutrophilic casts (microabscesses) admixed with cellular debris. As the process becomes more chronic, interstitial fibrosis and tubular atrophy develop with an infiltrate of lymphocytes, macrophages, and plasma cells; there may be

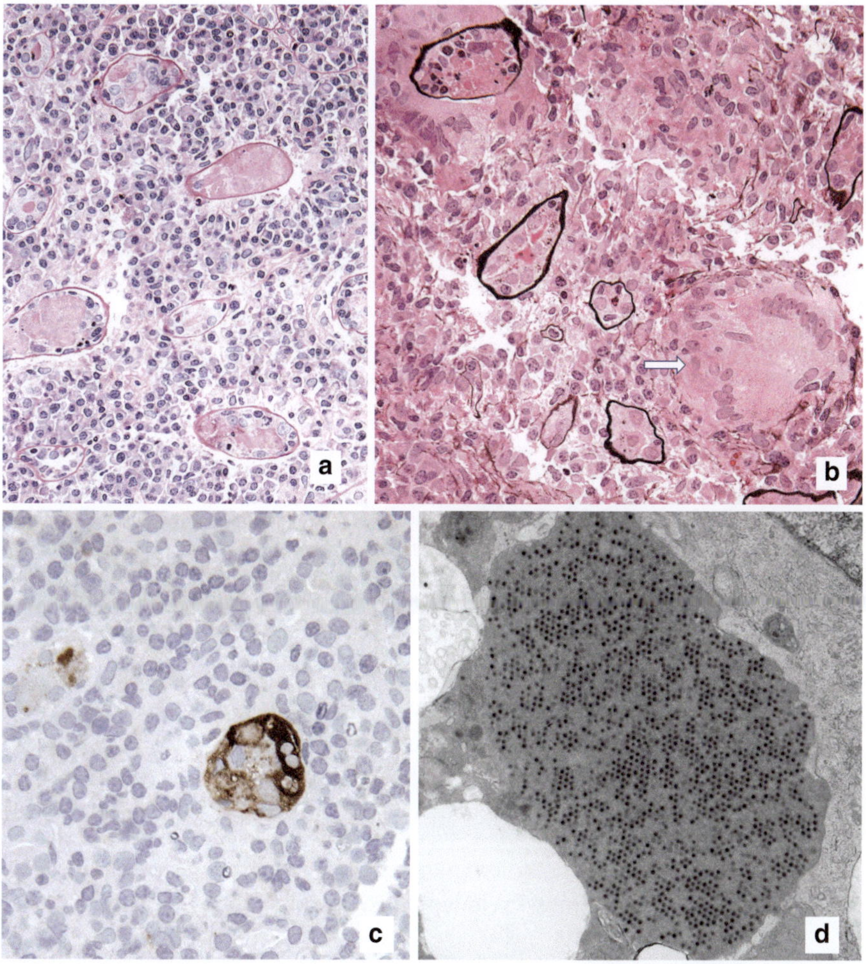

Fig. 9 Adenovirus infection. (**a**) There are tubular cell necrosis and focal tubular inflammation with a dense interstitial plasma cell rich inflammatory infiltrate. (Periodic-acid Schiff ×400). (**b**) In addition to tubular cell necrosis and a mononuclear interstitial infiltrate, there is a non-necrotizing interstitial granuloma (arrow). (Jones methenamine silver ×400). (**c**) Immunohistochemical staining for adenovirus showing virus in intact and necrotic tubular cells with dense surrounding inflammation. (×600). (**d**) Electron microcopy revealing viral particles forming organized paracrystalline arrays in the cytoplasm of a necrotic tubular cell. (×25,000)

notable eosinophils. Tubular atrophy may take the form of "thyroidization", in which tubules are dilated with flattened epithelium and luminal proteinaceous casts. Chronic active pyelonephritis is not uncommon, where neutrophils and tubular injury occur in concert with atrophy, fibrosis, and infiltrating mononuclear leukocytes. When bacteria seed the kidney from a systemic infection (hematogenous spread), inflammation starts in the cortex including glomerular involvement. In bacterial pyelonephritis, urine analysis and culture are best used to identify the organism. Special stains aid in identifying acid fast organisms, spirochetes, and fungal organisms and therefore should be used

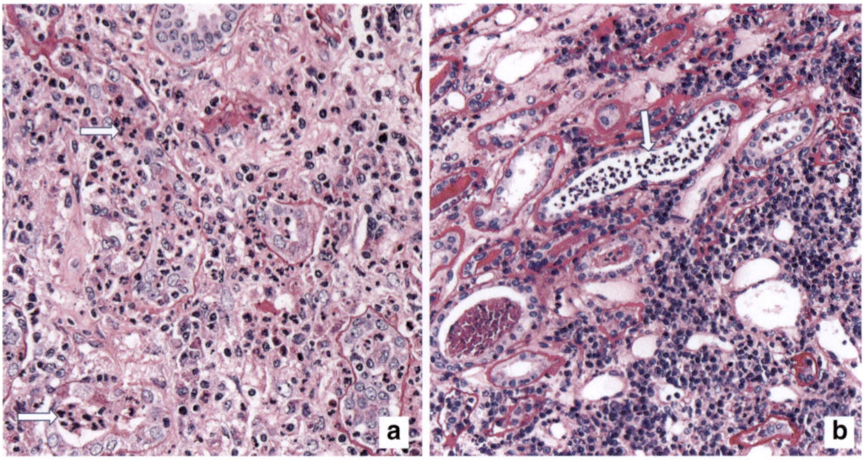

Fig. 10 Bacterial infectious interstitial nephritis (pyelonephritis). (**a**) Acute infection with numerous neutrophils in the interstitium, tubular walls and tubular lumens forming microabscesses (arrows). (Periodic-acid Schiff ×400). (**b**) Chronic active infection. There are a focal dense plasma cell infiltrate with tubular atrophy and interstitial fibrosis reflecting chronic injury, and active infection characterized by a tubular lumen containing neutrophils (microabscess, arrow). (Periodic-acid Schiff ×400)

whenever there is concern for these types of infection. Obstruction and reflux may be predisposing factors for kidney infection. When these are present, it is common for tubules to be dilated with luminal and extra-tubular Tamm-Horsfall protein, which may elicit a granulomatous or inflammatory response independent of infection or drug-induced injury.

3.2.1 Xanthogranulomatous Pyelonephritis, Malakoplakia, Megalocytic Interstitial Nephritis

There are unique forms of chronic IN related to intrarenal bacterial infection, usually with gram negative organisms, and a host defect in macrophage bacterial phagocytosis or degradation (Fig. 11). Xanthogranulomatous pyelonephritis (XGP) is a unilateral process typically occurring with obstructive nephrolithiasis and infection by *E. coli* or *Proteus mirabilis*. There are abundant lipid-laden macrophages (foam or xanthoma cells) admixed with lymphocytes, plasma cells, typical macrophages, variable granuloma formation, and focal multinucleated giant cells. This process starts in the pelvis and may extend to the entire kidney. With ongoing infection, neutrophils are present and there may be focal necrosis. Unlike XGP, malakoplakia may involve other organs, occurs in any part of the kidney, is bilateral in 40% of cases, and is identified more often in immunocompromised patients. There is a sheet-like infiltrate of macrophages (von Hansemann histiocytes) that have granular eosinophilic and PAS-positive cytoplasm and larger PAS-positive rounded inclusions (Michaelis-Gutmann bodies) that contain calcium and iron, likely

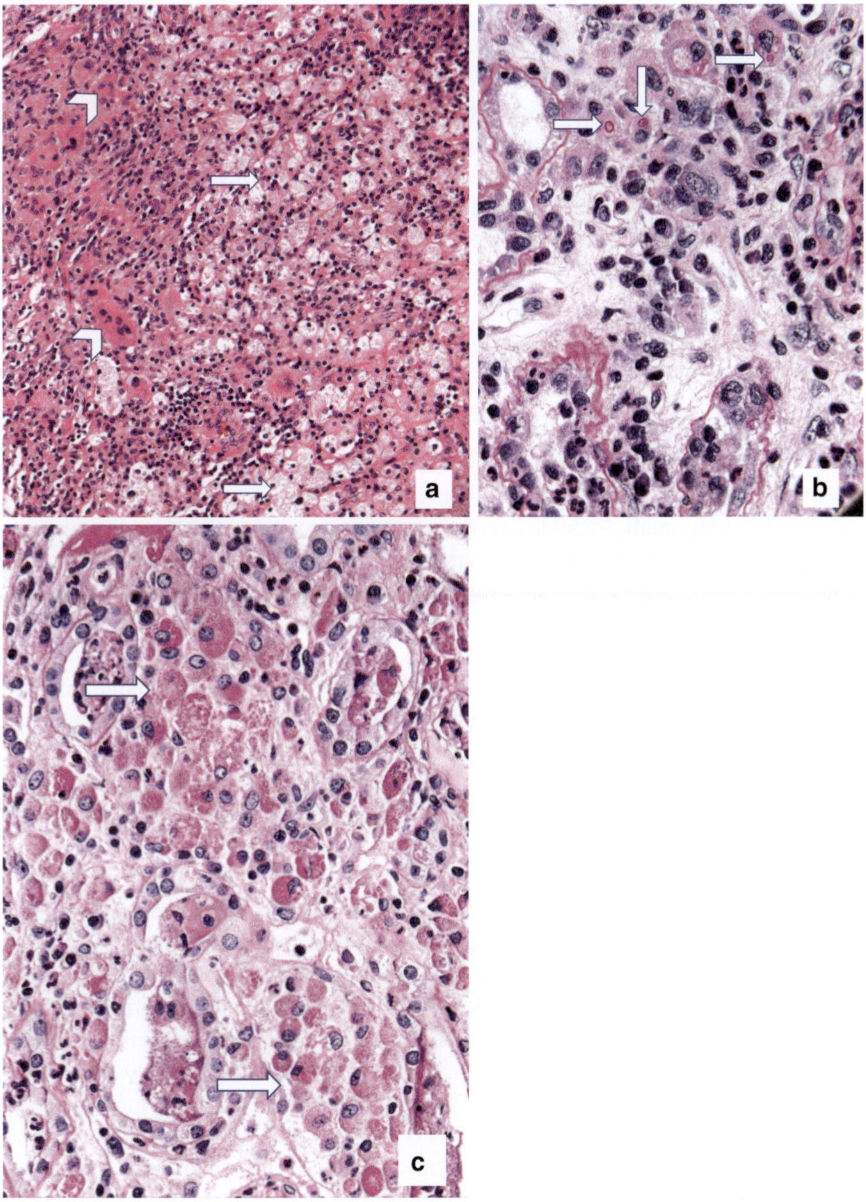

Fig. 11 Infection-related forms of injury associated with defective macrophage bacterial killing or degradation. (**a**) Xanthogranulomatous pyelonephritis. There are foamy macrophages (xanthoma cells) on the right side (arrows) while multinucleated giant cells (arrowheads) are on the left side with an additional lymphocytic infiltrate. (Hematoxylin and eosin ×100). (**b**) Malakoplakia. The interstitium is infiltrated by lymphocytes and macrophages (also known as von Hansemann histiocytes), the latter containing cytoplasmic Michaelis-Gutmann bodies (arrows). (Periodic-acid Schiff ×600). (**c**) Megalocytic interstitial nephritis. There is a prominent interstitial infiltrate of macrophages which have abundant cytoplasm with fine PAS positive granular material (arrows) but no Michaelis-Gutmann bodies. (Periodic-acid Schiff ×400)

representing remnants of partially digested bacterial fragments. In contrast, megalocytic interstitial nephritis is bilateral in 80% of cases and usually involves the cortex with glomerular sparing. There is widespread infiltration with large macrophages containing granular PAS-positive cytoplasm but without Michaelis-Gutmann bodies. Due to the bilateral kidney involvement, patients present with an elevated serum creatinine and enlarged kidneys on imaging, mimicking amyloidosis or lymphoma. Experimental models suggest that this may be a less severe form or earlier stage of malakoplakia. In these forms of infectious IN, there is extensive macrophage staining for CD68.

4 Granulomatous Interstitial Nephritis

Granulomatous IN has a large differential diagnosis, which includes infectious, allergic, and autoimmune etiologies. The interstitial granulomas may be well or ill-defined, large or small, localized or diffuse, with or without multinucleated giant cells and may be an active and/or chronic process with interstitial edema or fibrosis, respectively (Fig. 12). Granulomas may be randomly present in the cortex or localized to the corticomedullary junction or in perivascular areas. There may be a paucity of other interstitial inflammation or an associated lymphocytic infiltrate and, other than with the infrequent case of intrarenal tuberculosis, the granulomas are rarely necrotizing. Most cases of granulomatous IN are due to a variety of medications or sarcoidosis with fewer cases related to other autoimmune diseases such as tubulointerstitial nephritis with uveitis and Sjogren's syndrome. Reactive granulomas can be observed secondary to irritating material (THP, crystals) or glomerular rupture in crescentic glomerulonephritis, in immune reconstitution syndrome with HIV infection, and as a reaction to intravesicular Bacillus Calmette-Guerin instillation,. In up to 10% of cases, no etiology for granulomatous IN is identified.

As treatment of medication or autoimmune mediated granulomatous IN often includes immunosuppression, exclusion of an infectious etiology is crucial. Intrarenal fungal infections may evoke granulomas, although these are rare in the absence of immunosuppression in developed countries. Fungal organisms may be identified by routine light microscopic stains used in kidney biopsy pathology, including Period acid Schiff (PAS) and Jones methenamine silver. A more targeted fungal stain is Gomori methenamine silver (GMS) (Fig. 13). Granulomatous IN can be caused by mycobacterium avium complex (MAC) bacteria. Tuberculosis typically causes necrotizing granuloma formation although with immunosuppression, including active HIV infection, the granulomas may be non-necrotizing. Ziehl-Neelon or Kinyoun acid fast bacteria (AFB) stains and a more sensitive IF antibody stain will identify MAC bacteria (Fig. 14). Culture of the kidney biopsy tissue is more sensitive than staining to detect these infections.

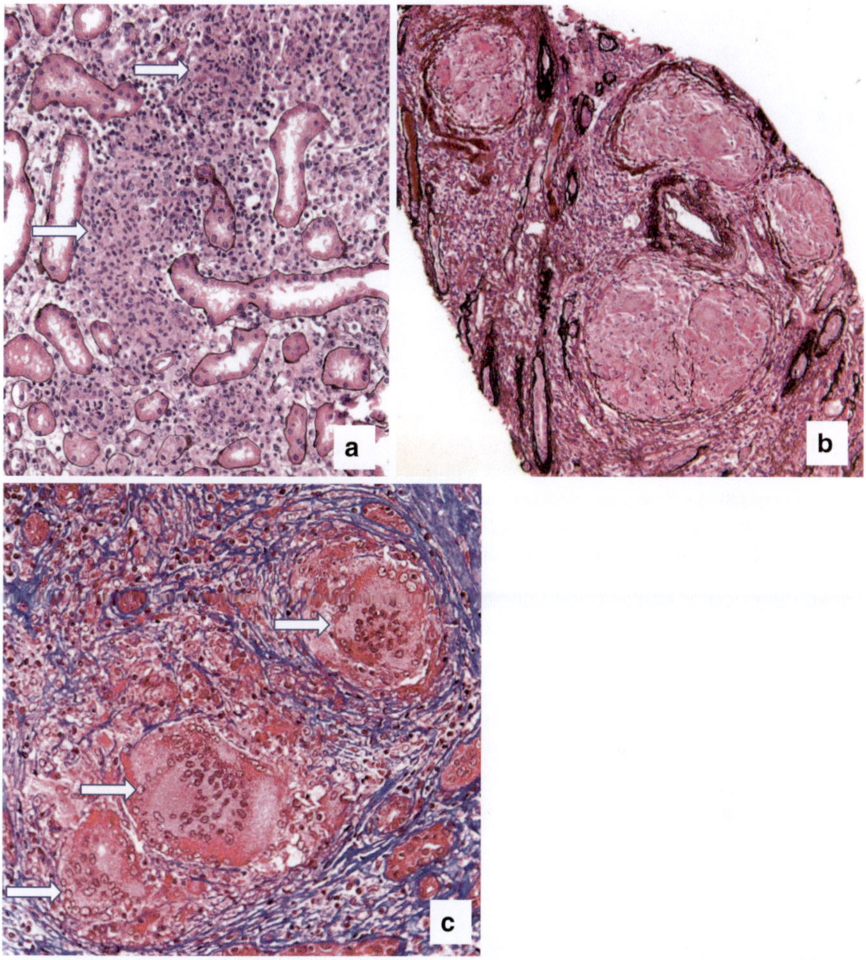

Fig. 12 Granulomatous interstitial nephritis. (**a**) The interstitium contains ill-defined granulomas (arrows) without necrosis, giant cells or tubular inflammation, although there is acute tubular cell injury. (Jones methenamine silver ×200). (**b**) There are large extensive non-necrotizing granulomas obliterating the normal cortical architecture. (Jones methenamine silver ×100). (**c**) Interstitial granulomas with prominent giant cells (arrows) and considerable associated interstitial fibrosis. (Masson's trichrome ×200)

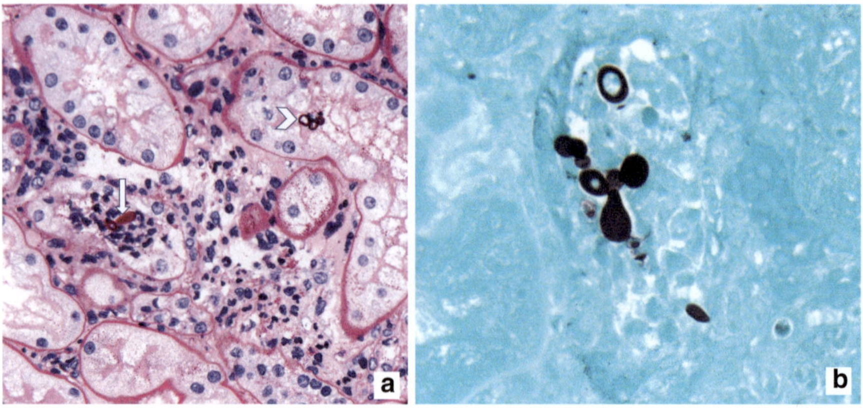

Fig. 13 Tubulointerstitial nephritis due to fungal infection. (**a**) There is a mixed inflammatory infiltrate including neutrophils around and within a tubule which has a luminal fungal organism (cryptococcus, arrow) staining positively with PAS. Note there is a tubule with a fungal organism in the lumen (arrowhead) but no associated intratubular inflammation. (Periodic-acid Schiff ×600). (**b**) The fungal organisms are highlighted in black with a Gomori methenamine silver stain. (×800)

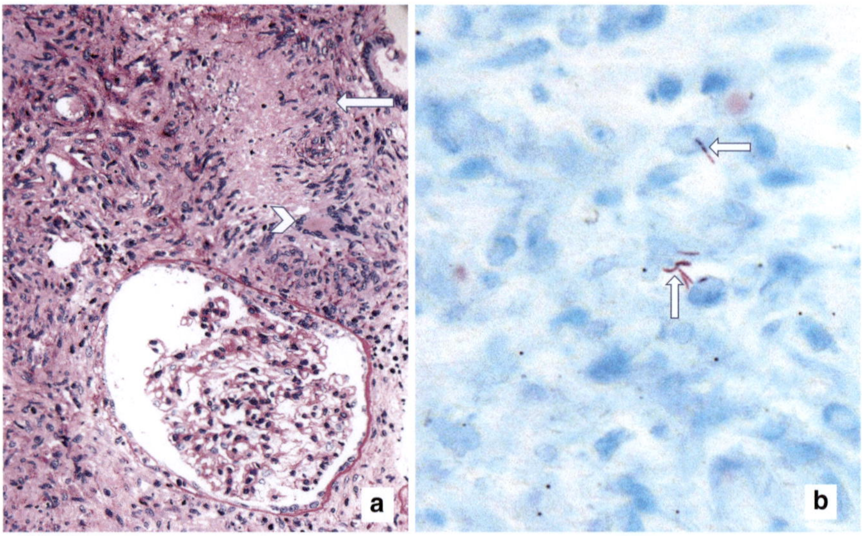

Fig. 14 Kidney with tuberculosis infection. (**a**) There is a necrotizing granuloma (arrow) containing a giant cell (arrowhead). (Periodic-acid Schiff ×200). (**b**) Acid fast stain highlighting the bacillus organisms in red (arrows). (×800)

5 Autoimmune Tubulointerstitial Nephritis

Autoimmune IN may be lymphocyte or plasma cell rich with varied histology and may or may not be associated with extra-glomerular immune complex deposition depending on the underlying disease. Plasma cells are particularly prominent in IgG4-related disease, Sjogren's syndrome, and anti-LRP2 nephropathy, and less often in lupus-related IN (Table 2).

Table 2 Etiologies of interstitial nephritis that may be plasma cell rich

Disease	Histologic features	IF and EM features	Associated findings
IgG4 -related disease	Abundant IgG4 plasma cells a diagnostic feature, expansile, storiform fibrosis with "bird's eye" pattern, glomerular sparing	Frequent TBM immune complex deposits of IgG/IgG4, C3, kappa, lambda +/− C1q, IgA or IgM	May be membranous nephropathy
Systemic lupus erythematosus	Mixed mononuclear inflammation often with T cells	Extra-glomerular deposits, "full house" IF, fingerprint deposits, TRIs	Usually associated with proliferative glomerulonephritis
Sjogren's syndrome	70% with prominent plasma cells, often many T cells, may be macrophages, granulomas, B cell aggregates	Rarely associated with TBM immune complex deposits of IgG and C3	Immune complex glomerulonephritis occurs usually without interstitial nephritis
Anti-LRP2 nephropathy	Mixed mononuclear inflammation, typically lymphocyte rich, variable TBM thickening	IgG and C3 deposits in TBMs +/− apical brush border IgG staining	IHC to identify LRP2. May be membranous nephropathy with LRP2 negative deposits
Viral infection (polyoma, adenovirus, CMV)	Mixed mononuclear inflammation, may be neutrophils particularly with necrosis, tubulitis, sloughed necrotic tubular cells, tubular cell inclusions	May be TBM immune complex deposits of IgG, IgM, C3	IHC used to identify specific virus
Chronic pyelonephritis	Mixed mononuclear inflammation, neutrophils in active infection, may be tubular thyroidization, may be focal or prominent in the medulla	Non-contributory	May be associated with obstruction or reflux
Crescentic glomerulonephritis	Mixed mononuclear inflammation, plasma cells may be IgG4 positive	Pauci-immune or linear IgG in GBMs may be present	Interstitial karyorrhexis or necrosis, medullary capillaritis are clues to ANCA-associated disease

(continued)

Table 2 (continued)

Disease	Histologic features	IF and EM features	Associated findings
Castleman's disease, multicentric plasma cell type	Associated lymphocytes, may have marked increase in IgG4 positive plasma cells in ANCA-associated disease	IHC for human herpesvirus 8 usually negative	May be HIV infection, membranous nephropathy, mesangial proliferative glomerulonephritis, amyloidosis
HIV infection	Some CD8+ cells, macrophages	Non-contributory	May be related to HIV itself, drugs, other infections, dysimmunity, or malignancy; 20% of unknown cause

Abbreviations: *IF* immunofluorescence, *EM* electron microscopy, *TBM* tubular basement membrane, *TRIs* tubuloreticular inclusions, *LRP2* LDL Receptor-Related Protein 2, *IHC* immunohistochemistry, *GBM* glomerular basement membrane

6 Immune Complex-Mediated Tubulointerstitial Nephritis

Immune complexes may be generated in autoimmune disease and less often infections such as polyomavirus, drug exposures, and malignancy. In TIN secondary to immune complexes, they usually deposit in extra-glomerular locations with IF and EM findings providing clues to underlying disease (Table 3). The interstitial inflammation can vary from minimal to extensive and may be plasma cell rich.

In systemic lupus erythematosus, TIN is typically associated with active glomerulonephritis but uncommonly occurs with preferential or isolated tubulointerstitial involvement. Lupus-related TIN was found to have a predominance of CD4+ cells in some studies, while others have identified more tubulointerstitial CD8+ cells, the latter prominently in intratubular lymphocytes. Other studies have identified more CD8+ cells with additional B cell rich lymphoid follicles and aggregates of T and B cells; the latter contained $CD138^{+}CD20^{low/-}$ plasmablasts and is associated with TBM immune complex deposition (Fig. 15). There can be "full house" IF with TBM, interstitial and/or peritubular capillary wall deposits staining for IgG, IgA, IgM, C1q and C3. These are seen as electron dense deposits by EM, and rarely may have a "fingerprint" substructure, a feature thought to be diagnostically relevant for lupus nephritis. The presence of tubuloreticular inclusions, identified by EM, is also strongly suggestive of, but not diagnostic for lupus nephritis.

Primary TIN can result from antigen-specific antibodies, located in the proximal tubules.

This disease, initially termed anti-brush border antibody (ABBA) disease, is now more specifically called anti-LRP2 nephropathy as proximal tubular cell injury is due to circulating antibodies against the brush border LDL Receptor-Related Protein 2, also known as megalin. This results in TIN which is usually lymphocyte predominant but can have a prominent plasma cell component and TBMs can be variably thickened. By IF, there is segmental to global granular TBM and Bowman's capsule staining for

Table 3 Interstitial nephritis with tubulointerstitial immune complex deposits

	Histologic features		Ancillary studies		
Disease	*Inflammatory infiltrate*	*Plasma cells*	*Special stains*	*IF findings*	*EM findings*
Systemic lupus erythematosus	Mixed interstitial inflammation, typically T cell predominant	Variable, can be plasma cell rich	Non-contributcry	Prominent full house glomerular and extra-glomerular deposits, "tissue ANA"	Electron dense deposits, "fingerprint" substructure, TRIs
Idiopathic hypocomplementemic interstitial nephritis	Mixed interstitial inflammation	Variable	IgG4 IHC demonstrating <10 IgG4+ plasma cells per HPF (40×)	Prominent Ig and complement staining in TBMs, often "full house" and C1q	Electron dense deposits in tubulointerstitium lacking substructure; TRI's should prompt exclusion of SLE
Anti-LRP2 nephropathy	Mixed interstitial inflammation, typically lymphocyte rich, variable TBM thickening	Variable	Staining of TBM's with anti-LRP2 antibody	Ig's and C3 staining in TBMs, some with apical brush border IgG staining	Typical electron dense deposits in TBM's and some along apical brush border
IgG4 -related disease	Expansile, mixed interstitial inflammation, storiform fibrosis	Plasma cell rich	IgG4 IHC demonstrating >10 IgG4+ plasma cells per HPF (40×)	Ig's and C3 staining in TBMs and interstitium, some with C1q	Typical electron dense deposits in TBMs and interstitium
Sjogren's syndrome	Mixed tubulointerstitial inflammation, prominent T cells	70% with prominent plasma cells	Non-contributory	IgG and C3 staining rarely described in TBMs	Typical electron dense deposits in TBMs
Viral infection	Mixed infiltrate, may be neutrophils with necrosis	Variable, can be plasma cell rich	IHC for viral antigens (see Table 1)	IgG and C3 staining in TBMs	Typical electron dense deposits in TBMs, viral particles

Abbreviations: *IF* immunofluorescence, *EM* electron microscopy, *ANA* anti-nuclear antibody, *TRI* tubuloreticular inclusion, *TBM* tubular basement membrane, *Ig* immunoglobulin, *LRP2* LDL Receptor-Related Protein 2, *IHC* immunohistochemistry

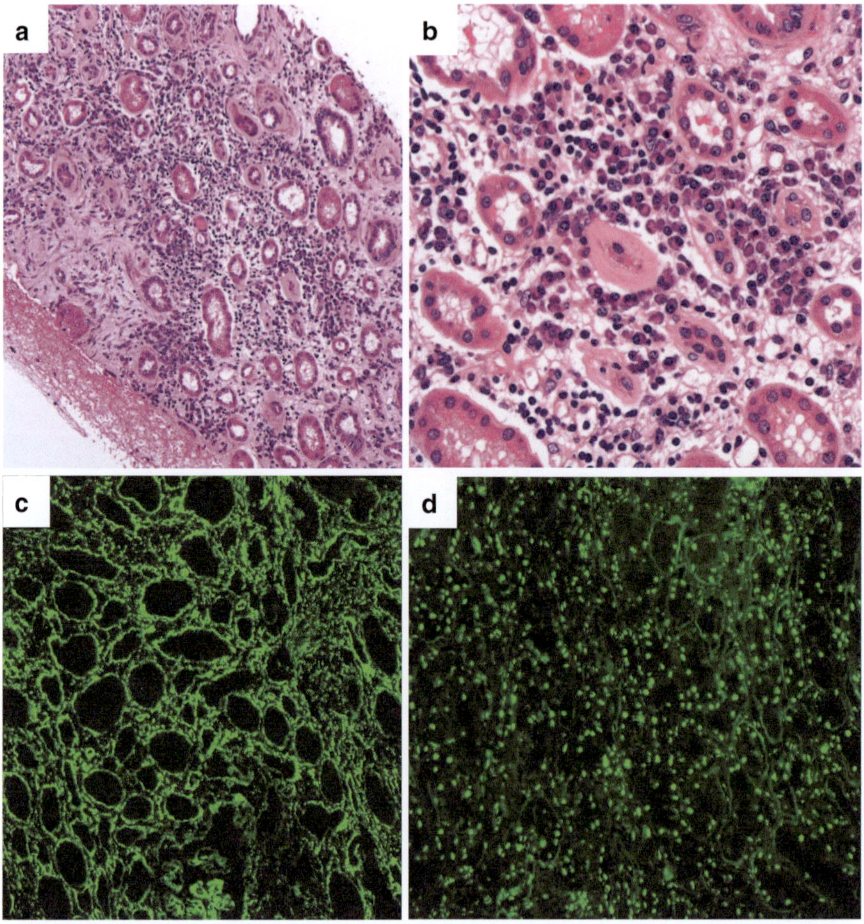

Fig. 15 Systemic lupus erythematosus-related interstitial nephritis. (**a**) There is a diffuse interstitial inflammatory infiltrate. (Hematoxylin and eosin ×100). (**b**) The interstitial inflammation is plasma cell rich and associated with edema. (Hematoxylin and eosin ×400). (**c**) Immunofluorescence showing granular staining for IgG in the tubular basement membranes, interstitium and peritubular capillary walls. (×200). (**d**) All parenchymal cell nuclei are staining for IgG in the pattern of a "tissue positive" ANA. (×200). (**e**) Electron microscopy showing numerous circumferential electron dense deposits (arrows) in a segmentally thickened tubular basement membrane. (×1200). (**f**) Electron dense deposits with a prominent "fingerprint" substructure in a tubular basement membrane. (×20,000). (**g**) Electron microscopy of an endothelial cell showing a tubuloreticular inclusion (arrow). (×40,000)

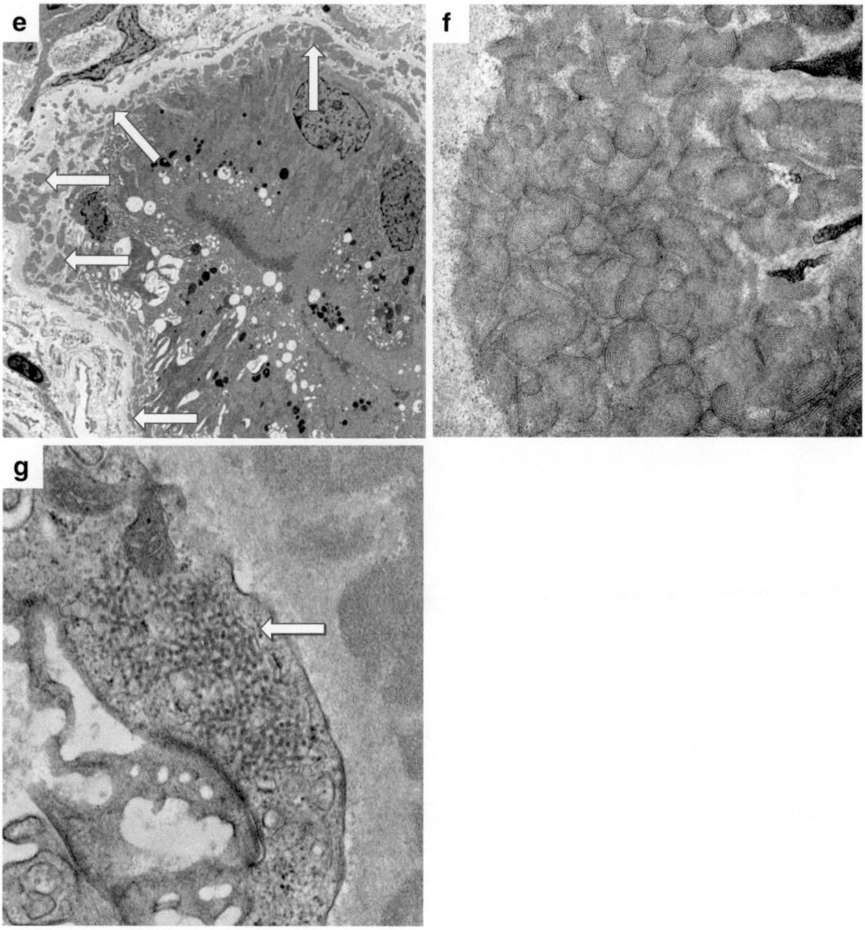

Fig. 15 (continued)

IgG and C3 staining with a subset of cases also showing segmental granular staining for IgG along the proximal tubular apical border (Fig. 16). These deposits correspond to electron dense deposits by EM, localized along the basolateral aspect of the TBMs and the apical surface of tubular epithelial cells. The diagnosis can be confirmed by IF staining with an antibody against LRP2 as well as colocalization of LRP2 and IgG.

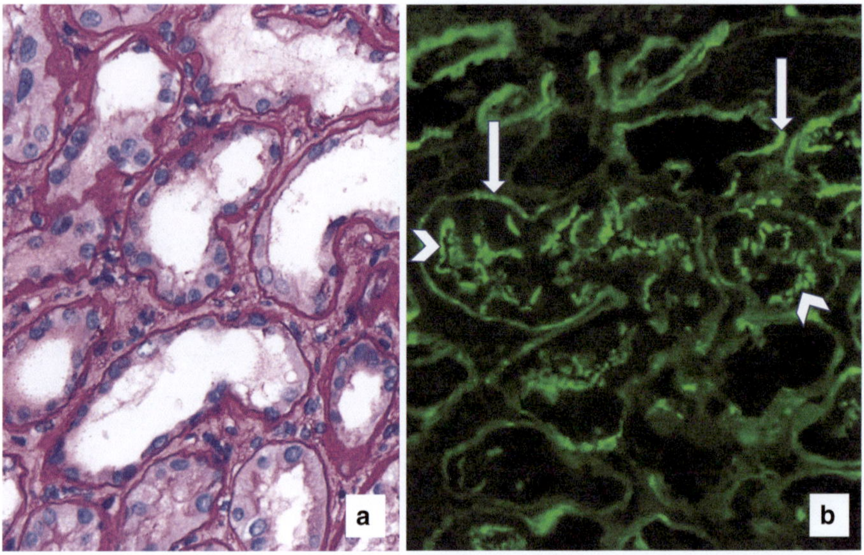

Fig. 16 Anti-LRP2 nephropathy. (**a**) Proximal tubules showing acute epithelial cell injury with mild interstitial edema and inflammation. (Periodic-acid Schiff ×400). (**b**) Immunofluorescence reveals staining for IgG in tubular basement membrane deposits (arrows) and in the apical brush border of proximal tubules (arrowheads) (×400)

7 Other Autoimmune Tubulointerstitial Nephritis

TIN associated with primary Sjogren's syndrome may be associated with IgG and C3 immune complex deposits and there has been a suggestion that anti-brush border antibodies may be related to the disease. However, the inflammation more often occurs without such deposits. There usually is a chronic active TIN and acute tubular injury may occur. In 70% of biopsies from patients with Sjogren's disease there is a prominent plasma cell component, which is dominant in 25% of cases. CD4+ cells predominate although CD68 (M1) and CD163 (M2) macrophages have been reported as prominent cell types, and occasionally granulomas or B cell nodules are seen.

IgG4-related disease is a presumed autoimmune or chronic allergic fibroinflammatory condition that can affect any organ and form mass-like lesions. Light microscopy typically reveals dense interstitial inflammation, which is plasma cell rich and often contains prominent eosinophils. The characteristic finding is that of a whirling, storiform (bird's eye) pattern of interstitial fibrosis similar to findings of other involved organs, although a small subset of IgG4-related TIN cases show an acute interstitial nephritis pattern without this fibrosis (Fig. 17). Immunohistochemical

Fig. 17 IgG4-related disease. (**a**) There is extensive storiform fibrosis causing obliteration of the cortical architecture. (Jones methenamine silver ×200). (**b**) Extensive interstitial plasma cell infiltration. (Hematoxylin and eosin ×400). (**c**) Positive IgG4 immunohistochemical stain in many plasma cells, involving more than 10/40× high power field. (×600). (**d**) Immunofluorescence showing granular deposits staining for IgG in the interstitium and tubular basement membranes (×200). (**e**) Electron microscopy reveals corresponding typical electron dense deposits in a tubular basement membrane. The deposits range in size from small and discrete to large and confluent (arrows). (×7500)

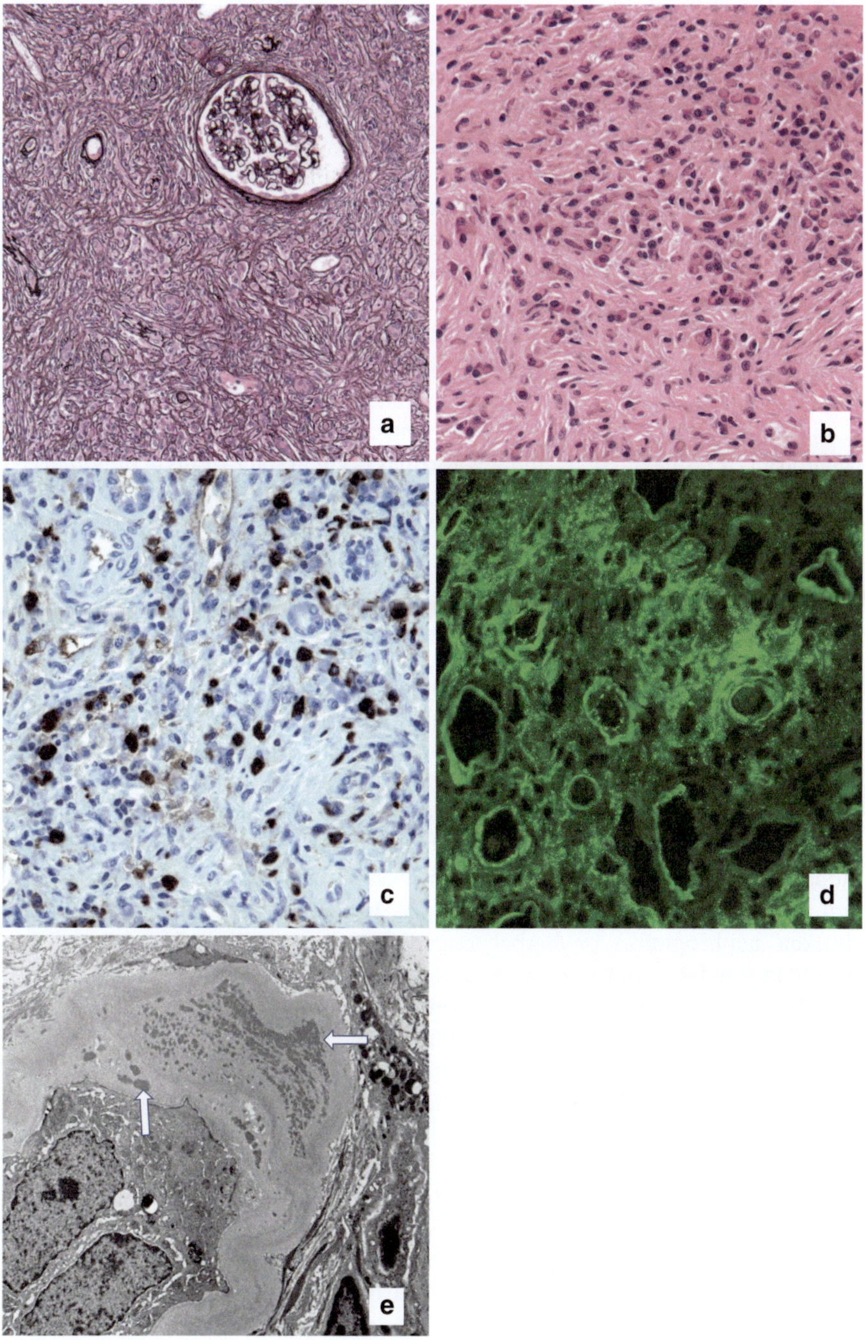
a
b
c
d
e

staining for CD138 or IgG highlights the plasma cells and the IgG4-positive plasma cells, which then can be quantified. For the kidney, it has been suggested that >10 IgG4 positive plasma cells per high power field (40× lens) may have acceptable specificity for a diagnosis of IgG4-related TIN, with the exceptions noted below. In >80% of cases, TBMs contain immune complex deposits, which also stain for nonspecific IgG, kappa and lambda light chains, and C3, with variable staining for C1q and other immunoglobulins by IF. By EM, discrete electron dense deposits are found in TBMs and have been reported on interstitial collagen fibers. A lesion associated with hypocomplementemia and tubulointerstitial immune complex deposits has been termed idiopathic hypocomplementemic interstitial nephritis; however, on careful review these likely are cases of IgG4 related disease. There are settings in which the number of IgG4 plasma cells meets criteria for IgG4-related disease but without the storiform fibrosing pattern. These include chronic pyelonephritis, diabetic kidney disease, and autoimmune diseases such as lupus nephritis, ANCA vasculitis, and anti-LRP2 nephropathy. Plasma cell rich infiltrates also may occur in some forms of drug-induced IN and associated with HIV infection or multicentric Castleman's disease.

8 Chronic Interstitial Nephropathies

There are some settings in which chronic IN occurs without preceding acute injury and can be considered chronic tubulointerstitial nephropathies (Fig. 18). In these instances, the tubulointerstitial scarring is disproportionate to the degree of glomerular or vascular sclerosis and often has a paucity of interstitial inflammation. This pattern of injury occurs with nephrotoxicity due to a small number of medications including calcineurin inhibitors and lithium, the former inducing a pattern of striped fibrosis and arteriolar hyalinization with peripheral adventitial hyaline nodules. Exposure to aristolochic acid either in food (Balkan nephropathy) or herbal remedies (aristolochic acid nephropathy) results in tubular atrophy and interstitial fibrosis occurring over a few years to decades typically with minimal interstitial inflammation. Patients with asymptomatic leptospirosis may present with chronic kidney disease and a chronic TIN with minimal to moderate interstitial inflammation. In this setting, a high index of suspicion and clinical correlation are required to recognize the possible infectious etiology of the kidney disease. Chronic interstitial nephritis in agricultural communities, a progressive chronic kidney disease occurring in poor agricultural regions also termed Mesoamerican nephropathy and CKDu, is characterized by tubulointerstitial fibrosis as the primary process with a variable interstitial and infrequent intratubular inflammatory infiltrate. Proximal tubular cell dysmorphic lysosomes have been described in cases of Mesoamerican nephropathy/CKDu, as well as in calcineurin inhibitor toxicity. Methenamine silver staining will often demonstrate proximal tubular silver positive granular cytoplasmic inclusions most prominently in cells of atrophic tubules. EM

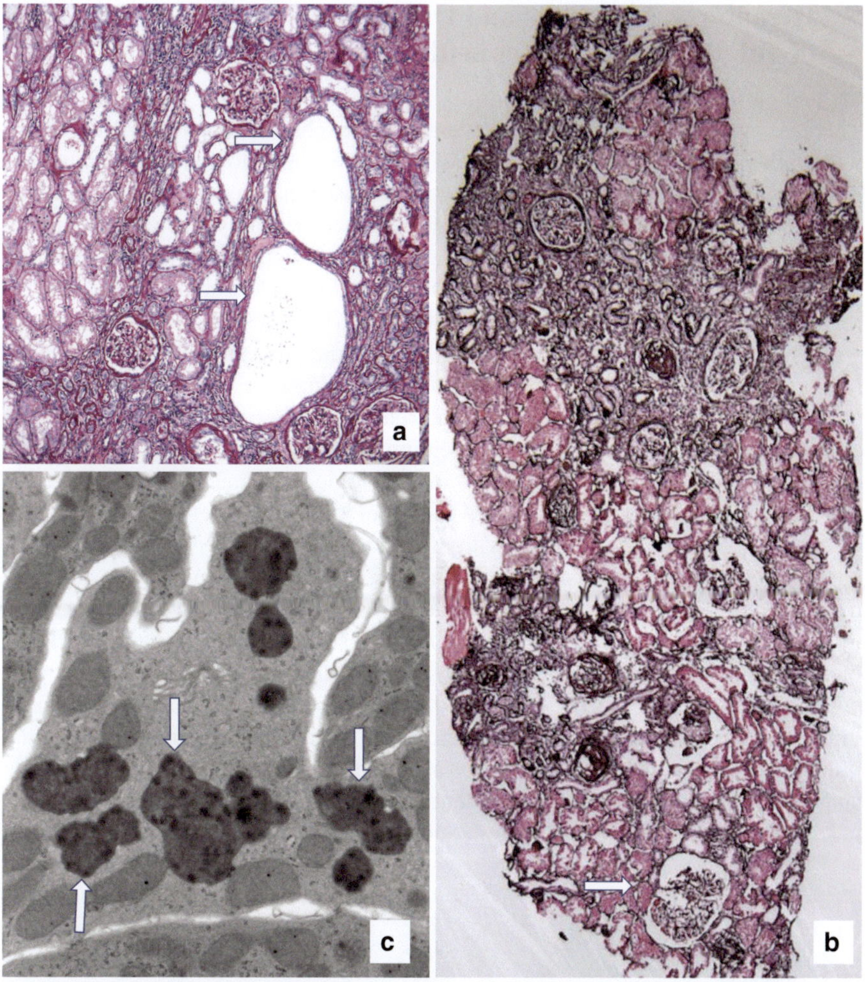

Fig. 18 (**a**) Lithium nephrotoxicity. There is focal cortical tubular atrophy with interstitial fibrosis associated with a very mild patchy lymphocytic interstitial infiltrate. Note the two cystically dilated tubules (arrows), which are characteristic of lithium nephrotoxicity. (Periodic-acid Schiff ×100). (**b**, **c**) Chronic interstitial nephritis in agricultural communities (Mesoamerican nephropathy/CKDu). The cortex shows focal areas of tubular atrophy and interstitial fibrosis with minor inflammation. There is one enlarged glomerulus (arrow) and other glomeruli show varying ischemic injury. (**c**, Jones methenamine silver ×40). Electron microscopy demonstrates proximal tubular cell large dysmorphic lysosomes containing dispersed electron dense aggregates. (**c**, ×8000)

reveals these granules to be dysmorphic lysosomes, which can be considerably enlarged with irregular contours and contain smaller dispersed electron densities.

9 Hereditary, Metabolic and Other Types of Tubulointerstitial Nephritis

There is a number of genetic disorders that result in chronic tubulointerstitial injury with variable inflammation appearing as TIN. Autosomal dominant tubulointerstitial kidney disease (ADTKD) is a collection of diseases caused by different specified or sometimes unknown mutations and is characterized by non-specific tubular atrophy with interstitial fibrosis and often with minimal inflammation. There are several involved genes, which engage different pathways leading to a similar histologic picture with few clues in specific settings. Mutations in *REN* are associated with enlarged juxtaglomerular apparatus. *UMOD* mutations may result in accumulation of Tamm-Horsfall protein in the thick ascending limb and distal tubular cell, appearing by EM as intracellular medium electron dense granular material in an expanded hyperplastic endoplasmic reticulum; this is the one form of ADTKD that can be diagnosed on kidney biopsy by its histologic appearance. The diagnosis of ADTKD depends on eliciting a family history of kidney disease.

Nephronophthisis, a ciliopathy with mutations in one of the *NPHP* gene family, has progressive tubulointerstitial scarring with or without tubular cysts and may have interstitial inflammation later in the course of disease. Karyomegalic IN is most often genetic due to mutations in *FAN1* resulting in dysregulation of DNA interstrand cross-link repair. This causes focally injured tubular epithelium with enlarged dysmorphic nuclei, attenuated cytoplasm, and sloughing into tubular lumens often associated with tubulointerstitial scarring and variable interstitial inflammation (Fig. 19). This also can be acquired due to drugs including ifosfamide and nivolumab; the IN is more prominent in the drug-induced form. Interestingly, a recent report linked a *UMOD* mutation to karyomegalic IN. Patients with

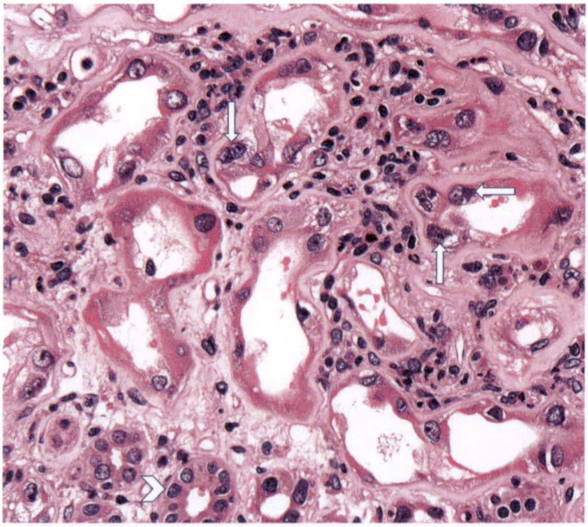

Fig. 19 Karyomegalic interstitial nephritis. There are focal tubular cells with enlarged abnormally shaped nuclei and variably attenuated cytoplasm (arrows). Compare these to normal tubular cell nuclei (arrowhead). The interstitium has a mild to moderate lymphocyte predominant infiltrate without tubular inflammation. (Hematoxylin and eosin ×600)

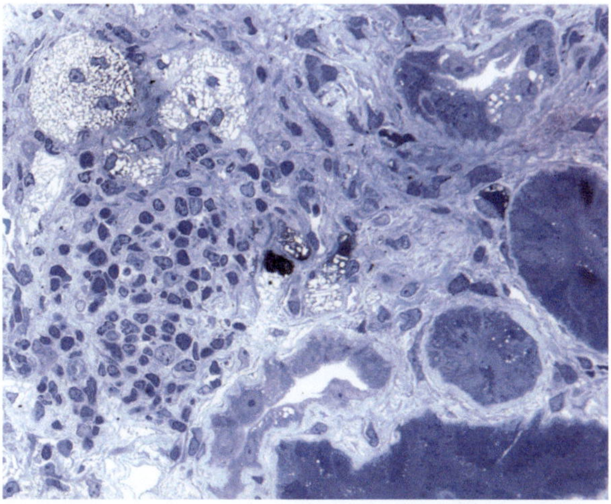

Fig. 20 Cystinosis. The cortical interstitium has an infiltrate of lymphocytes and macrophages, the latter containing cytoplasmic geometric rectangular to rhomboid crystals. Rare tubular cells also have fewer numbers of crystals in the cytoplasm. (Methylene blue ×600)

nephropathic cystinosis will develop chronic IN with interstitial macrophages containing cysteine crystals, which are best visualized in plastic sections and by EM as acicular or rhomboid empty cytoplasmic structures (Fig. 20).

IN occurs in some patients with metabolic disorders that may be genetic or acquired. Oxalate nephropathy may be primary or secondary and is characterized by oxalate deposition in tubular lumens and often in the interstitium with acute tubular injury, variable interstitial inflammation and development of tubulointerstitial scarring (Fig. 21). Uric acid nephropathy occurs when uric acid deposits in tubular lumens as clear crystals in a "sheaves of wheat" pattern or as amorphous material, preferentially in the medulla (Fig. 22). Tubules may rupture resulting in interstitial uric acid and a reactive macrophage or granulomatous response requiring differentiation from other forms of granulomatous IN.

Disorders inducing tubular cell injury may have an accompanying interstitial inflammatory component which may mimic IN. In patients with monoclonal immunoglobulin deposition disease, acute TIN reflects injury from the deposition of the monoclonal protein in the extracellular kidney compartments. This is a diffuse process throughout the parenchyma, is composed of mononuclear leukocytes often with some reactive neutrophils, and may be acute or chronic active with associated acute tubular injury. IF demonstrates linear staining of kidney structures for the monoclonal protein. Tubulotoxic casts may also evoke a tubulointerstitial inflammatory reaction appearing as IN or TIN. These include Bence Jones cast nephropathy (myeloma kidney), myoglobin casts in rhabdomyolysis, and drug-related casts or crystals.

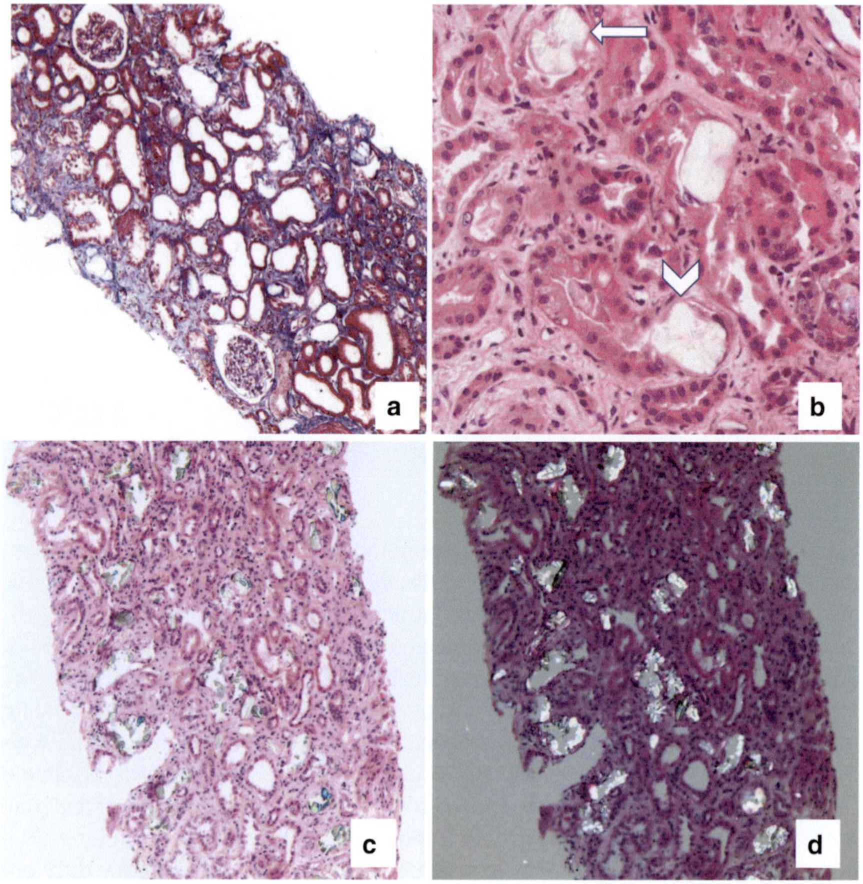

Fig. 21 Oxalate nephropathy. (**a**) The cortex has extensive acute tubular injury with epithelial cell flattening and severe luminal dilatation; oxalate crystals are not apparent with this magnification and stain. (Masson's trichrome ×200.) (**b**) Areas of tubular injury are associated with intratubular crystalline deposits which are angulated and can assume a "fan-like" appearance (arrow), with focal tubular basement membrane rupture (arrowhead). (Hematoxylin and eosin ×400). (**c**) There is an interstitial moderate mixed interstitial inflammatory infiltrate with numerous crystalline deposits located within the lumens of severely injured tubules. (Hematoxylin and eosin ×200). (**d**) The crystalline deposits show birefringence when viewed with polarized light. (Hematoxylin and eosin ×200)

10 Mimics of Tubulointerstitial Nephritis

Interstitial and tubulointerstitial inflammatory infiltrates may occur in some disease process that are not reflective of TIN. Patients with CLL, other lymphomas or leukemia may have kidney infiltration of malignant hematologic cells either in aggregates or diffusely. The cells are either monomorphic or have an atypical appearance indicative of malignant transformation and an appropriate hematopathology

Fig. 22 There is uric acid deposition in a "sheaves of wheat" pattern of crystallization, which has extended into the interstitium and elicited a granulomatous and giant cell reaction. (Jones methenamine silver ×400)

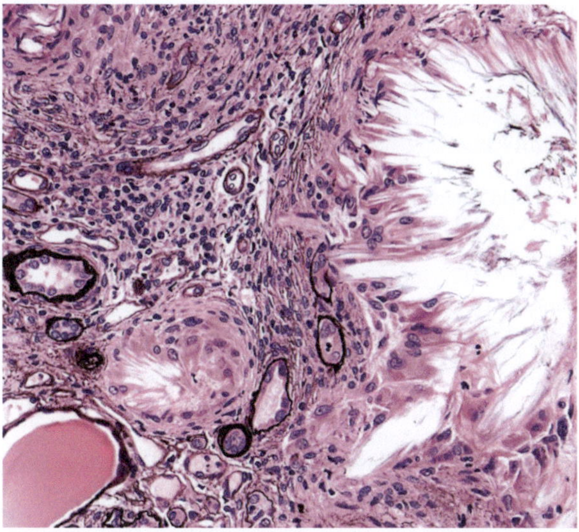

evaluation is required for a diagnosis. Extramedullary hematopoiesis infrequently occurs in the kidney interstitium in patients with hematologic malignancies and often is associated with a glomerulopathy.

Suggested Reading

al-Sulaiman MH, al-Khader AA, Mousa DH, al-Swailem RY, Dhar J, Haleem A. Renal parenchymal malacoplakia and megalocytic interstitial nephritis: clinical and histological features. Report of two cases and review of the literature. Am J Nephrol. 1993;13(6):483–8. https://doi.org/10.1159/000168668.

Alexander MP, Nasr SH, Kurtin PJ, Casey ET, Hernandez LP, Fidler ME, et al. Renal extramedullary hematopoiesis: interstitial and glomerular pathology. Mod Pathol. 2015;28(12):1574–83. https://doi.org/10.1038/modpathol.2015.117.

Alroy J, Sabnis S, Kopp JB. Renal pathology in Fabry disease. J Am Soc Nephrol. 2002;13(suppl 2):S134–S38.

Austin HA 3rd, Muenz LR, Joyce KM, Antonovych TA, Kullick ME, Klippel JH, et al. Prognostic factors in lupus nephritis. Contribution of renal histologic data. Am J Med. 1983;75(3):382–91. https://doi.org/10.1016/0002-9343(83)90338-8.

Bajema IM, Wilhelmus S, Alpers CE, Bruijn JA, Colvin RB, Cook HT, et al. Revision of the International Society of Nephrology/Renal Pathology Society classification for lupus nephritis: clarification of definitions, and modified National Institutes of Health activity and chronicity indices. Kidney Int. 2018;93(4):789–96. https://doi.org/10.1016/j.kint.2017.11.023.

Baker RJ, Pusey CD. The changing profile of acute tubulointerstitial nephritis. Nephrol Dial Transplant. 2004;19(1):8–11. https://doi.org/10.1093/ndt/gfg464.

Belliere J, Colombat M, Kounde C, Recher C, Ribes D, Huart A, et al. Kidney involvement in patients with chronic myelomonocytic leukemia or BCR-ABL-Negative myeloproliferative neoplasms. Kidney Int Rep. 2021;6(3):737–45. https://doi.org/10.1016/j.ekir.2020.12.005.

Belliere J, Meyer N, Mazieres J, Ollier S, Boulinguez S, Delas A, et al. Acute interstitial nephritis related to immune checkpoint inhibitors. Br J Cancer. 2016;115(12):1457–61. https://doi.org/10.1038/bjc.2016.358.

Berney-Meyer L, Hung N, Slatter T, Schollum JB, Kitching AR, Walker RJ. Omeprazole-induced acute interstitial nephritis: a possible Th1-Th17-mediated injury? Nephrology (Carlton). 2014;19(6):359–65. https://doi.org/10.1111/nep.12226.

Bhasin B, Ürekli HM, Atta MG. Primary and secondary hyperoxaluria: understanding the enigma. World J Nephrol. 2015;4(2):235–44. https://doi.org/10.5527/wjn.v4.i2.235.

Bijol V, Mendez GP, Nosé V, Rennke HG. Granulomatous interstitial nephritis: a clinicopathologic study of 46 cases from a single institution. Int J Surg Pathol. 2006;14(1):57–63. https://doi.org/10.1177/106689690601400110.

Bitik B, Gonul II, Haznedaroglu S, Goker B, Tufan A. Granulomatous interstitial nephritis associated with primary Sjögren's syndrome. Z Rheumatol. 2017;76(5):458–60. https://doi.org/10.1007/s00393-017-0269-5.

Blank U, Essig M, Scandiuzzi L, Benhamou M, Kanamaru Y. Mast cells and inflammatory kidney disease. Immunol Rev. 2007;217:79–95. https://doi.org/10.1111/j.1600-065X.2007.00503.x.

Bledsoe JR, Della-Torre E, Rovati L, Deshpande V. IgG4-related disease: review of the histopathologic features, differential diagnosis, and therapeutic approach. APMIS. 2018;126(6):459–76. https://doi.org/10.1111/apm.12845.

Boffa JJ, Esteve E, Buob D. Renal involvement in IgG4-related disease. Presse Med. 2020;49(1):104017. https://doi.org/10.1016/j.lpm.2020.104017.

Bracamonte E, Leca N, Smith KD, Nicosia RF, Nickeleit V, Kendrick E, et al. Tubular basement membrane immune deposits in association with BK polyomavirus nephropathy. Am J Transplant. 2007;7(6):1552–60. https://doi.org/10.1111/j.1600-6143.2007.01794.x.

Brentjens JR, Sepulveda M, Baliah T, Bentzel C, Erlanger BF, Elwood C, et al. Interstitial immune complex nephritis in patients with systemic lupus erythematosus. Kidney Int. 1975;7(5):342–50. https://doi.org/10.1038/ki.1975.47.

Buettner M, Xu H, Bohme R, Seliger B, Jacobi J, Wiesener M, et al. Predominance of TH2 cells and plasma cells in polyoma virus nephropathy: a role for humoral immunity? Hum Pathol. 2012;43(9):1453–62. https://doi.org/10.1016/j.humpath.2011.11.006.

Buglioni A, Hasadsri L, Nasr SH, Hogan MC, Moyer AM, Siddique K, et al. Mitochondriopathy manifesting as inherited tubulointerstitial nephropathy without symptomatic other organ involvement. Kidney Int Rep. 2021;6(9):2514–8.

Deshpande V, Zen Y, Chan JK, Yi EE, Sato Y, Yoshino T, et al. Consensus statement on the pathology of IgG4-related disease. Mod Pathol. 2012;25(9):1181–92. https://doi.org/10.1038/modpathol.2012.72.

Devuyst O, Olinger E, Weber S, Eckardt KU, Kmoch S, Rampoldi L, et al. Autosomal dominant tubulointerstitial kidney disease. Nat Rev Dis Primers. 2019;5(1):60. https://doi.org/10.1038/s41572-019-0109-9.

Eddy AA. Drug-induced tubulointerstitial nephritis: hypersensitivity and necroinflammatory pathways. Pediatr Nephrol. 2020;35(4):547–54. https://doi.org/10.1007/s00467-019-04207-9.

El Karoui K, Vuiblet V, Dion D, Izzedine H, Guitard J, Frimat L, et al. Renal involvement in Castleman disease. Nephrol Dial Transplant. 2011;26(2):599–609. https://doi.org/10.1093/ndt/gfq427.

Gaillard F, Ismael S, Sannier A, Tarhini H, Volpe T, Greze C, et al. Tubuloreticular inclusions in COVID-19-related collapsing glomerulopathy. Kidney Int. 2020;98(1):241. https://doi.org/10.1016/j.kint.2020.04.022.

Gerhardt RE, Loebl DH, Rao RN. Interstitial immunofluorescence in nephritis of Sjögren's syndrome. Clin Nephrol. 1978;10(5):201–7.

Greenhill AH, Norman ME, Cornfeld D, Chatten J, Buck B, Witzleben CL. Acute renal failure secondary to acute pyelonephritis. Clin Nephrol. 1977;8(3):400–3.

Györkey F, Min KW, Sincovics JG, Györkey P. Systemic lupus erythematosus and myxovirus. N Engl J Med. 1969;280(6):333. https://doi.org/10.1056/nejm196902062800620.

Herrera GA, Veeramachaneni R, Turbat-Herrera EA. Electron microscopy in the diagnosis of BK-polyoma virus infection in the transplanted kidney. Ultrastruct Pathol. 2005;29(6):469–74. https://doi.org/10.1080/01913120500323399.

Hess R, Oberbeck J, Grussenmeyer T, Schoeffel-Keller A, Haessler C, Braun DG, et al. PAb1614, a monoclonal antibody reactive with the tumor antigens of SV40, JC, BK, and polyoma virus, and other JC virus tumor antigen cross-reactive antibodies of the PAb1601-1636 panel. Intervirology. 1994;37(1):47–52. https://doi.org/10.1159/000150356.

Hever A, Nast CC. Polyoma virus nephropathy with simian virus 40 antigen-containing tubular basement membrane immune complex deposition. Hum Pathol. 2008;39(1):73–9. https://doi.org/10.1016/j.humpath.2007.05.006.

Hiromura K, Kurosawa M, Yano S, Naruse T. Tubulointerstitial mast cell infiltration in glomerulonephritis. Am J Kidney Dis. 1998;32(4):593–9. https://doi.org/10.1016/s0272-6386(98)70022-8.

Holdsworth SR, Summers SA. Role of mast cells in progressive renal diseases. J Am Soc Nephrol. 2008;19(12):2254–61. https://doi.org/10.1681/asn.2008010015.

Hultin S, Nahar K, Menzies AM, Long GV, Fernando SL, Atkinson V, et al. Histological diagnosis of immune checkpoint inhibitor induced acute renal injury in patients with metastatic melanoma: a retrospective case series report. BMC Nephrol. 2020;21(1):391. https://doi.org/10.1186/s12882-020-02044-9.

Hvala A, Kobenter T, Ferluga D. Fingerprint and other organised deposits in lupus nephritis. Wien Klin Wochenschr. 2000;112(15–16):711–5.

Joss N, Morris S, Young B, Geddes C. Granulomatous interstitial nephritis. Clin J Am Soc Nephrol. 2007;2(2):222–30. https://doi.org/10.2215/CJN.01790506.

Joyce E, Glasner P, Ranganathan S, Swiatecka-Urban A. Tubulointerstitial nephritis: diagnosis, treatment, and monitoring. Pediatr Nephrol. 2017;32(4):577–87. https://doi.org/10.1007/s00467-016-3394-5.

Kambham N, Markowitz GS, Tanji N, Mansukhani MM, Orazi A, D'Agati VD. Idiopathic hypocomplementemic interstitial nephritis with extensive tubulointerstitial deposits. Am J Kidney Dis. 2001;37(2):388–99. https://doi.org/10.1053/ajkd.2001.21320.

Korkes F, Favoretto RL, Bróglio M, Silva CA, Castro MG, Perez MD. Xanthogranulomatous pyelonephritis: clinical experience with 41 cases. Urology. 2008;71(2):178–80. https://doi.org/10.1016/j.urology.2007.09.026.

Krishnan N, Perazella MA. Drug-induced acute interstitial nephritis: pathology, pathogenesis, and treatment. Iran J Kidney Dis. 2015;9(1):3–13.

Kwon HJ, Yoo KH, Kim IY, Lee S, Jang HR, Kwon GY. Megalocytic interstitial nephritis following acute pyelonephritis with Escherichia coli bacteremia: a case report. J Korean Med Sci. 2015;30(1):110–4. https://doi.org/10.3346/jkms.2015.30.1.110.

Larsen CP, Trivin-Avillach C, Coles P, Collins AB, Merchant M, Ma H, et al. LDL receptor-related protein 2 (Megalin) as a target antigen in human kidney anti-brush border antibody disease. J Am Soc Nephrol. 2018;29(2):644–53. https://doi.org/10.1681/asn.2017060664.

Lee CJ, Suh KS, Kim KH, Chang YK, Na KR, Lee KW. The clinicopathologic significance of endothelial tubuloreticular inclusions in glomerular diseases. Ultrastruct Pathol. 2013;37(6):386–94. https://doi.org/10.3109/01913123.2013.814738.

Li L, Parwani AV. Xanthogranulomatous pyelonephritis. Arch Pathol Lab Med. 2011;135(5):671–4. https://doi.org/10.1043/2009-0769-RSR.1/10.5858/2009-0769-RSR.1.

Li P, Cheng D, Wen J, Ni X, Li X, Xie K, et al. The immunophenotyping of different stages of BK virus allograft nephropathy. Ren Fail. 2019;41(1):855–61. https://doi.org/10.1080/0886022X.2019.1617168.

Lin ZS, Liu XL, Cui Z, Wang SX, Yu F, Zhou FD, et al. Acute tubulointerstitial nephritis with germinal centers in antineutrophil cytoplasmic antibody-associated vasculitis: a case report and literature review. Medicine (Baltimore). 2019;98(48):e18178. https://doi.org/10.1097/MD.0000000000018178.

Lumlertgul N, Siribamrungwong M, Jaber BL, Susantitaphong P. Secondary oxalate nephropathy: a systematic review. Kidney Int Rep. 2018;3(6):1363–72. https://doi.org/10.1016/j.ekir.2018.07.020.

Melica G, Matignon M, Desvaux D, Audard V, Copie-Bergman C, Lang P, et al. Acute interstitial nephritis with predominant plasmacytic infiltration in patients with HIV-1 infection. Am J Kidney Dis. 2012;59(5):711–4. https://doi.org/10.1053/j.ajkd.2011.12.017.

Mihatsch MJ. Polyomavirus nephropathy: a brief review with special emphasis on clinico-pathological aspects. Prilozi. 2012;33(2):5–22.

Moledina DG, Perazella MA. The challenges of acute interstitial nephritis: time to standardize. Kidney360. 2021;2(6):1051–5. 20517290

Muriithi AK, Leung N, Valeri AM, Cornell LD, Sethi S, Fidler ME, et al. Biopsy-proven acute interstitial nephritis, 1993-2011: a case series. Am J Kidney Dis. 2014;64(4):558–66. https://doi.org/10.1053/j.ajkd.2014.04.027.

Muriithi AK, Nasr SH, Leung N. Utility of urine eosinophils in the diagnosis of acute interstitial nephritis. Clin J Am Soc Nephrol. 2013;8(11):1857–62. https://doi.org/10.2215/cjn.01330213.

Nast CC. Medication-induced interstitial nephritis in the 21st century. Adv Chronic Kidney Dis. 2017;24(2):72–9. https://doi.org/10.1053/j.ackd.2016.11.016.

Nossent J, Raymond W, Ognjenovic M, Kang A, Chakera A, Wong D. The importance of tubuloreticular inclusions in lupus nephritis. Pathology. 2019;51(7):727–32. https://doi.org/10.1016/j.pathol.2019.07.007.

Oliveira B, Jayawardene S, Shah S. Single-centre experience of granulomatous interstitial nephritis-time for a new approach? Clin Kidney J. 2017;10(2):249–54. https://doi.org/10.1093/ckj/sfw119.

Özcan ŞG, Alay MT, Kalaycı Yiğin A, Trabulus S, Seyahi N. MO056 karyomegalic interstitial nephritis: an entity associated with different genetic mutations. Nephrol Dial Transplant. 2021;36(Supplement_1). https://doi.org/10.1093/ndt/gfab080.0028.

Paueksakon P, Fogo AB. Drug-induced nephropathies. Histopathology. 2017;70(1):94–108. https://doi.org/10.1111/his.13064.

Perazella MA, Markowitz GS. Drug-induced acute interstitial nephritis. Nat Rev Nephrol. 2010;6(8):461–70. https://doi.org/10.1038/nrneph.2010.71.

Raissian Y, Nasr SH, Larsen CP, Colvin RB, Smyrk TC, Takahashi N, et al. Diagnosis of IgG4-related tubulointerstitial nephritis. J Am Soc Nephrol. 2011;22(7):1343–52. https://doi.org/10.1681/asn.2011010062.

Regusci A, Lava SAG, Milani GP, Bianchetti MG, Simonetti GD, Vanoni F. Tubulointerstitial nephritis and uveitis syndrome: a systematic review. Nephrol Dial Transplant. 2021. https://doi.org/10.1093/ndt/gfab030.

Rejeb I, Jerbi M, Jilani H, Gaied H, Elaribi Y, Hizem S, et al. New familial cases of karyomegalic interstitial nephritis with mutations in the FAN1 gene. BMC Med Genet. 2021;14(1):160. https://doi.org/10.1186/s12920-021-01009-7.

Roberts IS, Brenchley PE. Mast cells: the forgotten cells of renal fibrosis. J Clin Pathol. 2000;53(11):858–62. https://doi.org/10.1136/jcp.53.11.858.

Rosales IA, Collins AB, do Carmo PA, Tolkoff-Rubin N, Smith RN, Colvin RB. Immune complex tubulointerstitial nephritis due to autoantibodies to the proximal tubule brush border. J Am Soc Nephrol. 2016;27(2):380–4. https://doi.org/10.1681/asn.2015030334.

Ruebner RL, Fadrowski JJ. Tubulointerstitial nephritis. Pediatr Clin N Am. 2019;66(1):111–9. https://doi.org/10.1016/j.pcl.2018.08.009.

Ryuzaki M, Tokuyama H, Uchiyama K, Nakaya H, Hasegawa K, Miyashita K, et al. Acute interstitial nephritis with karyomegalic epithelial cells after nivolumab treatment-two case reports. Clin Med Insights Case Rep. 2019;12:1179547619853647. https://doi.org/10.1177/1179547619853647.

Sathick IJ, Zand L, Kamal AN, Norby SM, Garovic VD. Acute interstitial nephritis: etiology, pathogenesis, diagnosis, treatment and prognosis. Nephrol Res Rev. 2013;5(1):13–20. https://doi.org/10.4081/nr.2013.e4.

Schlagenhaufer F. Uber eigentumliche Staphylomykosen der Nieren und des pararenalen Bindegewebes. Frankf Zt Pathol. 1916;19:139–48.

Shah S, Carter-Monroe N, Atta MG. Granulomatous interstitial nephritis. Clin Kidney J. 2015;8(5):516–23. https://doi.org/10.1093/ckj/sfv053.

Shen SS, Truong LD, Scarpelli M, Lopez-Beltran A. Role of immunohistochemistry in diagnosing renal neoplasms: when is it really useful? Arch Pathol Lab Med. 2012;136(4):410–7. https://doi.org/10.5858/arpa.2011-0472-RA.

Spanou Z, Keller M, Britschgi M, Yawalkar N, Fehr T, Neuweiler J, et al. Involvement of drug-specific T cells in acute drug-induced interstitial nephritis. J Am Soc Nephrol. 2006;17(10):2919–27. https://doi.org/10.1681/ASN.2006050418.

Steele TH. Hyperuricemic nephropathies. Nephron. 1999;81(Suppl 1):45–9. https://doi.org/10.1159/000046298.

Tokumoto M, Fukuda K, Shinozaki M, Kashiwagi M, Katafuchi R, Yoshida T, et al. Acute interstitial nephritis with immune complex deposition and MHC class II antigen presentation along the tubular basement membrane. Nephrol Dial Transplant. 1999;14(9):2210–5. https://doi.org/10.1093/ndt/14.9.2210.

Tzen CY, Tsai JD, Wu TY, Chen BF, Chen ML, Lin SP, et al. Tubulointerstitial nephritis associated with a novel mitochondrial point mutation. Kidney Int. 2001;59(3):846–54. https://doi.org/10.1046/j.1523-1755.2001.059003846.x.

Vervaet BA, Nast CC, Jayasumana C, Schreurs G, Roels F, Herath C, et al. Chronic interstitial nephritis in agricultural communities is a toxin-induced proximal tubular nephropathy. Kidney Int. 2020;97(2):350–69. https://doi.org/10.1016/j.kint.2019.11.009.

Wang H, Xu J, Zhang X, Ren YL, Cheng M, Guo ZL, et al. Tubular basement membrane immune complex deposition is associated with activity and progression of lupus nephritis: a large multicenter Chinese study. Lupus. 2018;27(4):545–55. https://doi.org/10.1177/0961203317732407.

Winer RL, Cohen AH, Sawhney AS, Gorman JT. Sjögren's syndrome with immune-complex tubulointerstitial renal disease. Clin Immunol Immunopathol. 1977;8(3):494–503. https://doi.org/10.1016/0090-1229(77)90013-7.

Yang D, Keys B, DJ Conti, Foulke L, Stellrecht K, Cook L, et al. JC polyomavirus nephropathy, a rare cause of transplant dysfunction: case report and review of literature. Transpl Infect Dis. 2017;19(2). https://doi.org/10.1111/tid.12654.

Zaidan M, Lescure FX, Brochériou I, Dettwiler S, Guiard-Schmid JB, Pacanowski J, et al. Tubulointerstitial nephropathies in HIV-infected patients over the past 15 years: a clinico-pathological study. Clin J Am Soc Nephrol. 2013;8(6):930–8. https://doi.org/10.2215/cjn.10051012.

Zhang P, Cornell LD. IgG4-related tubulointerstitial nephritis. Adv Chronic Kidney Dis. 2017;24(2):94–100. https://doi.org/10.1053/j.ackd.2016.12.001.

Zhang PL, Pancioli T, Li W, Kanaan HD. Electron microscopic findings can support multiple etiologies of nephrotoxicity in renal tubules. Ultrastruct Pathol. 2020;44(4–6):481–8. https://doi.org/10.1080/01913123.2020.1839152.

Zhang Y, Ahmed H, Haririan A, Ugarte R, Papadimitriou JC, Drachenberg CB. Granulomatous inflammation in BK polyomavirus-associated nephropathy. Transpl Infect Dis. 2018;20(5):e12939. https://doi.org/10.1111/tid.12939.

Part VI
Treatment

Management of Tubulointerstitial Nephritis

Beatriz Sanchez-Alamo, Clara Cases-Corona, and Gema Fernández-Juárez

1 Introduction

Acute interstitial nephritis (AIN) is one of the common causes of acute kidney injury (AKI). AIN has been linked to a variety of etiologies such as drugs (>75%), infections (5–10%) and systemic diseases (10–15%) while others are idiopathic cases (5–10%). Management hinges importantly on identifying the cause of AIN and directing therapy at the cause. Since drug-induced AIN (DI-AIN) is the most common etiology of AIN, this chapter will focus on its management but will also cover some other causes.

2 Identifying and Removing the Culprit Drug

It is currently recognized that drugs are the most common cause of AIN and there is a general agreement in that the withdrawal of the presumed causative drug is the core fundament of the treatment of DI-AIN. Although this may seem straightforward, in daily practice, we know that AIN is under recognized and under diagnosed because it is sometimes not even suspected by the clinicians. In fact, one study found that only 25% of PPI-mediated DI-AIN cases were suspected before biopsy. However, this entity must be taken into account since it represents 15–20% of cases of AKI .

Even when DI-AIN may be suspected, identification of the putative drug is actually very challenging for several reasons, among others due to large amount of possible candidate drugs implicated in DI-AIN (Table 1), the time from starting the

B. Sanchez-Alamo · C. Cases-Corona · G. Fernández-Juárez (✉)
Hospital Universitario Fundación Alcorcón, Madrid, Spain
e-mail: gema.fernandezjuarez@salud.madrid.org

M. G. Atta, M. A. Perazella (eds.), *Tubulointerstitial Nephritis*,
https://doi.org/10.1007/978-3-030-93438-5_22

Table 1 Main causes of DI-AIN

Drug class	Examples	Time	Syntoms	Characteristics
NSAIDs	*Non-selective COX inhibitors*: Fenoprofen, ibuprofen, naproxen *COX-2 inhibitors*: Celecoxib and rofecoxib	Longer latency periods (6–18 months)	Fewer extra renal syntoms More frequent: Edema and cognitive heart failure, hiponatremia and hyperkalemia. Nephrotic syndrome	Less intense interstitial inflammation and tubilitis and esosinophils are not predominant
Antibiotics	*Beta-lactams*: Penicilins, cephalosporines, methicillin *Non-beta-lactams*: Rifampicin, ciprofloxacin, sulfonamide	Days after drug intake	Hypersensitivity manifestations (skin rash, fever, and eosinophilia) Less frequent with fluoroquinolone antibiotic	Rifampicin: Most often when drug is used intermittently. Dose-dependent
Antiviral	Abacavir Indinavir Aciclovir Atazanavir		Eosinophiluria Crystalluria	
PPIs	Omeprazole, lansoprazole, pantoprazole, esomeprazol	1 week to 9 months. Commonest 10–11 weeks	Fever, skin rash and eosinophilia <10%	Less severe AKI but lower probability of recovery by 6 months
5-Aminosalicylates	Sulfasalazine, mesalamine, olsalazine	During the initial year of therapy	Rare rash	
Antineoplastic agents	Immune checkpoint inhibitors (ipilimumab, nivolumab, pembrolizumab) Lenalidomide	1 to 24 months	Extrarenal manifestations such as hypophysitis or colitis may precede AKI	

drug to acute kidney injury is quite ranged, and the lack of precise screening methods to discriminate the offending drug. As an example, in the study by Fernández-Juárez et al., it was not possible to identify the offending drug in 30% of the patients. Reasons for this were the polypharmacy these patients received and the lack of a clear chronological association between treatment and the onset of DI-AIN.

On the other hand, it is remarkable the significant growth of self-medication with over-the-counter medicines such as NSAIDs for chronic pain or PPIs for gastric disorders. In most of the countries, these drugs do not require a prescription for their distribution and therefore patients perceive these drugs as secure with low side-effect profile and patients take them during months or even years increasing the risk for side adverse effects. In many situations, only an in-depth focused interview can uncover the uptake of this kind of drugs.

This is of special importance in the elderly. Indeed, elderly patients are at a particularly high risk for DI-AIN for their inherent fragility and because they are usually treated with polypharmacy. On the other hand, it has been postulated that elderly kidneys may have a greater vulnerability to drugs and their effects and besides many of these elderly patients already have an impaired kidney function.

Despite the efforts to identify the responsible drug, sometimes the culprit drug cannot be withdrawn or substituted due to its inherent benefits. This situation occurs frequently in AIN induced by chemotherapeutic drugs, specifically by immune checkpoint inhibitors (ICI). This group of drugs has shown promising results in the treatment of tumors with limited responses to conventional chemotherapeutic treatment such as melanoma, non-small-cell lung carcinoma, renal cell carcinoma and Hodgkin lymphoma.

ICIs are rapidly changing the standard of care for people with cancer, especially for those patients who have not responded to other lines of treatment or who have achieved a partial response. However, there are still many challenges to overcome in terms of managing their toxicities because ICIs have been related to a higher incidence of AKI. Initial studies noted a small incidence of AKI (2–3%), but recent data reported a higher incidence closer to 13–29% with the use of these agents in routine practice. It occurs more frequently in patients who received combination therapy with ipilimumab and nivolumab. The big question that exists is the safety of ICI rechallenge after an episode of AKI since additional kidney events can result in further loss of kidney function and may influence the overall prognosis.

The incidence of occurrence of a flare after ICI re-exposure has been widely described. Different series have reported an incidence of recurrent AKI of around 20% upon ICI re-challenge . Interestingly most of the patients were on low dose corticosteroids at re-challenge. The rationale to select lower doses of corticosteroids is that higher doses may diminish the response to ICI, but there is evidence that prednisone below 10 mg per day does not affect progression-free survival or overall survival. In contrast, the kidney prognosis after the re-challenge is not clear because the results are mixed in the literature. All in all re-challenge might be possible but it requires close attention and kidney function monitoring.

3 Treatment with Corticosteroids

Treatment of AIN remains a challenge for clinicians since there is no clinical trial that has shown evidence on specific therapies for this disease. The clinical evidence for these recommendations is scarce since most of the studies are retrospective and usually include a small sample size (Table 2). Even though there are significant numbers of studies supporting the role of steroids in the treatment of AIN and especially when they are promptly started. The rationale for this approach is that early

Table 2 Summary of published series of DI-AIN

Author	Year	Retrospective	Hospitals	Patients	DI-AIN	Other AIN Types	Limbs	Dosage of steroids	Results
Clarkson et al.	2004	Yes	1	60	92%	8% idiopathic	16 steroids 26 conservative treatment	IV Methylprednisolone 500 mg 2–4 days Oral prednisolone 0.75 mg/kg tapered over 3–6 weeks	No differences between groups in median serum creatinine at 1 year.
Gonzalez et al.	2008	Yes	10	61	100%		85% steroids 15% conservative treatment	IV Methylprednisolone 250–500 mg 3–4 days Oral prednisolone 1 mg/kg tapered over 8–12 weeks	Steroid group showed significantly better outcomes, 53% recovered their baseline renal function. Patients with incomplete recovery of renal function had a significantly longer interval between withdrawal of the offending drug and starting steroids treatment (34 ± 17 vs. 13 ± 10 days; $P < 0.05$).
Raza et al.	2012	Yes	1	49	67%	4 TINU 2 sarcoidosis 10 idiopathic	75% steroids	Oral prednisolone 1 mg/kg	Steroid-treated patients showed a higher improve in eGFR and a reduced tendency for needing dialysis.

Author	Year	Retrospective	Hospitals	Patients	DI-AIN	Other AIN Types	Limbs	Dosage of steroids	Results
Muriithi et al.	2014	Yes	1	133	71%	38 (29%) other	86% steroids	21% initial IV Methylprednisolone Oral prednisone 7.5 mg	Treatment with steroids affected neither recovery status at 6 months nor the ultimate outcome over long-term follow-up. Steroid treatment had no effect on kidney disease outcomes.
Ramachandran et al.	2015	Prospective Randomized	1	29	100%		100% steroids	Group 1: oral prednisolone 1 mg/kg for 3 weeks followed by rapid tapering in the next 3 weeks. Group 2: IV methyl prednisolone 30 mg/kg (maximum 1 g) as slow intravenous infusion over 60 min for 3 consecutive days followed by oral prednisolone 1 mg/kg for 2 weeks and tapered in next 3 weeks.	Early steroid therapy, both oral and pulse steroid, is equally effective in achieving remission in DI-AIN.

(continued)

Table 2 (continued)

Author	Year	Retrospective	Hospitals	Patients	DI-AIN	Other AIN Types	Limbs	Dosage of steroids	Results
Valluri et al.	2015	Yes	Several	171	72.5%	9.9% sarcoid/ TINU 7%autoimmune conditions 8.2% infection 2.3% unclear	63% steroids	Unknown	There was no significant difference in the proportion of the steroid-treated and the conservatively managed groups experiencing complete renal recovery (48% vs. 41%) or becoming dialysis dependent (10% in both groups).
Prendecki et al.	2017	Yes	1	187	25%	48% unknown/ other 13% TB 9% Sarcoidosis 3% TINU 2% Sjögren	84% steroids 16% conservative	All treated with oral prednisolone except for three patients receiving methylprednisolone prior to oral prednisolone.	Treatment with steroids was beneficial. They observed a greater improvement in eGFR and fewer patients progressing to end-stage renal disease
Chowdry et al.	2018	Prospective Randomized	1	31	100%		100% steroids	Group A: oral prednisolone 1 mg/kg for 2 weeks Group B: pulse methylprednisolone 30 mg/kg for 3 days (maximum 1 g) followed by oral prednisolone 1 mg/kg for 2 weeks, tapered over 2 weeks.	58.06% achieved CR and 41.93% achieved PR. Group A, 9 (56.2%) achieved CR and 7 (43.7%) achieved PR. Group B: 9 (60%) achieved CR and 6 (40%) achieved PR. There was no significant difference between the two groups

Author	Year	Retrospective	Hospitals	Patients	DI-AIN	Other AIN Types	Limbs	Dosage of steroids	Results
Fernandez-Juárez et al.	2018	Yes	13	182	100%		100% steroids	88 IV pulse corticosteroids. Initial dose of prednisone: 0.86 ± 0.2 mg/kg per day.	After 6 months of follow-up, the mean recovered GFR was 346 ± 26 ml/min. 75 patients (41%) achieved complete recovery of kidney function, 83 patients (46%) achieved partial recovery, and 24 patients (13%) did not recover kidney function.
Surendra et al.	2019	Yes	1	83	100%		100% steroids	500 mg of methylprednisolone for 3 consecutive days followed by prednisolone of 0.5–1 mg/kg tapered over 4–6 weeks	47% were CR and 53% PR. Diabetes was associated with poor response to steroids and significant progression of CKD. Initial serum creatinine and initial requirement of RRT not predicted the response to steroids and final recovery. Lack of fibrosis and neutrophils predominance in biopsy was associated with favorable response to steroid therapy.

Abbreviations: IV intravenous, *CR* complete response, *PR* partial response, *CKD* chronic kidney disease, *RRT* renal replacement therapy, *TINU* Tubulointerstitial nephritis and uveitis, *eGFR* estimated glomerular filtration rate corticosteroids would reduce the inflammatory infiltrates of the kidney interstitium, thus preventing the risk of subsequent fibrosis.

In regard to DI-AIN, the mainstay of treatment is, as above, to withdraw the offending agent, but it has been suggested that a course of corticosteroids should be included to hasten the recovery of kidney function, especially for those with no evidence of kidney function recovery after a 7–10 day period since suspension of the involved drug.

Clarkson and colleagues published a retrospective study on 60 patients diagnosed with AIN (92% DI-AIN), although clinical follow-up data were only available in 42 patients. They found no difference in kidney function at 6 and 12 months of follow-up between patients treated with corticosteroids (60%) and those who merely received supportive treatment (40%). Madrid Interstitial Nephritis Group studied 61 patients with kidney biopsy proven DI-AIN. Most patients received corticosteroids (85%). After a mean follow-up of 19 months, kidney function showed a greater improvement in those treated (serum creatinine 2.1 mg/dl) compared to those not treated (serum creatinine 3.7 mg/dl) $p < 0.05$), and the number of patients who required kidney replacement therapy was significantly lower (3.8% vs 44.4%, $p < 0.001$). Interestingly, in this study there was a significant correlation between the delay in the onset of corticosteroid treatment after drug withdrawal and the final kidney function ($r = 0.45$, $p < 0.005$). Specifically, the benefit was greatest for patients, who received early treatment with steroids, in particular during the first week after stopping the causative drug.

There are important differences in both studies. In the first study in which corticosteroids did not show a benefit on kidney function, baseline kidney function was worse in those patients treated with corticosteroids when compared to the non-treated patients (Baseline serum creatinine 7.9 mg/dL vs. 6.2 mg/dL). Additionally, corticosteroid treatment was started later and the mean time elapsed between the onset of symptoms, and the kidney biopsy was 4 weeks (IQR: 2–6 weeks).

Later studies showed similar findings. In the study conducted by Muriithi et al., 86% of the patients received steroids and the rest received conservative treatment. After 6 months, serum creatinine in both groups was similar (1.4 mg/dl vs 1.5 mg/dl). An interesting observation in this study is the fact that patients achieving partial or complete remission started corticosteroid treatment earlier (at 8 and 11 days, respectively) whereas patients not attaining remission commenced treatment considerably later (at 35 days) ($P = 0.05$).

In view of the published results, the following studies focused on directly addressing the question of when it is optimal to introduce corticosteroid therapy. This has been reflected in a study including 182 patients with biopsy-proven cases of DI-AIN treated with corticosteroids. Those patients starting treatment with corticosteroids during the first 2 weeks showed better kidney outcomes. In contrast, treatment started beyond 4 weeks exhibited little benefit on the final kidney function. More in detail, the mean time to start corticosteroid treatment was 9 days in the group that had complete recovery, 12 days in the group that had partial recovery and 29 days in the group that had no recovery ($P = 0.008$) .

4 Corticosteroid Use Versus Conservative Management

4.1 DI-AIN

The possible pharmacologic agents involved are numerous. The first cases of DI-AIN were related to antibiotics. Initial reports related this condition to sulfonamides, followed by the penicillins in the 1950s and later to methicillin. These reports presented DI-AIN as a benign condition in which withdrawal of the drug usually results in recovery and in a rapid improvement of kidney function.

However, this progression has not been observed in subsequent series involving other drugs. In a cohort of 182 patients, 41% of the patients managed to recover at least 75% of their baseline GFR, 46% recovered between 25% and 75% of their baseline GFR, and 13% recovered less than 25% of your basal GFR.

Many single factors have been postulated to explain the incomplete or poor kidney recovery. The first factor is the misrecognition of the responsible drug, which renders it impossible for its withdrawal. The second component is the ongoing kidney inflammatory reaction due to AIN, which might not be solved despite the withdrawal of the drug. The third and final consideration is that the recognition of the entity and the withdrawal of the drug, has occurred too late, and therefore the acute inflammatory infiltrate has led to irreversible chronic infiltration and tubulointerstitial fibrosis. In fact, the presence of fibrosis of more than 50% on kidney biopsy was a negative predictive factor for kidney outcomes .

Therefore, the dilemma is not to decide whether to choose between conservative treatment and corticosteroids, but rather to decide in which situations conservative management will be sufficient and in which situations it will be necessary to add corticosteroids to the treatment. According to the available evidence, early initiation of corticosteroids improves kidney prognosis. Hence, the delay between the withdrawal of the drug and the start of corticosteroids should not be postponed beyond 7 or 10 days. Another important aspect to be considered is the time elapsed between the onset of kidney damage, the diagnosis of kidney damage, the histological confirmation of the damage, and the withdrawal of the drug. When these periods are long, probably the time of drug withdrawal and the start of corticosteroids should coincide, to avoid delay in the start of corticosteroid treatment.

Finally, kidney biopsy is the one and essential tool to establish the accurate diagnosis of AIN. It can additionally provide prognostic information on the time of evolution of the damage, although its performance and subsequent review should not be a justification for extending decision-making deadlines. The presence of significant interstitial fibrosis/tubular atrophy (>50%) also helps predict patients that will not likely benefit from corticosteroid therapy and suffer complications without much benefit.

5 Intravenous Versus Oral Route of Corticosteroids

Many physicians frequently use pulse intravenous methylprednisolone prior to starting high dose oral corticosteroids in some kidney diseases where there is predominant inflammatory infiltration in glomeruli or tubule-interstitium, such as vasculitis or systemic lupus erythematosus. One of the fundamental reasons for the use of pulse methylprednisolone may be related to its rapid and strong anti-inflammatory effect.

Although there are no clinical trials that have demonstrated an additional effect to oral corticosteroid treatment in these pathologies, its use is widely accepted and is even recommended in clinical guidelines . The same situation applies to AIN. In this scenario, IV corticosteroids may accelerate recovery and potentiate the effect in the kidney interstitium.

To compare the efficacy of IV and oral corticosteroids in the treatment of DI-AIN, Ramachandran and coworkers performed a randomized study. A total of 29 patients with biopsy-proven AIN with a history of drug intake were randomized; 16 patients received oral prednisolone 1 mg/kg for 3 weeks and 13 patients received pulse methylprednisolone 30 mg/kg for 3 days followed by oral prednisolone 1 mg/kg for 2 weeks and then tapering over 3 weeks. There were no significant differences between the two-regimens used at the end of the study.

A subsequent randomized clinical trial conducted by Chowdry and colleagues showed similar results. In this study, oral and IV corticosteroids were compared. Accordingly, 31 patients with DI-AIN were treated with oral prednisolone 1 mg/kg for 2 weeks and then corticosteroids were tapered over 2 weeks. Fifteen patients additionally received pulse methylprednisolone (30 mg/kg) for 3 days (maximum 1 g) prior to oral prednisone. There were no significant differences between the two groups. Both oral and IV doses of corticosteroids were equally effective in the treatment of drug-induced AIN.

6 Length of Corticosteroid Therapy

The different available studies have shown large disparities in the duration of the treatment with corticosteroids ranging from a month to 6 months. However, the length of the therapy is not a trivial matter because the use of corticosteroids might produce a wide range of adverse effects. Therefore, a strict balance of the risks, including toxicity, and benefits of the treatment must be considered. A strict control of the dose and the duration of the treatment must be conducted to avoid administering more doses than necessary or for longer than necessary.

Despite its importance, the duration of the treatment with corticosteroids has not been discussed in depth. The study conducted by Fernandez and coworkers discussed the length of the duration of the treatment, concluding that the greatest kidney function recovery was obtained when the entire treatment lasted 8 weeks at maximum, out of which, 3 weeks would correspond to high-dose corticosteroids therapy followed by a tapering period of up to 5–6 weeks.

Similar results have been observed in other studies. As for González and colleagues, the results did not show a statistically significant difference in the duration of corticosteroid treatment between those with a complete or an incomplete recovery of baseline kidney function (75 ± 37 and 78 ± 42 days respectively) .

On the other hand, the evolution of kidney function within the first weeks after the start of corticosteroid treatment is fundamental to determine the final recovery of the glomerular filtration rate. In fact, the biggest impact in kidney function recovery is obtained during the first 4 weeks of treatment. Beyond this time point, the extent of kidney recovery is moderated, and in some cases, it is not even achieved.

7 Length of Corticosteroid Taper

Overall, treatment strategies recommend induction with high doses of corticosteroids subsequently followed by oral prednisone to be gradually tapered. Tapering duration has been scarcely studied. In fact, most studies describe their local experience and do not compare different strategies.

The optimal schedule for corticosteroid withdrawal has not been determined and therefore the length of taper is a matter of discussion. Clarkson and colleagues tapered the treatment with corticosteroids over 3–6 weeks in their study, whereas González and coworkers reduced the dose of corticosteroids more slowly (8–12 weeks). It is however remarkable that the González study employed a higher dose of corticosteroids and the length of corticosteroids tapering was similar among those who achieved complete or partial recovery .

As with other pathologies, during the corticosteroids -tapering period there is still a therapeutic effect and a subsequent improvement in kidney function. According to this, we could consider prolonging the treatment until the glomerular filtration rate reaches the baseline. However, several studies have confirmed that prolonging the global treatment for more than 8 weeks or the tapering period for more than 5 weeks does not provide an additional recovery in kidney function.

On the other hand, in other immunological diseases, steroids still must be tapered slowly to avoid relapses. With respect to DI-AIN, it seems less likely for this pathology the occurrence of a flare or relapse; in such a case, we should suspect other etiologies and rule out the possibility of an underlying autoimmune disease or a Dress syndrome.

8 Alternative Therapies for AIN

Clinicians must consider alternatives to corticosteroids for therapy of AIN when the drug is contraindicated or associated with complications, complicated by relapse during/after taper, or failed corticosteroid therapy.

In those refractory or relapsed AIN cases, the initial approach is to reconsider the initial diagnosis, avoiding successive immunological treatments. In case of refractory disease with a poor recovery of kidney function, despite drug withdrawal or therapy with corticosteroids, we should consider several aspects. Firstly, it is pertinent to ensure that the appropriate drug has been withdrawn. Secondly, it is highly recommended to identify if there is another putative cause, rather than the suspected drug, for example an underlying disease. Finally, when chronic kidney damage has already been established, and the acute infiltrate has already given way to chronic infiltrate and tubulointerstitial fibrosis, the damage is no longer reversible and therefore kidney recovery could not be possible. Thus, corticosteroids should be avoided in those with advanced fibrosis. Despite considering all of the above, there are still patients with immunosupresive treatment and for whom corticosteroids are not an adequate treatment, and they require another type of treatment.

Unfortunately, the treatment landscape for these patients is not standardized. In fact, there is not enough evidence in the literature for employing other immunosuppressive agents. Clinical cases treated with other immunosuppressive agents such as cyclophosphamide, cyclosporine, or mycophenolate are seldomly mentioned in the literature. In this setting, a recent report of eight patients with corticosteroid-dependency, recurrent AIN documented an interesting beneficial effect of mycophenolate mofetil.

As mentioned above, a challenging situation occurs when the drug cannot be withdrawn, as occurs with ICI induced AIN.

With this approach, serum creatinine should be monitored every 2 weeks, with corticosteroid re-initiation at the first sign of AKI from AIN with no other identified cause.

Faieta and colleagues reported one case of refractory ICI-induced AIN treated successfully treated with mycophenolate mofetil. The patient was diagnosed with DI-AIN related to nivolumab, a PD-1 inhibitor, in the context of the treatment of a metastatic clear cell renal cell carcinoma. The patient was initially treated with corticosteroids for this condition but suffered three relapses. Finally, doctors decided to initiate therapy with pulse 500 mg IV methylprednisolone and daily one gram of mycophenolate mofetil. The patient recovered kidney function and has been stable for 2 years.

9 Conclusions

In some selected cases we might consider initial high doses of steroids followed by MMF in those cases where steroids are contraindicated (Fig. 1).

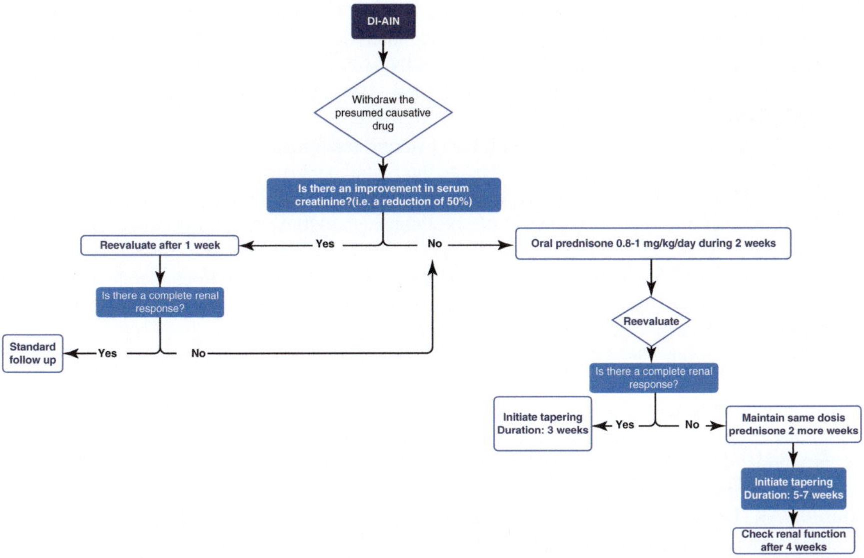

Fig. 1 Treatment algorithm for DI-AIN

Suggested Reading

Atkins MB, Clark JI, Quinn DI. Immune checkpoint inhibitors in advanced renal cell carcinoma: experience to date and future directions. Ann Oncol. 2017;28(7):1484–94. https://doi.org/10.1093/annonc/mdx151.

Chowdry AM, Azad H, Mir I, Najar MS, Ashraf BM, Muzafar WM, Ahmed WI. Drug-induced acute interstitial nephritis: prospective randomized trial comparing oral steroids and high-dose intravenous pulse steroid therapy in guiding the treatment of this condition. Saudi J Kidney Dis Transpl. 2018;29:598–607.

Clarkson MR, Giblin L, O'Connell FP, O'Kelly P, Walshe JJ, Conlon P, et al. Acute interstitial nephritis: clinical features and response to corticosteroid therapy. Nephrol Dial Transplant. 2004;19:2778–83.

Cortazar FB, Kibbelaar ZA, Glezerman IG, et al. Clinical features and outcomes of immune checkpoint inhibitor-associated AKI: a multicenter study. J Am Soc Nephrol. 2020;31:435–46.

Davison AM, Jones CH. Acute interstitial nephritis in the elderly: a report from the UK MRC glomerulonephritis register and a review of the literature. Nephrol Dial Transplant. 1998;13(Suppl 7):12–6. https://doi.org/10.1093/ndt/13.suppl_7.12.

Duru N, van der Goes MC, Jacobs JW, et al. EULAR evidence-based and consensus-based recommendations on the management of medium to high-dose glucocorticoid therapy in rheumatic diseases. Ann Rheum Dis. 2013;72(12):1905–13. https://doi.org/10.1136/annrheumdis-2013-203249.

Faieta A, Dancik T. Refractory acute interstitial nephritis in the setting of Nivolumab therapy. Case Rep Nephrol. 2021;2021:6640154. Published 2021 Mar 1. https://doi.org/10.1155/2021/6640154.

Fernandez-Juarez G, Perez JV, Caravaca-Fontán F, et al. Duration of treatment with corticosteroids and recovery of kidney function in acute interstitial nephritis. Clin J Am Soc Nephrol. 2018;13(12):1851–8. https://doi.org/10.2215/CJN.01390118.

Fried T. Acute interstitial nephritis. Postgrad Med. 1993;93(5):105–20. https://doi.org/10.1080/00325481.1993.11701663.

González E, Gutiérrez E, Galeano C, et al. Early steroid treatment improves the recovery of renal function in patients with drug-induced acute interstitial nephritis. Kidney Int. 2008;73:940–6.

Herrmann SM, Perazella MA. Immune checkpoint inhibitors and immune-related adverse renal events. Kidney Int Rep. 2020;5(8):1139–48. Published 2020 Apr 29. https://doi.org/10.1016/j.ekir.2020.04.018.

Isik B, Alexander MP, Manohar S, et al. Biomarkers, clinical features, and Rechallenge for immune checkpoint inhibitor renal immune-related adverse events. Kidney Int Rep. 2021;6(4):1022–31. Published 2021 Feb 2. https://doi.org/10.1016/j.ekir.2021.01.013.

Moledina DG, Parikh CR. Differentiating acute interstitial nephritis from acute tubular injury: a challenge for clinicians. Nephron. 2019;143(3):211–6. https://doi.org/10.1159/000501207.

Moledina DG, Wilson FP, Kukova L, Obeid W, Luciano R, Kuperman M, Moeckel GW, Kashgarian M, Perazella MA, Cantley LG, Parikh CR. Urine interleukin-9 and tumor necrosis factor-α for prognosis of human acute interstitial nephritis. Nephrol Dial Transplant. 2020:gfaa169. https://doi.org/10.1093/ndt/gfaa169.

Muriithi AK, Leung N, Valeri AM, et al. Biopsy-proven acute interstitial nephritis, 1993-2011: a case series. Am J Kidney Dis. 2014;64:558–66.

Muriithi AK, Leung N, Valeri AM, et al. Clinical characteristics, causes and outcomes of acute interstitial nephritis in the elderly. Kidney Int. 2015;87(2):458–64. https://doi.org/10.1038/ki.2014.294.

Naik RH, Annamaraju P. Interstitial Nephritis. [Updated 2020 Dec 14]. In: StatPearls [Internet]. Treasure Island (FL): StatPearls Publishing; 2021. Available from: https://www.ncbi.nlm.nih.gov/books/NBK564349/

Praga M, González E. Acute interstitial nephritis. Kidney Int. 2010;77(11):956–61. https://doi.org/10.1038/ki.2010.89.

Preddie DC, Markowitz GS, Radhakrishnan J, et al. Mycophenolate Mofetil for the treatment of interstitial nephritis. Clin J Am Soc Nephrol. 2006;1:718–22.

Prendecki M, Tanna A, Salama AD, et al. Long-term outcome in biopsy-proven acute interstitial nephritis treated with steroids. Clin Kidney J. 2017;10(2):233–9. https://doi.org/10.1093/ckj/sfw116.

Raghavan R, Eknoyan G. Acute interstitial nephritis - a reappraisal and update. Clin Nephrol. 2014;82(3):149–62. https://doi.org/10.5414/cn108386.

Ramachandran R, Kumar K, Nada R, Jha V, Gupta KL, Kohli HS. Drug-induced acute interstitial nephritis: a clinicopathological study and comparative trial of steroid regimens. Indian J Nephrol. 2015;25:281–6.

Ray S, Delaney M, Muller AF. Proton pump inhibitors and acute interstitial nephritis. BMJ. 2010;341:c4412.

Raza MN, Hadid M, Keen CE, Bingham C, Salmon AH. Acute tubulointerstitial nephritis, treatment with steroid and impact on renal outcomes. Nephrology (Carlton). 2012;17:748–53.

Ricciuti B, Dahlberg SE, Adeni A, Sholl LM, Nishino M, Awad MM. Immune checkpoint inhibitor outcomes for patients with non-small-cell lung cancer receiving baseline corticosteroids for palliative versus nonpalliative indications. J Clin Oncol. 2019;37:1927–34.

Sierra F, Suarez M, Rey M, et al. Systematic review: proton pump inhibitor associated acute interstitial nephritis. Aliment Pharmacol Ther. 2007;26:545–53.

Simpson IJ, Marshall MR, Pilmore H, et al. Proton pump inhibitors and acute interstitial nephritis: report and analysis of 15 cases. Nephrology (Carlton). 2006;11:381–38.

Surendra M, Raju S, Chandragiri S, Uppin MS, Raju N. Steroid therapy in drug induced acute interstitial nephritis- retrospective analysis of 83 cases. Saudi J Kidney Dis Transpl. 2019;30(1):157–65. PMID: 30804277.

Valluri A, Hetherington L, Mcquarrie E, et al. Acute tubulointerstitial nephritis in Scotland. QJM. 2015;108:527–32.
Wanchoo R, Karam S, Uppal NN, et al. Adverse renal effects of immune checkpoint inhibitors: a narrative review. Am J Nephrol. 2017;45(2):160–9. https://doi.org/10.1159/000455014.
Xie Y, Bowe B, Yan Y, Xian H, Li T, Al-Aly Z. Estimates of all cause mortality and cause specific mortality associated with proton pump inhibitors among US veterans: cohort study. BMJ. 2019;365:l1580.Published 2019 May 29. https://doi.org/10.1136/bmj.l1580.

Part VII
Prognosis/Outcomes

Prognosis and Outcomes of Acute Tubulointerstitial Nephritis

Dries Deleersnijder and Ben Sprangers

1 Introduction

The outcome of acute tubulointerstitial nephritis (ATIN) depends upon many factors, and therefore differs significantly between studies. First, the etiology and outcome of ATIN depends upon the time-frame and inclusion period of the study. For example, older studies included more methicillin-induced ATIN (methicillin is currently no longer used in clinical practice), while more recent studies have identified new medication-related culprits such as proton pump inhibitors (PPIs) and immune checkpoint inhibitors (ICPIs). Second, etiologies differ between geographical regions, and therefore also the outcomes of patients in these regional registries or case series differ. As an example, infection-related ATIN (e.g., Hantavirus infection, Leptospirosis, Yersinia infection) have a specific geographic distribution. Third, the age of the included patients, their comorbidities and pre-existing chronic kidney disease (CKD) all play a major role in disease outcome. For example, the elderly population more frequently has pre-existing CKD, has many comorbidities, is more frequently taking many medications and generally has a worse prognosis. Fourth, although kidney biopsy remains the gold standard for diagnosis of ATIN, many – mostly pediatric – registries included patients that had not undergone biopsy and were clinically diagnosed as having ATIN, which introduces risk of bias and complicates comparison of studies. Finally, definitions of renal recovery and CKD, as well as follow-up periods differ significantly between studies, which also hampers a systematic comparison. Ideally, studies should identify large patient cohorts with etiology-specific ATIN. However, ATIN remains a relatively rare entity compared to

D. Deleersnijder · B. Sprangers (✉)
Department of Microbiology, Immunology and Transplantation, Laboratory of Molecular Immunology, Rega Institute, KU Leuven, Leuven, Belgium

Division of Nephrology, University Hospitals Leuven, Leuven, Belgium
e-mail: ben.sprangers@uzleuven.be

M. G. Atta, M. A. Perazella (eds.), *Tubulointerstitial Nephritis*,
https://doi.org/10.1007/978-3-030-93438-5_23

other kidney diseases, and large etiology-specific cohorts with long follow-up periods are extremely difficult to construct in a reasonable time-frame. Therefore, this chapter will first discuss the outcomes of ATIN in general, derived from larger cohorts that included many disease etiologies. Next, we will focus on the outcomes of specific etiologies of ATIN, of which data is mostly derived from smaller case series.

2 Overall Renal Outcomes

Renal outcomes can be subdivided into acute outcomes (kidney function and need for acute renal replacement therapy [RRT]) and chronic long-term outcomes (renal recovery *vs.* CKD and end-stage kidney disease [ESKD]). Considering acute outcomes, patients with ATIN frequently present with acute kidney disease (AKD), which in some patients may progress to severe acute kidney injury (AKI) and oliguria requiring transient acute dialysis (Table 1). According to 12 studies, RRT in the acute disease setting was required in 3.3–58% of patients (median of 20.5%). Fortunately, kidney function recovers fully or partially in most patients, which is illustrated by the study of Clarkson et al., in which 35 of 60 adult patients (58%) with biopsy-proven ATIN required acute dialysis, but only two patients remained dialysis-dependent at 12 months follow-up. Despite this often impressive nadir of kidney function in the acute setting, the long-term prognosis of ATIN was historically considered to be favorable. However, many recent studies have now shown a less reassuring long-term prognosis (Table 1). At 6 months follow-up after the acute episode, full renal recovery (mostly defined as return of serum creatinine [sCr] to within 25% of baseline value and/or glomerular filtration rate [GFR] >60 mL/min and/or sCr <1.30 mg/dL) was found in only approximately 30–55% of patients with biopsy-proven ATIN. Partial recovery, mostly defined as >50% decrease of peak sCr value but not within 25% of baseline value, or sCr exceeding baseline value with 25–75% was found in approximately 25–45% of patients. No recovery, defined as not meeting previous criteria or RRT, was found in approximately 15–40% of patients. In studies that performed longer follow-up (outcome beyond 6 months, mostly 1–3 years), complete renal recovery was noted in approximately 45–55%, while incomplete recovery and CKD was present in approximately 40–55%. ESKD, defined as maintenance RRT or kidney transplantation was present in approximately 5–25% of patients (approximately 10%). In summary, at extended follow-up, only about half of patients will have recovered completely, while about 40% will have some degree of CKD, and 10% will require RRT, which illustrates that an episode of ATIN causes CKD in a significant proportion of the patient population.

Table 1 ATIN data in adult cohorts

Author Date Region	Age	Patients	Etiology (top 3)	Pre-existing CKD	Recovery/CKD	Acute dialysis	ESKD	Remarks
Kim et al. 2020 South Korea	Mean 55 yrs.	137 biopsy-proven ATIN	Not mentioned	No info	At 6 m FU: CKD: 69.4% (eGFR <60 mL/min)	No info	At mean 76.5 m FU: ESKD: 39.4% (not clearly defined)	Study compared ATN with ATIN
Rankin et al. 2020 Scotland	Mean 58 yrs.	120 biopsy-proven ATIN	Drugs (63%) Idiopathic (22%) Sarcoidosis (7%)	No info	At 1 yr. FU: CKD: 45% (GFR <60 mL/min OR sCr not decreased with 50% from biopsy value)	No info	At 1 yr. FU: eGFR <30 mL/min: 30% RRT: 4%	
Esteras et al. 2020 Scotland	Mean 58 yrs.	110 biopsy-proven ATIN	Drugs (53.6%) 1. PPI 2. NSAID, AB 3. Other 'Systemic disease' (14.5%) Idiopathic (9.1%)	Baseline CKD in 64.5% (not clearly defined) Mean baseline eGFR 66 mL/min	FU period unclear Recovery: 36.4% (sCr within ±0.3 mg/dL of baseline sCr) No recovery: 63.6% (not meeting criteria above)	7.3%	FU period unclear: RRT: 8.2%	FU until recovery, end of steroid treatment, death or lost-to-follow-up
Moledina et al. 2020 USA	Median 58 yrs.	51 biopsy-proven ATIN	Not mentioned	Median baseline eGFR 41 mL/min	At 6 m FU: Median eGFR 28 mL/min	6%	At 6 m FU: RRT: 14% Died: 3.9%	

(continued)

Table 1 (continued)

Author Date Region	Age	Patients	Etiology (top 3)	Pre-existing CKD	Recovery/CKD	Acute dialysis	ESKD	Remarks
Zheng et al. 2020 China	Mean 45 yrs.	81 biopsy-proven drug-induced ATIN	Drugs (100%) 1. β-lactam 2. Herbal medication 3. NSAID	Baseline CKD in 4.9% (not clearly defined)	At 6 m FU: Complete recovery: 64% (sCr within 25% of baseline) Partial recovery: 35% (sCr decrease with 50% from peak-value, but not within 25% of baseline) No recovery: 1% (not meeting criteria above or RRT) At 1 yr. FU: CKD: 42% (eGFR <60 mL/min)	22.2%	None	Study only included drug-induced ATIN
Zajjari et al. 2019 Morocco	Mean 47 yrs.	30 biopsy-proven ATIN	Drugs (43.3%) 1. NSAID 2. AB 3. PPI Auto-immune (33.3%): mostly sarcoidosis Others (13.2%)	Baseline CKD in 6.6% (eGFR <60 mL/min)	At 6 m FU: Complete recovery: 33.3% (sCr within 25% of baseline) Partial recovery: 26.7% (sCr decrease with 50% from biopsy-value, but not within 25% of baseline) No recovery: 40% (not meeting criteria above or RRT)	3.3%	At 6 m FU: RRT: 3.3%	

Yun et al. 2019 South Korea	Mean 58 yrs.	113 biopsy-proven ATIN	Idiopathic (68.1%) Drugs (22%) 1. Herbal medication 2. NSAID, AB 3. PPI Auto-immune (4.4%)	Baseline CKD in 11.5% (not clearly defined)	At 6 m FU: Recovery: 54.9% (sCr <1.3 mg/dL or >50% decrease from peak value) At last follow-up (median 33 m): Recovery: 73.5%	30.1%	FU period unclear: RRT or Tx: 25.7% Died: 17.7%	Better outcome in drug-induced ATIN
Wendt et al. 2019 Germany	Mean 52 yrs.	49 biopsy-proven ATIN, 39 patients included for outcome data	Not mentioned, in >70% use of drugs that are associated with ATIN	Mean baseline sCr in recovery group: 1.35 mg/dL Mean baseline sCr in no recovery group: 1.97 mg/dL	FU period unclear Complete recovery: 51.3% (reaching baseline sCr value) Partial recovery: 25.6% (coming off dialysis and/or sCr <2.26 mg/dL) No recovery: 23.1% (no improvement in renal function or remaining on RRT)	43.6%	FU period unclear ('end of FU'): RRT: 12.8%	

(continued)

Table 1 (continued)

Author Date Region	Age	Patients	Etiology (top 3)	Pre-existing CKD	Recovery/CKD	Acute dialysis	ESKD	Remarks
Su et al. 2018 China	Mean 47 yrs.	157 biopsy-proven ATIN	At diagnosis: Drugs (64.3%) Auto-immune (22.3%) Idiopathic (5.1%) At follow-up: Drugs (50.3%) Auto-immune (41.4%) Others (4.5%)	No info	At 6 m FU: Complete recovery: 45.9% (sCr within 25% of baseline) Partial recovery: 22.9% (sCr decrease with 50% from biopsy-value, but not within 25% of baseline) No recovery: 29.3% At 12 m FU: CKD: 54.8% (eGFR <60 mL/min) At median 38 m FU: CKD: 52.2% (eGFR <60 mL/min)	No info	FU period unclear: RRT: 20.4% (unclear whether acute or maintenance RRT) Died: 3.2%	Better outcome in drug-induced ATIN when compared to TINU/auto-immune etiology. Some patients were misclassified as drug-induced ATIN and later developed systemic manifestations of auto-immune etiology
Fernandez et al. 2018 Spain	Mean 67 yrs.	182 biopsy-proven drug-induced ATIN	Drugs (100%) 1. NSAID 2. AB 3. PPI	Baseline CKD: 41% (eGFR <60 mL/min) Mean baseline sCr 1.1 mg/dL (eGFR 68 mL/min)	At 6 m FU: Mean eGFR 34 mL/min Complete recovery: 41% (sCr within 25% of baseline) Partial recovery: 46% (sCr exceeded baseline with 25–75%) No recovery: 13% (exceeded baseline with >75% or RRT)	19%	At 6 m FU: RRT: 5.5%	Study only included drug-induced ATIN

Prendecki et al. 2017 UK	Median 52 yrs.	187 biopsy-proven ATIN	Idiopathic (48%) Drugs (25%) 1. AB 2. NSAID 3. PPI Auto-immune (14%)	No info	At 24 m FU: median eGFR 43 mL/min (steroid-treated) vs. 24 mL/min (not steroid-treated)	12.3%	At 6 m FU: RRT: Total: 5.9% Steroids: 3.2% No steroids: 20.6% At 24 m FU: RRT: Total: 8% Steroids: 5.1% No steroids: 24.1%	Comparison of steroid vs. no steroids and review of the literature
Effa et al. 2017 South-Africa	Mean 42 yrs.	54 biopsy-proven ATIN	Drugs (70.4%) 1. Rifampicin 2. TMP-SMX 3. Kanamycin Infection (14.8%) Idiopathic (7.4%)	No info	At 3 m FU: Complete recovery: 45.3% (sCr to baseline, or <1.13 mg/dL) Partial recovery: 42.6% (sCr decrease with 50% from peak-value, but not within 25% of baseline) No recovery: 7.6% (not meeting criteria above or RRT)	No info	At 3 m FU: RRT: 33.9% Died: 11%	Study in Cape Town, high prevalence of HIV and TBC. Better outcomes in drug-induced ATIN

(continued)

Table 1 (continued)

Author Date Region	Age	Patients	Etiology (top 3)	Pre-existing CKD	Recovery/CKD	Acute dialysis	ESKD	Remarks
Valluri et al. 2015 Scotland	Median 66 yrs.	171 biopsy-proven ATIN	Drugs (73%) 1. AB, PPI 2. NSAID Auto-immune (16.9%) Infection (8.2%)	Median baseline sCr 1.20 mg/dL	At 1 yr. FU: Complete renal recovery: 43% (sCr return to baseline) Incomplete recovery: 44% (sCr >0.3 mg/dL above baseline)	19%	At FU 1 yr.: RRT: 9.4%	
Muriithi et al. 2014 USA	Median 58 yrs.	133 biopsy-proven ATIN	Drugs (70%) 1. AB 2. PPI 3. NSAID Auto-immune (20%) Infection (4%)	Baseline CKD: 44% (eGFR <60 mL/min) Median baseline sCr 1.1 mg/dL (eGFR 63 mL/min)	At 6 m FU: Complete recovery: 47% (sCr within 25% of baseline) Partial recovery: 38% (sCr decrease with 50% from peak-value, but not within 25% of baseline) No recovery: 14% (not meeting criteria above or RRT) 'Outcome beyond 6 m FU': 'Normal' kidney function (sC 1.4 mg/dL) CKD: 42% (sCr >1.4 mg/dL)	22%	'Outcome beyond 6 m FU': RRT or Tx: 4%	
Raza et al. 2012 UK	Mean 64 yrs.	49 biopsy-proven ATIN	Drugs (67%) 1. AB 2. PPI 3. NSAID Idiopathic (20.4%) Auto-immune (12.2%)	Mean baseline sCr 1.13 mg/dL (eGFR 65 mL/min)	At mean FU 19 m: Median eGFR: 32.5 mL/min	22.4%	No info	Baseline sCr available from only 14 patients

Gonzalez et al. 2008 Spain	Mean 58 yrs.	61 biopsy-proven ATIN	Drugs (100%) 1. AB 2. NSAID 3. PPI and others	Baseline CKD: 36% (eGFR <60 mL/min) Mean baseline sCr 1.1 mg/d (eGFR 71 mL/min)	At mean 19 m FU: Complete recovery: 50.8% (sCr within 25% of baseline) Incomplete recovery: 49.2% (sCr >25% of baseline)	23%	At mean 19 m FU: RRT: 9.8%	Study only included drug-induced ATIN
Baker et al. 2004 UK	Mean 47 yrs.	33 patients, unclear whether biopsy-proven	Drugs (71.1%) Infection (15.6%) Idiopathic (7.8%)	No info	FU period unclear: Complete recovery: 64.1% (sCr <1.5mg/dL) Partial recovery: 23.4% (sCr >1.5 mg/dL) No recovery: 12.5% (RRT)	No info	FU period unclear: RRT: 12.5%	Study performs joint analysis with data from the series of Buysen et al. and Schwarz et al., total 128 ATIN cases
Clarkson et al. 2004 Ireland	Median 65 yrs.	60 biopsy-proven ATIN	Drugs (92%) 1. NSAID 2. AB 3. PPI Idiopathic (8%)	No info	At 1 yr. FU: Median sCr 1.59 mg/dL (ESKD patients excluded)	58%	At 1 yr. FU: Died: 3% ESKD: 7%	35 patients required acute dialysis, of which only two chronic RRT at 12 m

Abbreviations: *ATIN* acute tubulointerstitial nephritis, *FU* follow-up. *CKD* chronic kidney disease, *ESKD* end-stage kidney disease, *ATN* acute tubular necrosis, *RRT* renal replacement therapy, *sCr* serum creatinine, *Tx* kidney transplant, *TINU* tubulointerstitial nephritis with uveitis, *TMP-SMX* trimethoprim/sulfamethoxazole

3 Risk Factors for Adverse Renal Outcome

Patient baseline characteristics that predispose to worse renal outcomes include older age, female gender and hypertension. Clinical risk factors for worse outcome include the presence of hematuria and a higher degree of proteinuria. Histopathology is very important in predicting disease prognosis. A high percentage of acute interstitial inflammation on kidney biopsy without signs of disease chronicity, predicts renal recovery and better outcomes. In contrast, a high percentage of glomerulosclerosis and interstitial fibrosis and tubular atrophy (IFTA) predicts worse renal outcomes. The presence of granulomas on kidney biopsy (granulomatous interstitial nephritis) also predicts worse renal outcomes, as well as recurrent episodes of ATIN, which is more often seen in auto-immune ATIN when compared to drug-induced ATIN. Novel prognostic biomarkers that may predict renal outcomes (e.g., urine interleukin-9, prolonged low molecular weight proteinuria) are being investigated, but up until now no biomarkers have been rigorously validated.

4 Corticosteroids and Renal Outcome

Whether corticosteroid treatment results in better outcomes in ATIN patients is still a matter of debate as conflicting results have been reported. To date, no randomized controlled trials (RCTs) using corticosteroids in ATIN have been performed, because ATIN remains a rare kidney disease and not all patients undergo kidney biopsy, making inclusion of sufficient study participants with biopsy-proven ATIN very challenging. In addition, there is no standard approach to corticosteroid therapy in regard to timing, dose, route of administration (intravenous, oral, both), or duration. Data are therefore derived from observational studies and case series. One recent systematic review included eight retrospective studies in which treatment with corticosteroids was compared to non-corticosteroid therapy in drug-induced ATIN. A meta-analysis could not be performed due to study heterogeneity and risk of bias in the individual studies was considered very high. While 4 studies found a beneficial effect of corticosteroids on sCr, the other 4 studies found no significant effect. Corticosteroid-related adverse events were also underreported. The authors concluded that the effect of corticosteroid treatment in drug-induced ATIN is still uncertain and could not make any recommendations regarding its use. Renal outcomes are possibly better when corticosteroids are initiated early in the disease course of drug-induced ATIN, but focus should be on early discontinuation of the inciting drug. The availability of clinical, biochemical and/or histological markers to predict corticosteroid would be helpful in choosing patients appropriate for corticosteroid therapy.

5 Prognosis According to Age Category

5.1 Pediatric Patients

Limited data are available on outcome of ATIN in pediatric patients and case series generally included <30 biopsy-proven cases (Table 2). Furthermore, ATIN is frequently diagnosed without kidney biopsy, potentially biasing the biopsy-proven cohorts towards more severe cases that do not respond to cessation of a potentially causative drug. About 10% of pediatric patients with ATIN require transient acute dialysis. The long-term prognosis of pediatric patients with ATIN varies between studies. In 2 case series from Turkey that mostly included patients with clinically diagnosed ATIN (only about 25% biopsy-proven), all patients showed complete recovery of kidney function. However, when considering 5 case series that only included biopsy-proven cases, only 1 study noted complete renal recovery in all patients at extended follow-up. In the remaining 4 studies, chronic kidney disease (eGFR <80–90 mL/min) was present in 15%, 32%, 56%, and 70% of patients at a mean/median follow-up of 1–2.75 years, respectively. Importantly, in these series, the presence of uveitis or explicit diagnosis of tubulointerstitial nephritis with uveitis (TINU) as etiology of ATIN was reported in 28–65% of cases. Fortunately, evolution to ESKD remains extremely rare in the pediatric population. In summary, although long-term outcomes are better when compared to the adult population, a significant proportion of pediatric patients with biopsy-proven ATIN will develop a degree of chronic kidney disease.

5.2 Elderly Patients

Recent data suggest that the prevalence of ATIN is increasing in the elderly. Many studies have found an association between older age and worse renal outcomes. Data on ATIN in this patient population have recently been published by Muriithi and colleagues. The authors reported outcomes in 45 patients with biopsy-proven ATIN aged 65 years and older (median age 73 yrs.) and compared them to 88 patients aged 18–64 years (median age 49 yrs.). Elderly patients more often had baseline CKD, higher peak serum creatinine and more need for transient dialysis. Surprisingly however, complete or partial recovery within 6 months was observed in 86% of elderly patients and was not significantly different when compared to the younger cohort. Recovery was predicted by rapid initiation of steroids and antibiotic-induced ATIN compared with proton-pump inhibitor-induced AIN. In the older cohort, more patients had drug-induced ATIN (87% vs. 64% in younger cohort) and fewer patients with auto-immune-related ATIN (7% *vs.* 27% in younger cohort), which might partially explain the relatively good outcomes in the elderly. Importantly however, in this study, very few patients had follow-up beyond 6 months and 3 out of 4 patients that developed ESKD were in the elderly group.

Table 2 ATIN data in pediatric cohorts

Author Date Region	Age	Patients	Etiology	Recovery/CKD	Acute dialysis	ESKD	Remarks
Güngör et al. 2020 Turkey	Median 13 yrs.	38 cases, 10 biopsy-proven ATIN	Drugs (60.5%) 1. NSAID 2. β-lactam 3. PPI Infection (21.1%) Idiopathic (18.4%)	At 6 m FU: CKD: 0% Mean sCr 0.65 mg/dL (eGFR 104 mL/min)	10.5% (4 pts)	None	No CKD at 6 m FU Only 26% biopsy-proven ATIN
Roy et al. 2020 UK	Range 6–16 yrs.	10 biopsy-proven ATIN	TINU (60%) Idiopathic (20%) Sarcoidosis (10%)	At median 18.5 m FU: CKD: 70% (eGFR <90 mL/min) Median sCr 0.8 mg/dL (eGFR 80 mL/min)	10% (1 pt)	None	No drug-induced ATIN patients included in this study
Clavé et al. 2019 France	Median 13 yrs.	25 biopsy-proven ATIN	Drugs (32%) 1. NSAID 2. AB 3. Others TINU (28%) Idiopathic (28%)	At 6 m FU: Median eGFR 84 mL/min At 12 m FU: CKD: 32% (eGFR <90 mL/min) 5 mild CKD 2 moderate CKD 1 ESKD Median eGFR 93 mL/min	8% (2 pts)	At 12 m FU: Tx: 4% (1 pt)	ESKD secondary to MDMA-use
Howell et al. 2016 UK	Median 12 yrs.	27 biopsy-proven	Drugs (44%) Infection (30%) Idiopathic (48%)	At median 21 m FU: CKD: 56% (eGFR <80 mL/min) Median eGFR 75.7 mL/min	14.8% (4 pts)	None	65% of patients experienced uveitis and therefore possible underestimation of auto-immune etiology

Taktak et al. 2015 Turkey	Median 14 yrs.	19 cases, 5 biopsy-proven ATIN	Drugs (73.6%) Infection (15.7%) Others (10.6%)	At 6 m FU: Complete recovery: 100% (normalization of creatinine)	No info	None	Only 26% biopsy-proven ATIN
Jahnukainen et al. 2011 Finland	Mean 12 yrs.	26 biopsy-proven idiopathic ATIN	Idiopathic (100%)	At mean 2.75 yrs. FU: CKD: 15% (eGFR <90 mL/min) Persistent LMW proteinuria: 31%	3.8% (1 pt)	None	46% of patients experienced uveitis
Ellis et al. 1981 USA	Median 11 yrs.	13 biopsy-proven ATIN	Infection (76.9%) Idiopathic (15.4%) Drugs (7.7%) 1. Penicillin	Mean 69 days and 'extended FU': Complete recovery: 100%	7.7% (1 pt)	None	

Abbreviations: *ATIN* acute tubulointerstitial nephritis, *FU* follow-up, *CKD* chronic kidney disease, *ESKD* end-stage kidney disease, *RRT* renal replacement therapy, *sCr* serum creatinine; *Tx* kidney transplant, *TINU* tubulointerstitial nephritis with uveitis, *LMW* low molecular weight; *pt(s)* patient(s)

Considering the previously found association of older age with worse outcomes and the short follow-up period of this study, more studies with longer follow-up are required before concluding that the elderly indeed have a similar prognosis to younger adults.

6 Prognosis According to Specific Etiology

6.1 Drugs

6.1.1 Overall Outcomes

Drugs are the most frequent cause of ATIN, as they are implicated in approximately 65% of adult biopsy-proven ATIN cases. The classes of drugs that are most frequently associated with ATIN vary across case series. In general, antibiotics, PPIs, and non-steroidal anti-inflammatory drugs (NSAIDs) are most frequent. Drug-induced ATIN has a better prognosis when compared to auto-immune etiologies (e.g., TINU, Sjögren's syndrome, sarcoidosis, IgG4-related disease), possibly because drug exposure primarily represents a single episode of AKI. In contrast, auto-immune etiologies more frequently cause recurrent AKI-episodes, which may hamper renal recovery and induce fibrosis and CKD. Three larger case series have exclusively included patients with drug-induced ATIN. Gonzalez et al. included 61 patients (mean age 58 yrs., one third had baseline CKD) and reported a complete renal recovery in 51% of cases, while 10% required maintenance RRT at a median follow-up of 19 months. Fernandez et al. included 182 patients (mean age 67 yrs., at least 40% with baseline CKD) and reported a complete renal recovery in 41% of cases, while 5.5% required maintenance RRT at a median follow-up of 6 months. Zheng et al. included 81 patients (mean age 45 yrs., 4% with baseline CKD) and reported complete recovery in 64%, partial recovery in 35% and no recovery in 1% of patients at 6 months follow-up, although at 12 months 42% had CKD (eGFR <60 mL/min). In general, renal outcomes are better when the causal drug is discontinued early. For example, Muriithi et al. found that both longer duration of drug exposure and delay in initiation of steroid treatment were associated with poor renal recovery. Re-exposure to the inciting drug should be avoided to prevent disease recurrence.

6.1.2 Proton-Pump Inhibitors (PPIs)

PPIs are frequently cited as the culprit for interstitial nephritis and some case series have found PPIs to be the most frequent cause of drug-induced ATIN (in 35–64% of drug-induced cases) (Table 3), while other series mention antibiotics and NSAIDs as the most frequent etiologic agent. Two systematic reviews both found that PPI-users have an approximately three-fold higher risk of ATIN when compared to non-PPI-users. PPI therapy was also associated with a more modest but significantly increased risk of AKI, CKD and ESKD in general (hazard ratios approximately 1.5

Table 3 PPI-induced ATIN

Author Date Region	Age	Patients	Pre-existing CKD	Recovery/CKD	Acute dialysis	ESKD	Remarks
Muriithi et al. 2015 USA	Median 73 yrs.	8 biopsy-proven PPI-induced ATIN	Baseline CKD: 63% (not clearly defined) Median baseline sCr 1 mg/dL (eGFR 56 mL/min)	At 6 m FU: Complete recovery: 28.5% (sCr within 25% of baseline) Partial recovery: 43% (sCr >50% reduction from peak, not within 25% of baseline) No recovery: 28.5% (no criteria above or RRT) At 'ultimate outcome' FU: Normal: 57% Progressive CKD 43% ESKD: 0%	None	None	Case series drug-induced ATIN, subgroup analysis of PPI-pts Follow-up period of 'ultimate outcome' not clearly defined, 'normal' and 'progressive CKD' not clearly defined
Geevasinga et al. 2006 Australia	Median 74 yrs.	18 biopsy-proven PPI-induced ATIN	Baseline CKD: 94% (eGFR <60mL/min) Mean baseline eGFR 37 mL/min	At 6 m FU: Mean reduction eGFR of 11.5 mL/min	No info	At 6 m FU: ESKD: 11.1% (eGFR <15 mL/min)	Patients with severe baseline CKD No criteria of recovery defined

(continued)

Table 3 (continued)

Author Date Region	Age	Patients	Pre-existing CKD	Recovery/CKD	Acute dialysis	ESKD	Remarks
Simpson et al. 2006 New Zealand	Median 78 yrs.	15 cases of which 12 biopsy-proven PPI-induced ATIN	Mean baseline sCr 0.94 mg/dL	At FU range 3-18 m: CKD: 73% (eGFR <60 mL/min) Mean sCr 1.57 mg/dL	6.7% (1 pt)	None	No recovery defined No baseline eGFR, only sCr
Torpey et al. 2004 UK	Median 69 yrs.	8 biopsy-proven PPI-induced ATIN	No info	At median 24 m FU: Mean sCr 1.63 mg/dL	None	At median 24 m FU: ESKD: 12.5% (1 pt with sCr 3.54 mg/dL)	No recovery defined No info on baseline kidney function No eGFR provided

Abbreviations: *ATIN* acute tubulointerstitial nephritis, *FU* follow-up, *CKD* chronic kidney disease, *ESKD* end-stage kidney disease, *RRT* renal replacement therapy, *sCr* serum creatinine, *pt(s)* patient(s) for all). A proportion of the CKD-group might consist of patients with incompletely recovered kidney function after an episode of acute PPI-induced ATIN or AKI. In other patients, PPIs may directly induce chronic kidney injury without preceding AKI, likely also contributing to this group.

To date, renal outcome data on PPI-induced ATIN can be derived from small case series in which outcome parameters were not clearly defined and pre-existing CKD not consistently reported. Patients in these series were older (median age 68.5–78 yrs.). One case series included 15 cases (12 biopsy-proven cases) in which the mean baseline sCr-value of 0.94 mg/dL deteriorated to a mean value of 1.57 mg/dL at follow-up after the ATIN-episode (range of 3–18 months). One patient required acute dialysis and no patients progressed to ESKD at follow-up. A second case series included 18 biopsy-proven PPI-induced ATIN cases, of which 94% already had severe CKD at baseline (mean eGFR 37 mL/min). At 6 months follow-up, mean eGFR reduction was 11.5 mL/min when compared to baseline, and two patients (11%) that previously had eGFR >30 mL/min deteriorated to ESKD (eGFR <15 mL/min). Additional outcome data can be derived from 1 larger study on drug-induced ATIN in the elderly, which performed a subgroup analysis of patients with PPI-induced ATIN ($n = 8$). At baseline, 5 patients (63%) had CKD (median eGFR 56 mL/min) and at 6 months follow-up, 28.5% of patients showed complete recovery, 43% partial recovery and 28.5% no recovery, although no patients required acute dialysis or progressed to ESKD. In conclusion, PPI-induced ATIN occurs most frequently in older patients who frequently have CKD at baseline, and although acute dialysis and ESKD remain rare, these data show that many patients do not experience full renal recovery and often develop clinically significant CKD.

6.1.3 NSAIDs

NSAIDs are well known to cause AKI, most frequently through a hemodynamic/vasomotor effect caused by vasoconstriction of the afferent glomerular arteriole, but less frequently by ATIN. Similar to PPIs, no large observational studies of NSAID-induced ATIN have been published and outcome data can only be derived from small (primarily pediatric) case series (Table 4), or from subgroup analyses of larger studies in adults with ATIN. Clarkson et al. included 60 adult patients with ATIN and could not find a difference in sCr at 12 months when comparing NSAID-induced ATIN cases (44%) with other etiologies, which were also predominantly drug-related. Gonzalez et al. performed a subgroup analysis of 20 adult patients with NSAID-induced ATIN that were treated with steroids: 9 patients (45%) showed complete renal recovery, while 11 patients (55%) did not and 1 patient required maintenance RRT (5%), which does not differ substantially from the overall renal outcomes in adults with ATIN. When considering the small pediatric case series on NSAID-induced ATIN, most patients fully recovered to normal kidney function, few patients required acute dialysis and almost none evolved to ESKD with need for chronic RRT.

Table 4 NSAID-induced ATIN

Author Date Region	Age	Patients	Recovery/CKD	Acute dialysis	ESKD	Remarks
Clave et al. 2019 France	Median 12 yrs.	4 biopsy-proven NSAID-induced ATIN	At 24 m FU: Full recovery: 75% (3 pts) (GFR >90 mL/min) CKD: 25% (1 pt) (eGFR 68 mL/min)	None	None	
Misurac et al. 2013 USA	Median 15 yrs.	6 biopsy-proven NSAID-induced ATIN	Pooled analysis At median 9 m FU: Full recovery: 70% (eGFR <90mL/min) Mild CKD: 26% (eGFR >60 mL/min, <90 mL/min) Moderate CKD: 4% (eGFR <60 mL/min)	Pooled analysis 15%	None	6 ATIN patients are pooled in the analysis with 21 NSAID-induced ATN cases, which complicates analysis
Dixit et al. 2010 USA	Median 15 yrs.	5 biopsy-proven NSAID-induced ATIN	At 1-2 m FU: Full recovery: 100% (normalization of sCr) Mean sCr 0.71 mg/dL	40%	None	

Abbreviations: *ATIN* acute tubulointerstitial nephritis, *FU* follow-up, *CKD* chronic kidney disease, *ESKD* end-stage kidney disease, *sCr* serum creatinine, *pt(s)* patient(s)

6.1.4 Antibiotics

In two large studies published in 2008 and 2014, antibiotics were the most frequent cause of drug-induced ATIN. Penicillins are most frequently implicated in antibiotic-induced ATIN, with fluoroquinolones (FQs) and cephalosporins being second and third, respectively. No large studies focusing on penicillin-induced ATIN have been recently published, while older studies consist of small case series of patients mostly treated with methicillin. These studies are highly prone to bias, considering that ATIN was frequently diagnosed without kidney biopsy and some patients even had normal kidney function. In addition, outcome measures were not clearly defined, nor was follow-up period clearly reported. One study noted that 5 out of 14 patients with methicillin-induced ATIN required acute dialysis, and 5 out of 14 patients still experienced 'renal dysfunction' at a minimum of 1-year follow-up, although the authors noted that previous studies reported better renal outcomes.

Regarding the use of FQs, 1 study from the Mayo Clinic retrospectively identified 24 patients with biopsy-proven FQ-induced ATIN, with outcome data reported on 21 patients. Ciprofloxacin was most frequently implicated (71% of cases). A total of 15 patients (71%) showed complete recovery, 5 patients (24%) showed partial recovery and one patient (5%) showed no recovery after 6 months of follow-up. The median time to recovery was short (20.5 days). A total of 6 patients (25%) required acute dialysis.

6.2 *Malignancy*

6.2.1 ICPIs Therapy and Other Cancer Treatments

ICPIs are considered standard of care in the management of an ever-increasing number of advanced malignancies. ICPIs result in unopposed T cell activation and significant anti-cancer responses. Not surprisingly, ICPIs are associated with a wide range of immune-mediated side effects, termed immune-related adverse events (irAEs). Although renal irAEs are rare, they can be serious. It is important to note that most cases of AKI in ICI-treated cancer patients are prerenal. In recent years, several large case series have been published focusing on ICPI-associated acute kidney injury after exclusion of other causes of AKI in cancer patients treated with ICPI. The most common biopsy finding in patients with ICPI-associated AKI is ATIN. In the largest case series to date, Cortazar et al. included 138 patients with ICPI-associated AKI. Lower baseline eGFR, use of PPIs and combination of ICPI were associated with the development of AKI. Eighty-six percent of patients received corticosteroid treatment and complete, partial, and no recovery of kidney function was observed in 40%, 45%, and 15% of patients, respectively. Concomitant extrarenal irAEs were associated with worse renal outcomes, while corticosteroid treatment and use of ATIN-causing medication (NSAIDS, PPI, antimicrobial agents) were associated with better kidney outcomes. Absence of kidney recovery was associated with increased mortality. Whether the development of ICI-associated irAEs is associated with better cancer and patient outcomes is not well established at this time as conflicting results have been reported. A recent article by Lin et al. reported on the limited experience with infliximab-containing regimens in 10 patients with ICPI-associated AKI. Complete, partial and no renal recovery was obtained in 40%, 40% and 20%, respectively.

In a study from 2013 (before the ICPI era) by Airy et al. including cancer patients with biopsy-proven tubulointerstitial nephritis (TIN), ifosfamide, bacillus Calmette-Guérin-vaccination, tyrosine kinase inhibitors and pemetrexed were the most commonly implicated drugs. ATIN was associated with better renal outcomes than chronic TIN. Moreover, pemetrexed and ifosfamide were associated with worse renal outcomes.

6.2.2 Myelodysplastic Syndrome

In a study focusing on 19 patients with myelodysplastic syndrome undergoing a kidney biopsy, ATIN was present in 7 patients (37%), while glomerulopathy was present in the remaining cases. In the ATIN-cases no clear association with a causative medication was observed, although 2 patients were on long-term treatment with PPIs. The authors therefore concluded that there may be an association between MDS and ATIN. Of these seven patients, 1 patient achieved remission (eGFR 74 mL/min at 5 months), 5 patients evolved to CKD of which 2 patients required chronic dialysis and 1 patient developed ESKD and died of progression to acute myeloid leukemia. The kidney prognosis of MDS-associated ATIN therefore appears poor.

6.3 *Auto-immune/inflammatory Disorders*

6.3.1 Tubulointerstitial Nephritis with Uveitis (TINU)

Tubulointerstitial nephritis with uveitis is a rare clinical syndrome in which uveitis precedes, co-occurs or most often follows the onset of acute interstitial nephritis. The clinical course and severity of the uveitis does not seem to correlate with the nephritis. Although smaller case series of mostly pediatric patients suggested a good long-term renal prognosis, 2 larger studies that included adult patients with biopsy-proven TINU clearly showed less reassuring outcomes (Table 5). In the first study, Li et al. reported on a Chinese cohort of 31 adult patients with biopsy-proven TINU, of which 80% developed CKD (eGFR <60 mL/min) at 1-year follow-up. Disease relapse was associated with poor outcomes, as were older age, higher sCr level at biopsy, higher erythrocyte sedimentation rate, leukocyturia, and concomitant thyroid dysfunction. The second study by Legendre et al. reported on a French cohort of 41 adult patients with biopsy-proven TINU of which 32% developed CKD (eGFR <60 mL/min) at 1-year-follow-up. In this study, higher peak sCr levels and older age were also associated with lower eGFR at 1-year follow-up. Corticosteroid treatment did not result in better kidney function but was associated with fewer

Table 5 TINU in adult cohorts

Author Date Region	Age	Patients	Pre-existing CKD	Recovery/ CKD	Acute dialysis	ESKD	Remarks
Legendre et al. 2016 France	Median 47 yrs.	41 biopsy-proven TINU	Baseline CKD: 2.4% (1 pt, eGFR 58 mL/min)	At 1 yr. FU: CKD in 32% (eGFR <60 mL/min) Median eGFR 76 mL/min	10%	None	
Li et al. 2014 China	Mean 48 yrs.	31 biopsy-proven TINU	No info	At 1 yr. FU: CKD: 80% (GFR <60 mL/min)	16%	None	Relapse was seen in 36% of patients and predicted poor outcome

Abbreviations: *ATIN* acute tubulointerstitial nephritis, *FU* follow-up, *CKD* chronic kidney disease, *ESKD* end-stage kidney disease, *TINU* tubulointerstitial nephritis with uveitis, *pt* patient uveitis relapses. Although the difference in CKD at 1-year follow-up in both studies is quite striking and potentially related to differences in treatment and ethnicity between the two studies, it is clear that TINU may cause significant CKD in a substantial proportion of adult patients.

Fortunately, in pediatric patients, kidney prognosis of TINU appears to better. Jahnukainen et al. included 26 pediatric patients (mean age 12 yrs.) with idiopathic biopsy-proven ATIN, of which 12 (46%) developed uveitis and therefore can be reclassified as TINU. At a mean follow-up of 2.75 years, only 1 patient with uveitis (8%) developed CKD (eGFR <90 mL/min), which is substantially lower when compared to the adult cohorts. In contrast to studies in adult patients, no biochemical or histologic features could be identified as predictors of these adverse renal outcomes.

6.3.2 IgG4-Associated Renal Disease

In contrast to IgG4-assocated glomerular disorders, IgG4-associated tubulointerstitial nephritis (IgG4-TIN) is highly responsive to corticosteroid treatment. However, recovery of kidney function is often not complete. Studies have established that there is no clear correlation between histologic lesions and treatment response. Relapses are frequent (20–46%) in IgG4-related disease (IgG4-RD) and are predicted by baseline serum IgG4, IgE, and eosinophils.

6.3.3 Sjögren's Syndrome

Maripuri et al. described 24 patients with Sjögren's syndrome that underwent kidney biopsy, of which 17 (70.8%) had acute or chronic TIN as the primary lesion on histopathology. Only 12 patients were followed beyond 1 year (median follow-up 73.5 months) and five of these patients (42%) presented with eGFR <30 mL/min at biopsy (no baseline reported). Kidney function improved in 6 patients (50%), remained stable in 4 patients (33%) and deteriorated in 2 patients (17%). At final follow-up, 5 of these 12 patients (42%) had severe CKD (eGFR <30 mL/min). In many patients, chronic kidney injury remained unrecognized until severe CKD occurred and kidney biopsy was performed, which explains the poor renal outcomes in this study. The authors therefore advocate early detection and aggressive treatment of TIN in Sjögren's syndrome.

6.4 Infections

6.4.1 Leptospirosis

Kidney injury in leptospirosis infection can occur in the setting of acute systemic infection with multi-organ dysfunction, and is generally characterized by ATIN or acute tubular necrosis on kidney biopsy. The mortality rate of acute infection depends upon the studied population (overall *vs*. in-hospital *vs*. critically ill) and is generally estimated at approximately 15–20% in patients with AKI and is predominantly attributed to pulmonary hemorrhage. Abdulkader et al. reviewed the literature on leptospirosis-induced AKI and concluded that complete recovery of kidney function can be expected in young patients without comorbidities, although dysfunction in urinary concentration capacity may remain present.

6.4.2 Hantavirus

Hantavirus-infection can cause hemorrhagic fever with renal syndrome (HFRS), which is associated with severe AKI caused by ATIN. HFRS is typically caused by four hantaviruses: Puumala, Dobrava/Belgrade, Hantaan, and Seoul virus. In Europe, Puumala virus (PUUV) and Dobrava/Belgrade virus (DOBV) most frequently cause Hantavirus-infection and mortality of both infections is below 1%. In hospitalized patients with PUUV infection, a maximum of 6% of patients require acute dialysis. A recent smaller study included patients with DOBV-infection and AKI. This study reported that 4 out of 34 patients (12%) required transient acute dialysis (Table 6). Long-term prognosis of PUUV and DOBV Hantavirus infection is good and does not seem to correlate with the severity of the acute infection. One study found normalized kidney function (mean eGFR 84 mL/min) at 1-year follow-up of patients with DOBV-infection and kidney injury. Three other studies on patients with PUUV infection found normalized kidney function at 2 years, 5 years, 6 years and 10 years follow-up. A slightly increased eGFR, proteinuria and blood pressure at approximately 5 years follow-up was described in patients with previous PUUV-infection. However, these effects normalized at 10 years follow-up. So in general, full recovery from Hantavirus-induced ATIN can be expected.

6.4.3 Yersinia Pseudotuberculosis (Y. Pseudotuberculosis)

Most cases of AKI and ATIN caused by *Y. pseudotuberculosis* have been reported in Japan and Korea and generally occurred in the pediatric population. In two small studies of pediatric patients, microbiological diagnosis of *Y. pseudotuberculosis* was achieved by stool cultures, serology or a compatible clinical course, which introduces risk of bias. In most cases, ATIN was diagnosed clinically, and few kidney biopsies were performed. Although acute hemodialysis was required in 1 out of 6 patients and 2 out of 9 patients, both studies reported full recovery of kidney function in all patients at follow-up. Quality of evidence from these studies is very low and more research is warranted.

6.4.4 HIV

In HIV patients, ATIN was the third most common diagnosis on kidney biopsy following HIV-associated nephropathy (HIVAN) and focal segmental glomerulosclerosis, with the prevalence of HIVAN decreasing in recent years due to the

Table 6 Hantavirus infection-related ATIN

Author Date Region	Age	Hantavirus	Patients	Recovery/ CKD	Acute dialysis	ESKD	Remarks
Meier et al. 2018 Germany	Mean 41 yrs.	Serologically confirmed DOBV	34 DOBV cases, 6 biopsy-proven ATIN	At 1 yr. FU: Mean GFR 84 mL/min	11.8%	None	
Outinen et al. 2015 Finland	Median 40 yrs.	Serologically confirmed PUUV	Total of 556 PUUV cases, 459 patients had AKI (83%), 189 (34%) had severe AKI, biopsy rate not mentioned	At 5 yrs. FU: median sCr 0.84 mg/dL, only 1 pt. CKD	4% (of total)	None	No one had baseline CKD Risk of bias (biopsy rate not mentioned, analysis of AKI patients in general) No difference in renal outcome when AKI vs. non AKI group is compared
Miettinen et al. 2009 Finland	Mean 49 yrs.	Serologically confirmed PUUV	37 PUUV cases, biopsy rate not mentioned	At 6 yrs. FU: Mean eGFR 120 mL/min	No info	No info	At 6 yrs. FU: more tubular proteinuria, increased eGFR (hyperfiltration) and elevated systolic blood pressure
Miettinen et al. 2006 Finland	Mean 50 yrs.	Serologically confirmed PUUV	36 PUUV cases, biopsy rate not mentioned	At 5 yrs. FU: Mean eGFR 121 mL/min At 10 yrs. FU: Mean eGFR 113 mL/min	10.9%	None	Follow-up study of cohort from Mäkelä et al. At 5 yrs. higher proteinuria, hyperfiltration and elevated blood pressure when compared to controls, but no longer present at 10 yrs. Data from study of Mäkelä et al. ($n = 5$ out of 46 patients)

Abbreviations: *ATIN* acute tubulointerstitial nephritis, *FU* follow-up, *CKD* chronic kidney disease, *ESKD* end-stage kidney disease, *sCr* serum creatinine, *DOBV* Dobrava/Belgrade virus, *PUUV* Puumala virus, *AKI* acute kidney injury, *pt* patient introduction of highly active antiretroviral therapy. In a study by Parkhie et al., 11% of HIV patients undergoing a kidney biopsy had ATIN without evidence of HIVAN. Drugs were identified as the cause of ATIN in the majority (72%) of cases, which were most commonly associated with use of NSAIDS and sulfamethoxazole/trimethoprim. Also, the protease inhibitor atazanavir may cause both acute and chronic (granulomatous) interstitial nephritis, with a higher risk when used in combination with tenofovir. One study reviewed the outcomes of 8 cases of atazanavir-related interstitial nephritis: five patients experienced complete remission after cessation of treatment, 1 patient experienced partial remission and 2 patients experienced no remission after treatment cessation of which 1 required chronic hemodialysis. In all patients that experienced partial or no remission, kidney biopsy showed granulomatous interstitial nephritis.

6.5 Other Etiologies

6.5.1 Mesoamerican Nephropathy/CKDu

Mesoamerican nephropathy belongs to the group of CKD of unknown cause (CKDu) in agricultural communities, together with similar diseases such as Sri Lankan nephropathy and Uddanam nephropathy. These kidney diseases occur in agricultural workers in hot climates, clinically present with CKD with relatively unremarkable urinary examinations and are characterized by chronic tubulointerstitial disease with inflammation and interstitial fibrosis on kidney biopsy. The etiology remains unknown. In a report by Fischer et al., 49 of 586 (8.4%) agricultural workers with acute Mesoamerican nephropathy progressed to CKD (eGFR <60 mL/min in about 60% of these 49 patients), most of them already within 6 months after diagnosis. The presence of anemia and paresthesias at the time of diagnosis were identified as predictors of CKD progression. As these are young patients (median age 32 yrs.) without pre-existing CKD, these renal outcomes are concerning and more research is urgently needed to identify the underlying cause and to develop preventive and therapeutic strategies.

7 Conclusion

Current evidence suggests that long-term kidney outcomes of patients with ATIN are far less favorable than originally thought. As a rule of thumb, when adult patients are followed for 1–3 years after an episode of ATIN, about 50% will experience full renal recovery, 40% will develop CKD and 10% ESKD requiring RRT. Most important risk factors for adverse renal outcome are older age, signs of disease chronicity on kidney biopsy, and recurrent ATIN-episodes. Whether the use of corticosteroids improves long-term kidney outcomes remains controversial. Pediatric patients have a better long-term prognosis, although a significant proportion of patients will also develop CKD. Outcomes are also influenced by the underlying disease etiology. Drug-induced ATIN has a better prognosis when compared to auto-immune etiology, certainly if the inciting drug is discontinued early in the disease course and re-exposure is avoided. ATIN related to ICPIs is an emerging etiology with slightly worse kidney outcomes when compared with the overall ATIN-population, although corticosteroid use is associated with better outcomes. Auto-immune etiologies frequently cause CKD, and especially chronic TIN related to Sjögren's syndrome has been under-recognized in the past with very poor kidney outcomes. Finally, when considering infection-related ATIN, long-term kidney outcomes of Hantavirus-infections (PUUV and DOBV) are very good and full renal recovery can be expected in nearly all patients, even in those that initially require transient dialysis.

Suggested Reading

Abdulkader RC, Silva MV. The kidney in leptospirosis. Pediatr Nephrol. 2008;23(12):2111–20.

Airy M, Raghavan R, Truong LD, Eknoyan G. Tubulointerstitial nephritis and cancer chemotherapy: update on a neglected clinical entity. Nephrol Dial Transplant. 2013;28(10):2502–9.

Al-Aly Z, Maddukuri G, Xie Y. Proton pump inhibitors and the kidney: implications of current evidence for clinical practice and when and how to deprescribe. Am J Kidney Dis. 2020;75(4):497–507.

Appel GB. The treatment of acute interstitial nephritis: more data at last. Kidney Int. 2008;73(8):905–7.

Baker RJ, Pusey CD. The changing profile of acute tubulointerstitial nephritis. Nephrol Dial Transplant. 2004;19(1):8–11.

Berliner AR, Fine DM, Lucas GM, Rahman MH, Racusen LC, Scheel PJ, et al. Observations on a cohort of HIV-infected patients undergoing native renal biopsy. Am J Nephrol. 2008;28(3):478–86.

Buysen JG, Houthoff HJ, Krediet RT, Arisz L. Acute interstitial nephritis: a clinical and morphological study in 27 patients. Nephrol Dial Transplant. 1990;5(2):94–9.

Cheong HI, Choi EH, Ha IS, Lee HJ, Choi Y. Acute renal failure associated with Yersinia pseudotuberculosis infection. Nephron. 1995;70(3):319–23.

Clarkson MR, Giblin L, O'Connell FP, O'Kelly P, Walshe JJ, Conlon P, et al. Acute interstitial nephritis: clinical features and response to corticosteroid therapy. Nephrol Dial Transplant. 2004;19(11):2778–83.

Clavé S, Rousset-Rouvière C, Daniel L, Tsimaratos M. Acute tubulointerstitial nephritis in children and chronic kidney disease. Arch Pediatr. 2019a;26(5):290–4.

Clavé S, Rousset-Rouvière C, Daniel L, Tsimaratos M. The invisible threat of non-steroidal anti-inflammatory drugs for kidneys. Front Pediatr. 2019b;7:520.

Cortazar FB, Kibbelaar ZA, Glezerman IG, Abudayyeh A, Mamlouk O, Motwani SS, et al. Clinical features and outcomes of immune checkpoint inhibitor-associated AKI: a multicenter study. J Am Soc Nephrol. 2020;31(2):435–46.

Davidson B, Nel D, Jones ESW, Manning K, Spies R, Bohmer R, et al. Granulomatous interstitial nephritis on renal biopsy in human immunodeficiency virus positive patients: prevalence and causes in Cape Town. South Africa Nephrology (Carlton). 2019;24(7):681–8.

Dixit M, Doan T, Kirschner R, Dixit N. Significant acute kidney injury due to non-steroidal anti-inflammatory drugs: inpatient setting. Pharmaceuticals (Basel). 2010;3(4):1279–85.

Effa EE, Ekrikpo UE, Borkum M, Rayner BL, Heering P, Okpechi IG. Clinical profile and outcome of patients with biopsy-proven acute interstitial nephritis in Cape Town: a 10-year review. Clin Nephrol. 2017;88(8):97–104.

Ellis D, Fried WA, Yunis EJ, Blau EB. Acute interstitial nephritis in children: a report of 13 cases and review of the literature. Pediatrics. 1981;67(6):862–70.

Espi M, Teuma C, Novel-Catin E, Maillet D, Souquet PJ, Dalle S, et al. Renal adverse effects of immune checkpoints inhibitors in clinical practice: ImmuNoTox study. Eur J Cancer. 2021;147:29–39.

Esteras R, Fox JG, Geddes CC, Mackinnon B, Ortiz A, Moreno JA. Hematuria is associated with more severe acute tubulointerstitial nephritis. J Clin Med. 2020;9(7)

Evans RDR, Cargill T, Goodchild G, Oliveira B, Rodriguez-Justo M, Pepper R, et al. Clinical manifestations and long-term outcomes of IgG4-related kidney and retroperitoneal involvement in a United Kingdom IgG4-related disease cohort. Kidney Int Rep. 2019;4(1):48–58.

Farid S, Mahmood M, Abu Saleh OM, Hamadah A, Nasr SH, Garrigos ZE, et al. Clinical manifestations and outcomes of fluoroquinolone-related acute interstitial nephritis. Mayo Clin Proc. 2018;93(1):25–31.

Fernandez-Juarez G, Perez JV, Caravaca-Fontan F, Quintana L, Shabaka A, Rodriguez E, et al. Duration of treatment with corticosteroids and recovery of kidney function in acute interstitial nephritis. Clin J Am Soc Nephrol. 2018;13(12):1851–8.

Fischer RSB, Vangala C, Mandayam S, Chavarria D, Garcia-Trabanino R, Garcia F, et al. Clinical markers to predict progression from acute to chronic kidney disease in Mesoamerican nephropathy. Kidney Int. 2018;94(6):1205–16.

Galpin JE, Shinaberger JH, Stanley TM, Blumenkrantz MJ, Bayer AS, Friedman GS, et al. Acute interstitial nephritis due to methicillin. Am J Med. 1978;65(5):756–65.

Garcia-Carro C, Bolufer M, Bury R, Cataneda Z, Munoz E, Felip E, et al. Acute kidney injury as a risk factor for mortality in oncological patients receiving check-point inhibitors. Nephrol Dial Transplant. 2021;(epub ahead of print).

Geevasinga N, Coleman PL, Webster AC, Roger SD. Proton pump inhibitors and acute interstitial nephritis. Clin Gastroenterol Hepatol. 2006;4(5):597–604.

Gonzalez E, Gutierrez E, Galeano C, Chevia C, et al. Early steroid treatment improves the recovery of renal function in patients with drug-induced acute interstitial nephritis. Kidney Int. 2008;73(8):940–6.

Güngör T, Cakici EK, Yazilitas F, Eroglu FK, Özdel S, Kurt-Sukur ED, et al. Clinical characteristics of childhood acute tubulointerstitial nephritis. Pediatr Int. 2021;63(6):693–8.

Hara M, Suganuma A, Yanagisawa N, Imamura A, Hishima T, Ando M. Atazanavir nephrotoxicity. Clin Kidney J. 2015;8(2):137–42.

Howell M, Sebire NJ, Marks SD, Tullus K. Biopsy-proven paediatric tubulointerstitial nephritis. Pediatr Nephrol. 2016;31(10):1625–30.

Jahnukainen T, Ala-Houhala M, Karikoski R, Kataja J, Saarela V, Nuutinen M. Clinical outcome and occurrence of uveitis in children with idiopathic tubulointerstitial nephritis. Pediatr Nephrol. 2011;26(2):291–9.

Johnson RJ, Wesseling C, Newman LS. Chronic kidney disease of unknown cause in agricultural communities. N Engl J Med. 2019;380(19):1843–52.

Joyce E, Glasner P, Ranganathan S, Swiatecka-Urban A. Tubulointerstitial nephritis: diagnosis, treatment, and monitoring. Pediatr Nephrol. 2017;32(4):577–87.

Kim H, Jo SK, Ahn SY, Kwon YJ, Lee H, Oh J, et al. Long-term renal outcome of biopsy-proven acute tubular necrosis and acute interstitial nephritis. J Korean Med Sci. 2020;35(26):e206.

Kim YK, Cho MH, Hyun HS, Park E, Ha IS, Cheong HI, et al. Acute kidney injury associated with Yersinia pseudotuberculosis infection: forgotten but not gone. Kidney Res Clin Pract. 2019;38(3):347–55.

Koo JW, Park SN, Choi SM, Chang CH, Cho CR, Paik IK, et al. Acute renal failure associated with Yersinia pseudotuberculosis infection in children. Pediatr Nephrol. 1996;10(5):582–6.

Legendre M, Devilliers H, Perard L, Groh M, Nefti H, Dussol B, et al. Clinicopathologic characteristics, treatment, and outcomes of tubulointerstitial nephritis and uveitis syndrome in adults: a national retrospective strobe-compliant study. Medicine (Baltimore). 2016;95(26):e3964.

Li C, Su T, Chu R, Li X, Yang L. Tubulointerstitial nephritis with uveitis in Chinese adults. Clin J Am Soc Nephrol. 2014;9(1):21–8.

Lin JS, Mamlouk O, Selamet U, Tchakarov A, Glass WF, Sheth RA, et al. Infliximab for the treatment of patients with checkpoint inhibitor-associated acute tubular interstitial nephritis. Onco Targets Ther. 2021;10(1):1877415.

Mäkelä S, Ala-Houhala I, Mustonen J, Koivisto AM, Kouri T, Turjanmaa V, et al. Renal function and blood pressure five years after puumala virus-induced nephropathy. Kidney Int. 2000;58(4):1711–8.

Mandeville JT, Levinson RD, Holland GN. The tubulointerstitial nephritis and uveitis syndrome. Surv Ophthalmol. 2001;46(3):195–208.

Maripuri S, Grande JP, Osborn TG, Fervenza FC, Matteson EL, Donadio JV, et al. Renal involvement in primary Sjögren's syndrome: a clinicopathologic study. Clin J Am Soc Nephrol. 2009;4(9):1423–31.

Meier M, Kramer J, Jabs WJ, Nolte C, Hofmann J, Krüger DH, et al. Proteinuria and the clinical course of Dobrava-Belgrade hantavirus infection. Nephron Extra. 2018;8(1):1–10.

Miettinen MH, Mäkelä SM, Ala-Houhala IO, Huhtala HS, Kööbi T, Vaheri AI, et al. Ten-year prognosis of Puumala hantavirus-induced acute interstitial nephritis. Kidney Int. 2006;69(11):2043–8.

Miettinen MH, Makela SM, Ala-Houhala IO, Huhtala HS, Kööbi T, Vaheri AI, et al. Tubular proteinuria and glomerular filtration 6 years after puumala hantavirus-induced acute interstitial nephritis. Nephron Clin Pract. 2009;112(2):c115–20.

Misurac JM, Knoderer CA, Leiser JD, Nailescu C, Wilson AC, Andreoli SP. Nonsteroidal anti-inflammatory drugs are an important cause of acutekidney injury in children. J Pediatr. 2013;162(6):1153–9.

Moledina DG, Wilson FP, Kukova L, Obeid W, Luciano R, Kuperman M, et al. Urine interleukin-9 and tumor necrosis factor-alpha for prognosis of human acute interstitial nephritis. Nephrol Dial Transplant. 2021;36(10):1851–8.

Muriithi AK, Leung N, Valeri AM, Cornell LD, Sethi S, Fidler ME, et al. Biopsy-proven acute interstitial nephritis, 1993-2011: a case series. Am J Kidney Dis. 2014;64(4):558–66.

Muriithi AK, Leung N, Valeri AM, Cornell LD, Sethi S, Fidler ME, et al. Clinical characteristics, causes and outcomes of acute interstitial nephritis in the elderly. Kidney Int. 2015;87(2):458–64.

Nochaiwong S, Ruengorn C, Awiphan R, Koyratkoson K, Chaisai C, Noppakun K, et al. The association between proton pump inhibitor use and the risk of adverse kidney outcomes: a systematic review and meta-analysis. Nephrol Dial Transplant. 2018;33(2):331–42.

Nolan CM, Abernathy RS. Nephropathy associated with methicillin therapy. Prevalence and determinants in patients with staphylococcal bacteremia. Arch Intern Med. 1977;137(8):997–1000.

Outinen TK, Mäkelä S, Clement J, Paakkala A, Pörsti I, Mustonen J. Community acquired severe acute kidney injury caused by hantavirus-induced hemorrhagic fever with renal syndrome has a favorable outcome. Nephron. 2015;130(3):182–90.

Parkhie SM, Fine DM, Lucas GM, Atta MG. Characteristics of patients with HIV and biopsy-proven acute interstitial nephritis. Clin J Am Soc Nephrol. 2010;5(5):798–804.

Patel V, Elias R, Formella J, Schwartzman W, Christie A, Cai Q, et al. Acute interstitial nephritis, a potential predictor of response to immune checkpoint inhibitors in renal cell carcinoma. J Immunother Cancer. 2020;8(2):e001198.

Prendecki M, Tanna A, Salama AD, Tam FW, Cairns T, Taube D, et al. Long-term outcome in biopsy-proven acute interstitial nephritis treated with steroids. Clin Kidney J. 2017;10(2):233–9.

Qiu T, Zhou J, Zhang C. Acid-suppressive drugs and risk of kidney disease: a systematic review and meta-analysis. J Gastroenterol Hepatol. 2018;33(9):1566–73.

Quinto LR, Sukkar L, Gallagher M. Effectiveness of corticosteroid compared with non-corticosteroid therapy for the treatment of drug-induced acute interstitial nephritis: a systematic review. Intern Med J. 2019;49(5):562–9.

Raissian Y, Nasr SH, Larsen CP, Colvin RB, Smyrk TC, Takahashi N, et al. Diagnosis of IgG4-related tubulointerstitial nephritis. J Am Soc Nephrol. 2011;22(7):1343–52.

Rankin AJ, Cannon E, Gillis K, Crosby J, Mark PB, Geddes CC, et al. Predicting outcome in acute interstitial nephritis: a case-series examining the importance of histological parameters. Histopathology. 2020;76(5):698–706.
Raza MN, Hadid M, Keen CE, Bingham C, Salmon AH. Acute tubulointerstitial nephritis, treatment with steroid and impact on renal outcomes. Nephrology (Carlton). 2012;17(8):748–53.
Roy S, Awogbemi T, Holt RCL. Acute tubulointerstitial nephritis in children- a retrospective case series in a UK tertiary paediatric centre. BMC Nephrol. 2020;21(1):17.
Saeki T, Kawano M, Mizushima I, Yamamoto M, Wada Y, Nakashima H, et al. The clinical course of patients with IgG4-related kidney disease. Kidney Int. 2013;84(4):826–33.
Schwarz A, Krause PH, Kunzendorf U, Keller F, Distler A. The outcome of acute interstitial nephritis: risk factors for the transition from acute to chronic interstitial nephritis. Clin Nephrol. 2000;54(3):179–90.
Schwotzer N, Provot F, Ville S, Daniel L, Le FA, Kissling S, et al. Spectrum of kidney involvement in patients with myelodysplastic syndromes. Kidney Int Rep. 2021;6(3):746–54.
Shah S, Carter-Monroe N, Atta MG. Granulomatous interstitial nephritis. Clin Kidney J. 2015;8(5):516–23.
Simpson IJ, Marshall MR, Pilmore H, Manley P, Williams L, Thein H, et al. Proton pump inhibitors and acute interstitial nephritis: report and analysis of 15 cases. Nephrology (Carlton). 2006;11(5):381–5.
Stein C, Burtey S, Mancini J, Pelletier M, Sallée M, Brunet P, et al. Acute kidney injury in patients treated with anti-programmed death receptor-1 for advanced melanoma: a real-life study in a single-centre cohort. Nephrol Dial Transplant. 2021;36(9):1664–74.
Su T, Gu Y, Sun P, Tang J, Wang S, Liu G, et al. Etiology and renal outcomes of acute tubulointerstitial nephritis: a single-center prospective cohort study in China. Nephrol Dial Transplant. 2018;33(7):1180–8.
Taktak A, Uncu N, Acar B, Cayci S, Ensari A, Gür G, et al. Acute tubulointerstitial nephritis: a case series and long-term renal outcomes. Turk J Pediatr. 2015;57(6):566–71.
Torpey N, Barker T, Ross C. Drug-induced tubulo-interstitial nephritis secondary to proton pump inhibitors: experience from a single UK renal unit. Nephrol Dial Transplant. 2004;19(6):1441–6.
Valluri A, Hetherington L, Mcquarrie E, Fleming S, Kipgen D, Geddes CC, et al. Acute tubulointerstitial nephritis in Scotland. QJM. 2015;108(7):527–32.
Wallace ZS, Mattoo H, Mahajan VS, Kulikova M, Lu L, Deshpande V, et al. Predictors of disease relapse in IgG4-related disease following rituximab. Rheumatology (Oxford). 2016;55(6):1000–8.
Wendt R, Schliecker J, Beige J. Inflammatory leucocyte infiltrates are associated with recovery in biopsy-proven acute interstitial nephritis: a 20-year registry-based case series. Clin Kidney J. 2019;12(6):814–20.
Xie Y, Bowe B, Li T, Xian H, Yan Y, Al-Aly Z. Long-term kidney outcomes among users of proton pump inhibitors without intervening acute kidney injury. Kidney Int. 2017;91(6):1482–94.
Yang CW. Leptospirosis renal disease: emerging culprit of chronic kidney disease unknown etiology. Nephron. 2018;138(2):129–36.
Yun D, Jang MJ, An JN, Lee JP, Kim DK, Chin HJ, et al. Effect of steroids and relevant cytokine analysis in acute tubulointerstitial nephritis. BMC Nephrol. 2019;20(1):88.
Zajjari Y, Montasser D, Sobhi A, Aatif T, Azizi M, Alayoud A, et al. Acute interstitial nephritis in the military hospital of Morocco: clinical features and renal outcomes. Saudi J Kidney Dis Transpl. 2019;30(6):1407–14.
Zheng XZ, Gu YH, Su T, Zhou XJ, Huang JW, Sun PP, et al. Elevation of erythrocyte sedimentation rate and C-reactive protein levels reflects renal interstitial inflammation in drug-induced acute tubulointerstitial nephritis. BMC Nephrol. 2020;21(1):514.

Index

M. G. Atta, M. A. Perazella (eds.), *Tubulointerstitial Nephritis*, https://doi.org/10.1007/978-3-030-93438-5

MIX
Papier aus verantwortungsvollen Quellen
Paper from responsible sources
FSC® C105338
www.fsc.org

If you have any concerns about our products,
you can contact us on
ProductSafety@springernature.com

In case Publisher is established outside the EU,
the EU authorized representative is:
Springer Nature Customer Service Center GmbH
Europaplatz 3, 69115 Heidelberg, Germany

Printed by Libri Plureos GmbH
in Hamburg, Germany